Basic and Advanced

Visual Cardiology

Basic and Advanced Visual Cardiology

Illustrated Case Report Multi-Media Approach

TAKASHI WADA, M.D.
Consulting Cardiologist
Ohfuna Central General Hospital
Kamakura, Japan
Clinical Professor of Medicine
School of Medicine
Tokai University
Isehara, Japan

Lea & Febiger   1991   Philadelphia / London

Lea & Febiger
200 Chester Field Parkway
Malvern, Pennsylvania 19355-9725
U.S.A.
(215) 251-2230

Library of Congress Cataloging-in-Publication Data

Wada, Takashi.
    Basic and advanced visual cardiology: illustrated case report multi-media approach / Takashi Wada.
    p. cm.
    An updated and enlarged translation of a book published in Japanese.
    Includes index.
    ISBN 0-8121-1354-3
    1. Heart–Diseases–Case studies–Atlases. 2. Heart–Diseases–Diagnosis–Atlases. I. Title.
    [DNLM: 1. Heart Diseases–case studies. WG 200 W1165b]
RC682.W24 1991
616.1'2–dc20
DNLM/DLC
for Library of Congress   90-6353
                                                              CIP

Printed in Singapore by Singapore National Printers through Palace Press

Print Number: 6 5 4 3 2 1

Dedication

To the Memory of
My Teachers

Gordon B. Myers, M.D. (1904-1960)
Former Professor,
Chairman of the Department of Medicine
Wayne State University
Detroit General Hospital
Detroit, Michigan

Noboru Kimura. M.D. (1911-1983)
Former Professor and Chairman of Medicine
Kurume Medical School
Kyushu, Japan

Myron Prinzmetal, M.D. (1908-1987)
Former Clinical Professor of Medicine
University of California at Los Angeles
Los Angeles, California

Robert Berman, M.D. (1898-1988)
Former Consulting Cardiologist
Detroit Memorial Hospital
Detroit, Michigan

Foreword

This book is an updated and enlarged translation of a book already published in Japanese. Lea & Febiger has done a praiseworthy service to the cause of international scientific exchange by producing for the first time in publishing history an English translation of a Japanese cardiology book. They have chosen to publish this work because they believe the book's attractive multi-media teaching format makes learning cardiology a fascinating experience for physicians at any stage in their career, and it deserves to be made available to an international audience.

I consider it a privilege to be asked to assist in the translation and editing of this book because I am grateful to Dr. Wada for making me a better cardiologist and teacher. Dr. Wada has devoted most of his medical life to teaching, and has been one of Japan's most popular lecturers in cardiology. Dr. Wada founded the Medical Educational Association (MEA) in Tokyo for postgraduate training over the past 10 years. Despite his busy schedule, he spends nearly 500 additional hours per year on other teaching tours. When I was exposed to his third book on the physical examination of the cardiac patient about 25 years ago, I was so impressed with his imaginative methods of teaching that I envied those physicians and students who were taught by him, and looked forward to meeting him. Since then, I have become personally acquainted with Dr. Wada, and have been a co-lecturer at conferences in which we both discussed the same cases. I have been impressed by his ability not only to come up with a correct diagnosis but also to explain the physical signs and technological data in a clear, unique manner.

I have learned much from Dr. Wada because he has the kind of inquiring mind that leads to many new discoveries and unique explanations for symptoms, as well as findings in physical examinations, electrocardiography, and echocardiography.

It is not widely known outside Japan that Dr. Wada worked with Dr. Myron Prinzmetal and was co-author with him on the first article on Variant Angina (Am J Med. 27:375, 1959). I understand that Dr. Wada took all the electrocardiographic tracings himself, remaining at the patient's bedside for several days and nights to await the attacks because there were no transistorized electrocardiograms.

We are privileged, in this book, to have some of Dr. Wada's vast collection of illustrations, which he uses for his lectures. These illustrations are so beautifully mounted and clearly labelled that they serve as a model for teachers and publishers and show us that teaching can be an art as well as a science.

Jules Constant, M.D.
Buffalo, New York

Preface

With recent advances in echocardiography, cardiac computerized tomography, and magnetic resonance imaging, not only medical students but internists and cardiologists have to spend a tremendous number of hours reading appropriate texts. These texts often contain only a limited approach which may not be related to other conventional diagnostic methods, a method of study that is inefficient for the well-rounded cardiologist. *Basic and Advanced Visual Cardiology* includes the pertinent history, clinical findings, electrocardiograms, echoes, phonocardiograms, and chest x-rays on each patient. In addition to these conventional diagnostic procedures, it contains the newly developed diagnostic methods of cardiac CT and MRI in order to offer up-to-date cardiology for medical students, internists, and cardiologists.

This book first emphasizes the key pathophysiology and fundamental facts of the disease, then demonstrates a typical case followed by an atypical case. One of the aims of this book is to help the physician choose the best diagnostic method for a particular abnormality. This is, therefore, a completely new attempt to create an atlas of case reports in cardiology by a multi-media approach.

Long follow-up studies and pre- and postoperative findings will give the reader an understanding of the changes to be expected with specific diseases. The multi-media approach guides the reader so that he can choose the diagnostic methods in order of importance when a specific diagnosis is suspected.

Almost all illustrations are presented in their original sizes, except for the chest x-rays. The pertinent findings in each illustration are meticulously labelled in order to offer the reader the diagnostic clues at a glance.

In summary, *Basic and Advanced Visual Cardiology* is a completely new attempt to teach cardiology by illustrating both usual and unusual cases. It emphasizes the visual understanding of the many diagnostic methods so that learning cardiology becomes an interesting experience and requires less effort than reading a text. Therefore, this book is recommended as an enjoyable way for medical students, house-staff, internists, and cardiologists to learn cardiology. The reader should try to render his own interpretation of the illustrations before reading the text.

William Osler stated, "Listen to the patient. He is telling you the diagnosis." The author would like to add "Accumulate cases and analyze them carefully. In this way you may discover a new hypothesis."

Takashi Wada, M.D.
Kamakura, Japan

Acknowledgments

The author wishes to first express his appreciation for the help and encouragement given by his good friends Jules Constant, M.D., of the State University of New York at Buffalo, and Walter J. Russell, M.D., the former chief of Radiology at Radiation Effect Research Center in Hiroshima. Without their assistance in editing, this book would not have been published.

Particular thanks are in order for Shiaki Kawada, M.D., Professor of Cardiac Surgery, for his surgical photography, and Seiya Matsuyama, M.D., Professor of Radiology at Tokai University, who performed magnetic resonance imaging, digital subtraction angiography, and conventional angiography and, in addition to reviewing the manuscript, gave many suggestions. The author also extends his thanks to his colleague Nobuko Yanagisawa, M.D., who has been working with the author for the past 18 years and spent so much of her time in accumulating voluminous data and recording high-quality phonocardiograms. The author's thanks also go to Kenji Kikuda of the Yokogawa-Hewlett Packard Company, who so ably assisted in taking color Doppler echoes. Morihiro Honda, M.D., at International Good-Will Hospital, Kazuyo Matsukawa, M.D., Keiko Shinada, Hisako Suzuki, and Chieko Kubo at Ohfuna Central General Hospital all assisted in taking the echoes and ECGs. The author must mention Mitsue Aoyama, a photographer, who, for 30 years, has made beautiful slides and illustrations for the author. Thanks are also due to Junichi Yoshikawa, M.D., Chief of Cardiology at Kobe Municipal Central Hospital, and Shigeru Ogata, M.D., Chief of Cardiology at Tokyo Mishuku General Hospital, for reviewing the manuscript. The author is also grateful to Isao Masuoka, M.D., Medical Director at Ohfuna Central General Hospital, for his generous cooperation in preparing this book.

May the author take this opportunity to express his gratitude to all his teachers, colleagues, and friends in the USA who supported his postgraduate training during his stay from 1950 to 1957.

T.W.

Contents

Chapter 1. Ventricular Septal Defect

Pathophysiology and Clinical Clues

In order to understand the anatomical descriptions of the various types of ventricular septal defects (VSD) it is necessary to know that the course between the left ventricle (LV) and aorta (Ao) is different from the course between the right ventricle (RV) and pulmonary artery (PA). On the right side there is a muscular structure termed the crista supraventricularis between the RV and PA in the right ventricular outflow tract, or infundibulum. Ventricular septal defects may therefore be classified into three types (see Fig. 1-1).

> **Fig. 1-1. A and B, I:** The supracristal defect is immediately below the pulmonary valve. Since the sinus of Valsalva* lies immediately behind this defect, prolapse of the right cusp usually produces aortic regurgitation. However a prolapsed cusp may result in occlusion of the VSD. An aneurysmal dilatation of the sinus of Valsalva may obstruct the right ventricular outflow tract to produce a loud cardiac murmur. **II:** An infracristal defect can be seen between the right and non-coronary cusps of the Ao from the LV side. This lesion is also termed a membranous septal defect. The above two types are the most common types of VSD. The VSD in tetralogy of Fallot is also included in this group. A defect in the region of the membranous portion may also produce a LV to RA shunt. **III:** Defects in the muscular portion of the ventricular septum (IVS) are usually small and produce no symptoms, despite a loud murmur. A perforation of the muscular septum may develop after myocardial infarction, usually in patients with poor collaterals, as suggested by a history of no previous infarction or angina.
>
> *The sinuses of Valsalva are three bulges in the aortic root. These pouched dilatations prevent obstruction of coronary orifices by the left and right aortic cusps during systole. They also promote better coronary flow during diastole.

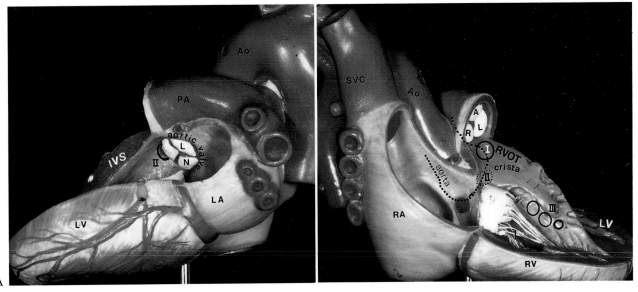

A   B

Since spontaneous closure of the VSD often occurs before adolescence, VSDs are infrequently observed in adults. Unless the defect is large, there are no characteristic clinical findings other than a cardiac murmur.

The clinical approach to diagnosing VSD is as follows (greater numbers of stars indicates greater degrees of diagnostic significance):

★★★★ Auscultation reveals a coarse regurgitant murmur, usually of pan- or holosystolic type, along the left lower sternal border.

★★ Chest x-rays may show a slight increase in pulmonary vascularity due to the left-to-right shunt (shunt vascularity).

★★ In the electrocardiogram (ECG), if the shunt is large there will be signs of biventricular volume overload often shown by large biphasic RS complexes in the mid-precordial leads (the Katz-Wachtel sign). There may be diastolic LV overloading manifested by tall QRS and T waves in the left ventricular leads.

★★ Echocardiogram (echo) will show enlargement of the LV, RV, and left atrium (LA) if the shunt is large. When the shunt is small, only Doppler echoes will be helpful in revealing the shunt noninvasively.

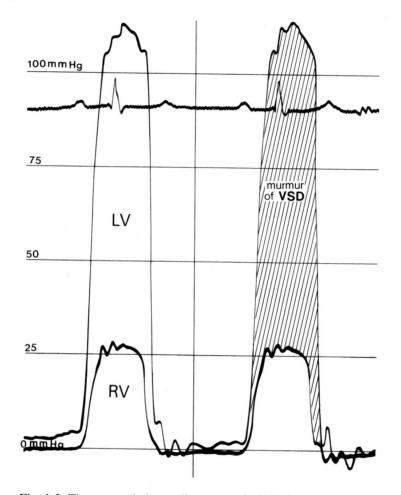

Fig. 1-2. The pan- or holosystolic murmur in VSD is due to the systolic pressure gradient between the LV and RV, represented by diagonal lines. It should be emphasized that there is no pressure gradient between the ventricles during diastole so there is no murmur through the VSD in diastole.

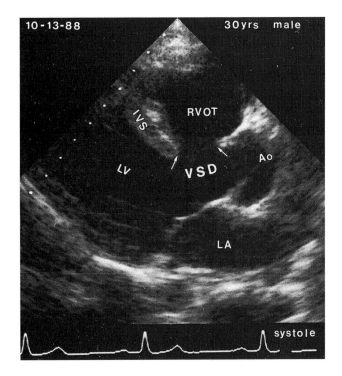

Fig. 1-3. This 30-year-old man had a heart murmur since childhood, with cyanosis and clubbing of his fingers and toes. His long axis two-dimensional (2D) echo shows a large VSD outlined by arrows and separating the anterior aortic wall from the IVS. A dilated RV outflow tract is seen. This is an Eisenmenger syndrome with a large VSD. Further details of his case are discussed in chapter 11.

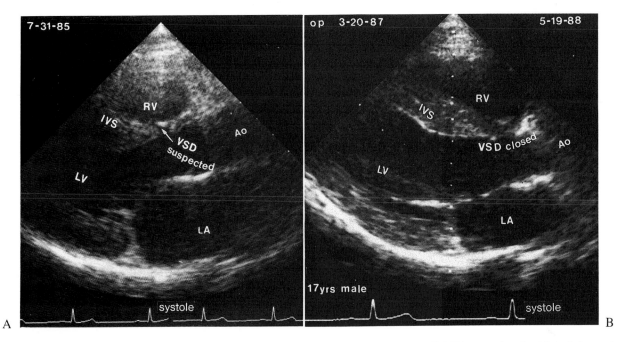

Fig. 1-4. A, These long-axis 2D-echoes are from a 17-year-old boy with a small VSD associated with a deformed right aortic cusp. A preoperative echo on the left shows a small separation suspicious of a small VSD (arrow). There is no definite discontinuity of the anterior aortic wall and the IVS to indicate a VSD. Therefore, the findings of this echo alone are inconclusive. **B,** On the right is his three-month postoperative echo showing no break in the IVS.

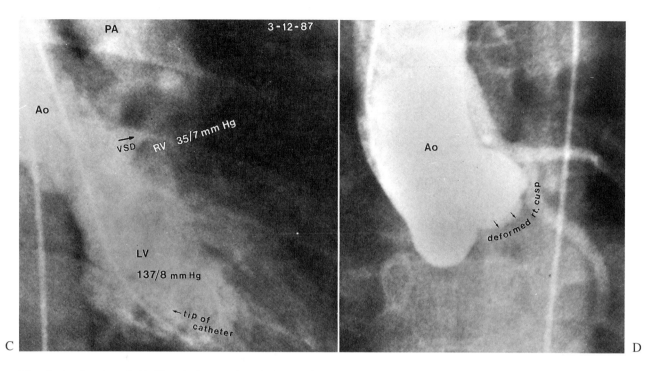

Fig. 1-4. *(Continued)* **C,** The angiogram is a right anterior oblique view of the same patient in A and B. The tip of the catheter is in the LV (arrow). Contrast medium has been injected into the LV and there is a small jet stream through the VSD into the RV just below the aortic valve. However, the LV to RV shunt is not sufficiently large to visualize the RV. **D,** Contrast medium has been injected into the Ao and although the deformed right cusp is visualized, no aortic regurgitation (AR) is seen. There was minimal AR on the cineangiogram.

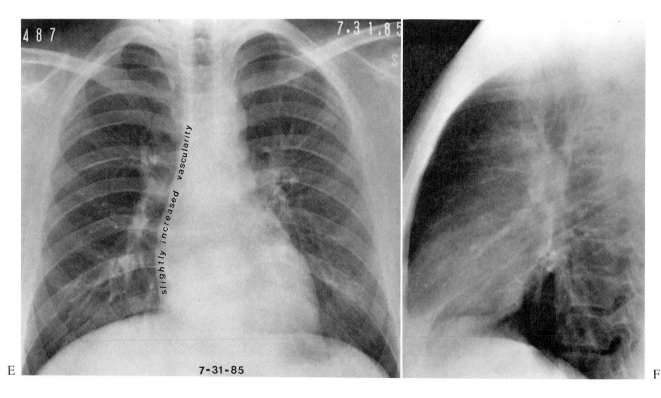

Fig. 1-4. *(Continued)* **E** and **F,** Preoperative chest x-rays of the same patient are unremarkable, although there may be slight increased pulmonary vascularity. His VSD was closed because of a deformed right aortic cusp; and a small degree of AR commonly becomes severe if the VSD is not closed.

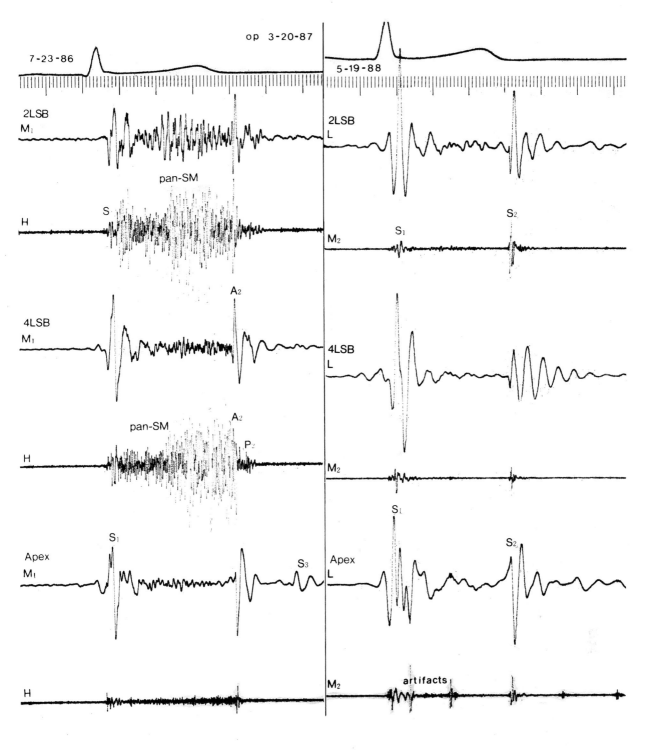

G

H

Fig. 1-4. *(Continued)* **G,** Phonocardiogram (PCG) on the left shows a loud pansystolic murmur (pan-SM) along the left sternal border from the 2nd to 4th left intercostal space (2LSB to 4LSB). The murmur is loudest at the 4LSB where the high frequency components show a crescendo configuration. The split second heart sound (S_2) is not sharp and the minimal vibration after the murmur may be a pulmonary component (P_2). There is an insignificant third heart sound (S_3) at the apex. **H,** The postoperative PCG on the right shows a resolving murmur and some artifacts at the apex.

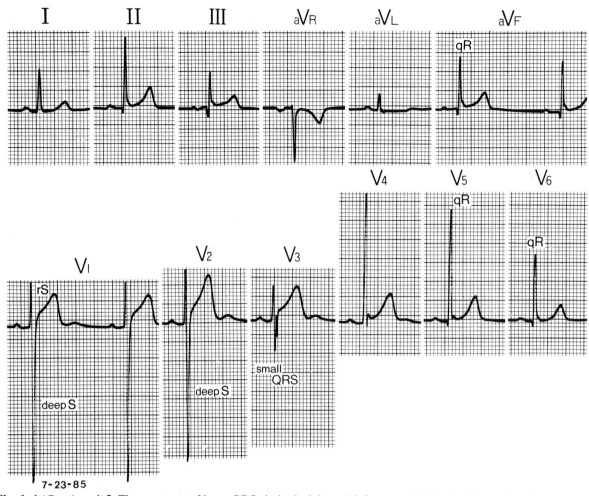

Fig. 1-4 *(Continued)* **I,** The presence of large QRSs in both right and left precordial leads with upright T waves in V_5 to V_6 may represent diastolic LV overloading.* Postoperative ECG showed some reduction of the QRS amplitudes. This may be a result of surgical intervention.

* A tall R wave and T wave in the left precordial leads are frequently seen in LV diastolic volume overloading as in aortic and mitral regurgitation.

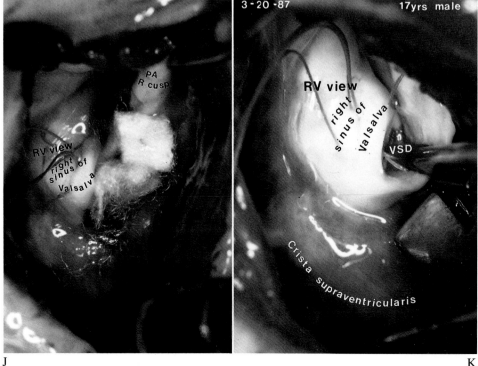

Fig. 1-4. *(Continued)* **J,** From the right ventricular outflow tract approach, a 3 × 10 mm slit-like VSD was found at the right sinus of Valsalva. **K,** A magnified view demonstrates the defect when the medial aspect of the VSD is retracted. The white region at the right ventricular outflow tract indicates a protruding sinus of Valsalva of the right aortic cusp behind the VSD.

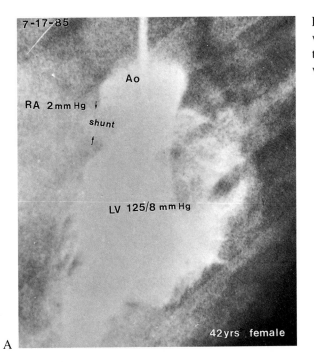

A

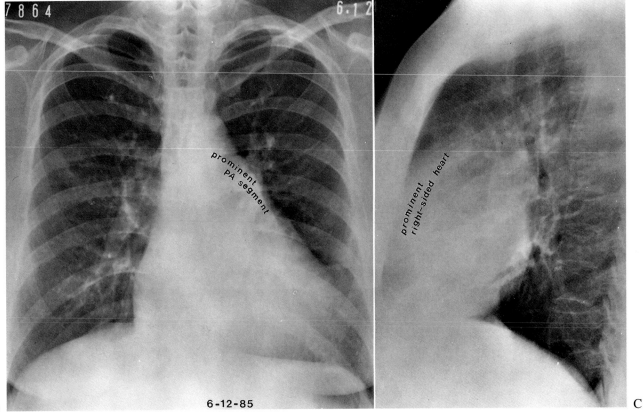

B

C

Fig. 1-5. A, Angiogram of a 42-year-old asymptomatic woman with a loud pansystolic murmur at her cardiac base. The left ventriculogram shows a LV to RA shunt. The pressure in the RA is within normal limits.

Fig. 1-5. *(Continued)* **B,** Chest x-rays show cardiomegaly and increased vascular markings (shunt vascularity) together with an exaggerated pulmonary artery segment. **C,** Her right atrium and ventricle are enlarged as shown in the lateral projection where the cardiac shadow contacts more than one third of the sternum.

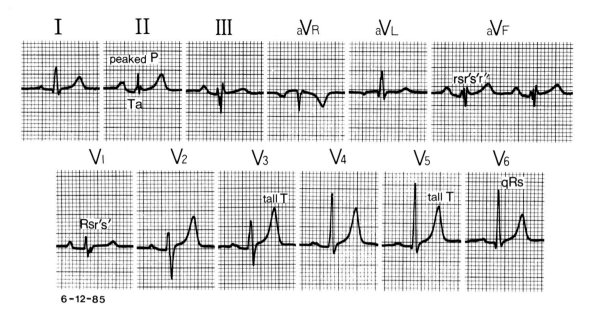

6-12-85

D

Fig. 1-5. *(Continued)* **D,** ECG of the same patient shows slightly peaked P waves in V_1. The QRS complex in aVF is equiphasic, making a QRS axis of 0°. The T waves in leads V_2 to V_6 are somewhat tall compared to their respective QRS complexes and may indicate diastolic LV overloading despite normal QRS amplitudes. An s wave in V_6 and the Rsr's' pattern with a peaked P wave in V_1 suggest some RV and right atrial overloading. The PR segment in lead II is depressed, probably due to a T_a wave.* In summary, LV and/or RV overloading is suggested but not definite.

* Repolarization of the atrium occurs opposite the P wave and is termed the T_a wave. When the P wave is positive, the T_a wave causes depression of the PR segment which extends into the ST segment and may produce ST segment depression. This is often seen when P waves are tall as in tachycardia and/or atrial overloading. The T_a wave usually is sagging in shape and it may be difficult to differentiate from true ST depression.

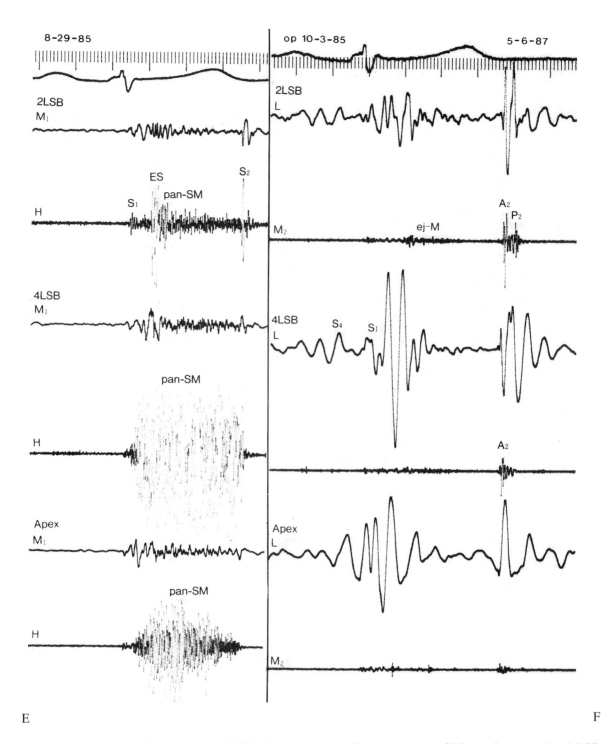

E   F

Fig. 1-5. *(Continued)* Preoperative PCG shows a pansystolic murmur (pan-SM) maximum at the 4 LSB radiating to both the 2LSB and apex, **E**. Other than a loud ejection sound (ES) at the 2LSB, heart sounds are normal. Note that the pansystolic murmur preceeds this ejection sound.* Surgery was performed 5 weeks later, and a PCG 7 months thereafter. **F** shows a slight splitting of the S_2 and a soft fourth heart sound (S_4) at the apex. The previously described pansystolic murmur and ejection sound have resolved, leaving only a soft ejection murmur (ej-M).

* If the murmur preceeds an ejection sound which is due to aortic valve opening, then the murmur must be occurring during isovolumic contraction (between mitral valve closure and aortic valve opening) and is therefore due to regurgitation either through a VSD or the mitral valve (mitral regurgitation).

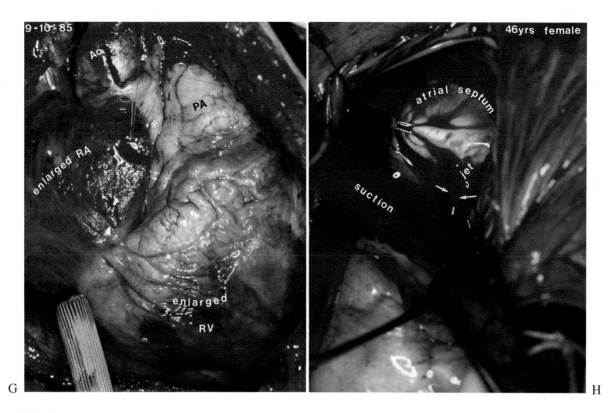

G

H

Fig. 1-5. *(Continued)* **G,** At surgery, both RA and RV were enlarged. **H,** The intra-atrial view of the RA shows a jet from the LV indicated by the arrows. A portion of the tricuspid ring is retracted to show the lesion clearly.

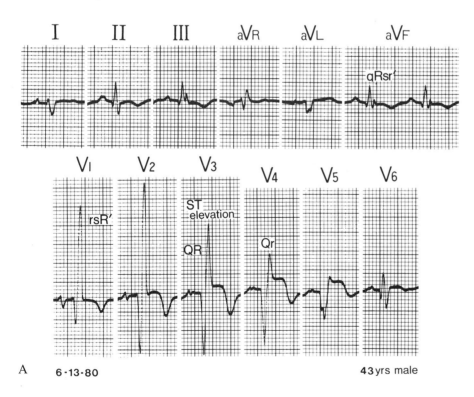

A   6·13·80   43 yrs male

Fig. 1-6. A, ECG of 43-year-old man who suddenly developed a loud heart murmur following myocardial infarction; a perforated ventricular septum was suspected. His ECG shows an rsR' pattern in V_1 to V_2; leads V_3 to V_6 showed wide Q waves of necrosis and ST elevations. These findings are indicative of right bundle branch-block due to acute anteroseptal myocardial infarction. In addition there is a large area of terminal P negativity in V_1 denoting left atrial overloading.

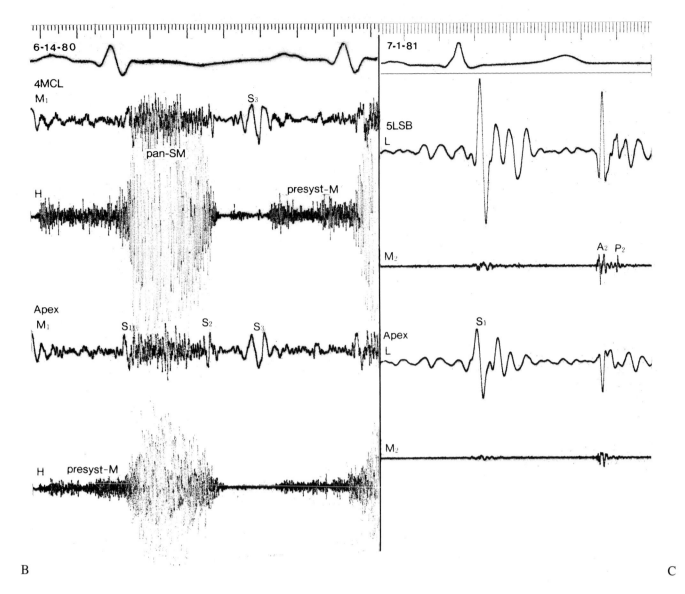

B   C

Fig. 1-6. *(Continued)* **B,** Preoperative PCG shows a loud pansystolic murmur (pan-SM) associated with a high-pitched presystolic murmur (presyst-M). This presystolic murmur indicates a diastolic pressure gradient and is typical of a perforated IVS associated with LV failure. **C,** The postoperative PCG shows resolution of the murmurs.

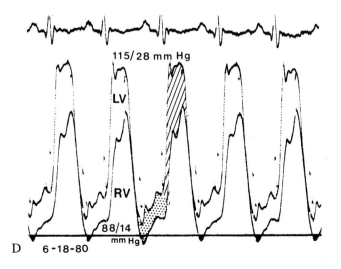

Fig. 1-6. *(Continued)* **D,** Preoperative catheterization showed pressures of 115/28 in the LV and 88/14 mm Hg in the RV indicating pressure gradients in systole and diastole producing both systolic and diastolic murmurs; see diagonal and dotted areas.

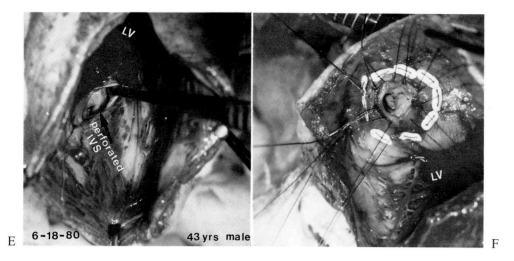

E 6-18-80   43 yrs male   F

Fig. 1-6. *(Continued)* **E** and **F**, At surgery, there was a 2 × 3 cm perforation in the lower portion of the IVS. A patch closure was made and postoperative recovery was uneventful.

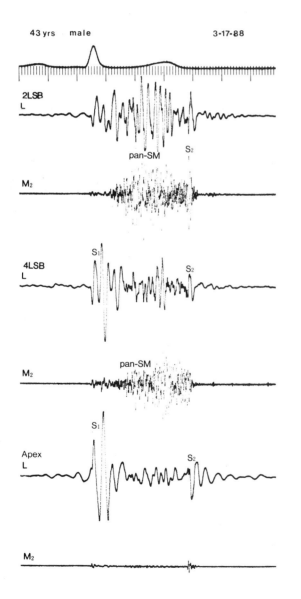

Fig. 1-7. A, PCG of a 43-year-old asymptomatic man who had a loud systolic murmur. He was told that he had a heart murmur since childhood. His chest x-rays and ECG were unremarkable. A crescendo pansystolic murmur (pan-SM) is maximum at the 4LSB without transmission to the apex. At the 2LSB, there is a crescendo-decrescendo murmur lasting until S_2. This murmur at the 2LSB is probably a pansystolic VSD murmur associated with a concomitant pulmonary ejection murmur.

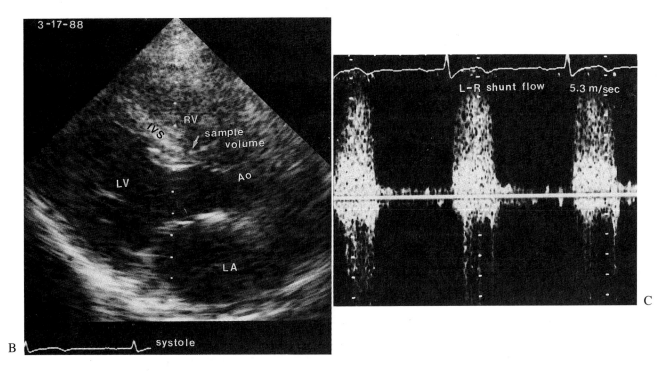

Fig. 1-7. *(Continued)* **B** and **C**, Long-axis 2D-echoes show findings suggesting a VSD; the Doppler echo shows a LV to RV shunt flow with a velocity of 5.3 m/sec, compatible with the presence of a VSD.

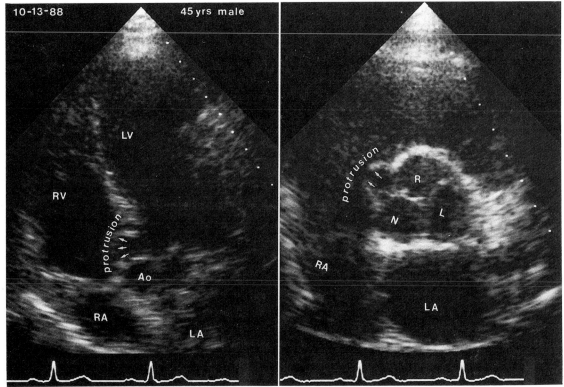

Fig. 1-8. These 2D-echoes are from a 45-year-old asymptomatic man who was told during his childhood that he had a loud heart murmur. The apical four-chamber view in **A** shows a pouch-like protrusion at the upper portion of the IVS in the RV cavity (arrows). A short-axis view of the Ao shows a similar deformity at the base of the right cusp, **B**. These findings suggest a closed VSD or a congenital diverticulum of the membranous portion of the IVS.*

*The superior portion of the interventricular septum just below the aortic valve is actually a transluscent membrane. Most congenital VSDs are at this site.

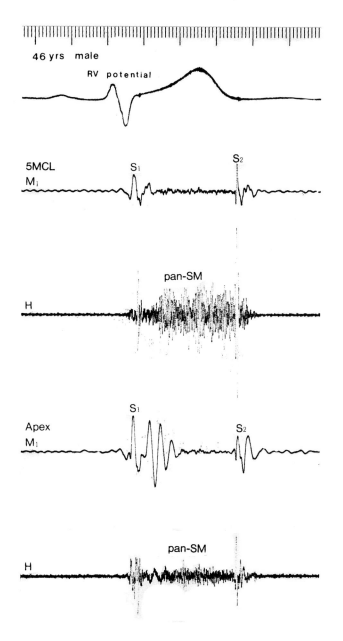

Fig. 1-9. The differentiation of a VSD murmur from a mitral regurgitation murmur may be difficult, especially when the MR murmur's maximum intensity is near the 4LSB. T. Sakamoto of Tokyo university has suggested obtaining a precordial ECG at the site of maximum intensity of the murmur, where the tracing will show an RV potential (rS pattern) if there is a VSD in contrast to an LV potential (qRs, qR or R pattern) in cases of MR. This PCG is from a 42-year-old man with a pansystolic murmur (pan-SM) loudest between the apex and the sternal border radiating to the 6th anterior axillary line, thus simulating MR. However, an electrode at the site of maximum intensity showed an rS pattern, indicating an RV potential suggesting a VSD. This easy maneuver is useful in making a bedside diagnosis.

Chapter 2 Persistent (Patent) Ductus Arteriosus (PDA) and Arteriovenous Shunt

Pathophysiology and Clinical Clues

The fetal circulation receives oxygen-saturated blood from the mother via the placenta. The main circulatory system is maintained via the RA to RV to PA to Ao through the persistent ductus arteriosus PDA. After birth and simultaneous with onset of respiration both the increase in pulmonary blood flow and the production of oxygen-sensitive vasoactive material complete the closure of the PDA in 1 to 2 weeks, resulting in a nonfunctioning ligament. When the PDA does not close, the shunt from the higher pressure of the Ao to the lower pressure of the PA prevails both in systole and diastole, causing a continuous murmur which is loudest at the second left intercostal space near the sternum (2LICS). The maximal intensity of this murmur is very important clinically in differentiating its cause from those of other continuous murmurs which are situated either higher or lower than the 2LICS.*

* PDA murmurs are transmitted better to the first left interspace than to the third left interspace. If the murmur is louder in the third than the first left interspace, the continuous murmur is more likely because of a coronary arterio-venous fistula or a coronary-pulmonary artery fistula in adults. In infants such a murmur may be due to an aortic-pulmonary septal defect. In the differential diagnosis of a continuous murmur, the location of its maximal intensity is important. When it is loudest above the clavicle, it is due to a venous hum, thyroid bruit, or more rarely, aneurysmal dilatation of the subclavian artery.

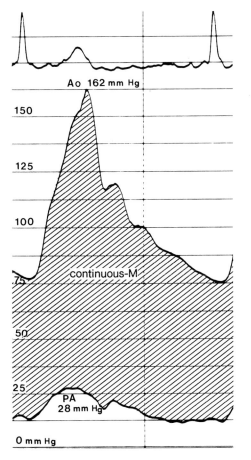

Fig. 2-1. This Ao and pulmonary artery (PA) pressure tracing is from a 28-year-old man with a PDA. His Ao pressure was 162/75 and his PA pressure was 28/12 mm Hg. The pressure gradients between the Ao and the PA are represented by oblique lines. Continuous pressure gradients cause continuous murmurs. Because of the shunt from Ao to PA to PV (pulmonary vein) to LA to LV, the LV receives more blood than in normal persons, and this may produce LV diastolic (volume) overloading. This is seen in the ECG as large amplitude qR and T waves in leads V_5 and V_6, together with deep S waves in leads V_1 and V_2. When the PA pressure is increased, as in the Eisenmenger syndrome, leads V_1 and V_2 may show tall R waves.

An approach to the diagnosis of PDA is as follows:

★★★★ The continuous murmur with maximal intensity at the second LICS and the next loudest area at the first LICS.

★★★ A chest x-ray showing some increase of the pulmonary vascularity with a prominent Ao and PA, resembling a "slanting figure 3".

★★ An ECG which is either normal or shows diastolic LV overloading.

★ Presence of the ductus is rarely identified on an echo except by Doppler.

The definitive diagnosis is often made by aortography and an increase in oxygen step-up in the pulmonary artery by right heart catheterization.

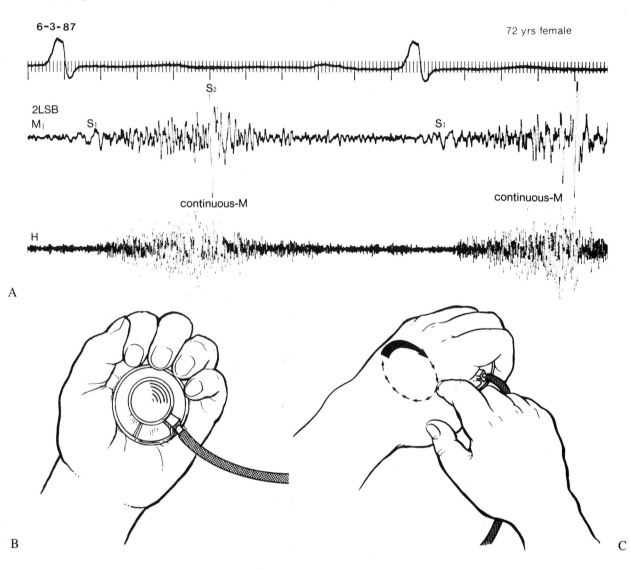

Fig. 2-2. A, PCG from a 72-year-old woman with a probable PDA shows a characteristic continuous murmur enveloping the S_2. The character of this murmur when loud has been described as "machinery". The use of a diaphragmatic stethoscope covered by the palm, **B**, while making a circular movement with tip of the other index finger on the back of the hand can simulate a continuous murmur. Start at the 6 o'clock position, **C**, and accelerate the speed of the finger at the 11 to 1 o'clock position to produce maximal intensity near the S_2. As the Ao pressure rises during systole the Ao to PA shunt flow increases and intensifies the murmur.

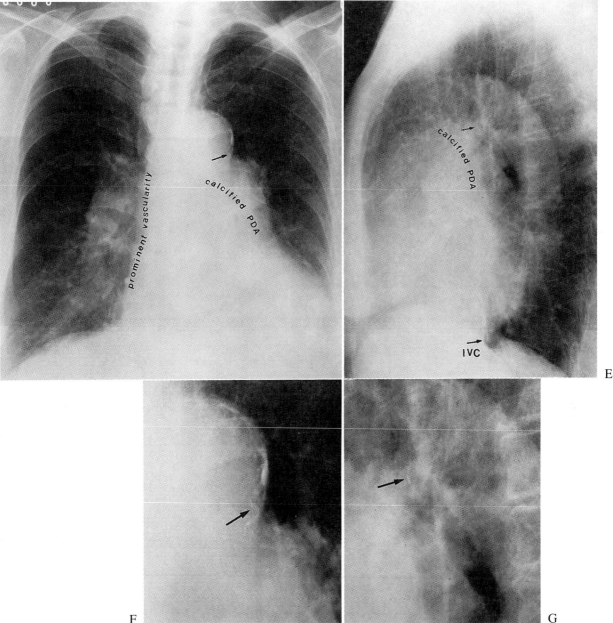

D

E

F

G

Fig. 2-2. *(Continued)* **D**, The chest x-rays of the same patient reveal a prominent aortic arch and a main PA resembling a slanting figure 3. The central arteries of the PA are enlarged with prominent peripheral vessels, indicating increased pulmonary blood flow due to the left to right shunt via a PDA. In addition to the calcification along the margin of the aortic arch, an arrow indicates a very fine calcification probably in the ductus. **E**, This can also be seen in the aortopulmonary window area of the lateral projection. This fine calcification in the PDA is better appreciated in the magnified radiographs shown in **F** and **G**. Also, an enlarged LV is suggested by the low site of crossing between the inferior vena cava (IVC) and the LV in the lateral view. Usually the IVC crosses the posterior border of the LV well above the diaphragm. The feature differentiating PDA from VSD by chest radiography is the fact that the shunt occurs between the Ao and PA in the former, and at the ventricular level in the latter. Therefore, although the frontal chest x-ray shows some increment of pulmonary vascularity in both PDA and VSD, there is increased flow into the Ao, and the aortic arch is prominent only in PDA. Another radiographic feature of PDA is the prominent main PA which, together with an enlarged Ao, resembles a slanting figure 3.*

---

* Occasionally, there is a fine line at the neck of the slanting figure 3 termed a ductus line. In some cases, a portion of the ductus may be observed at the junction of the aortic arch and the descending Ao as a small protrusion, called the infundibular sign. In other cases, there is some discontinuity of the lateral border of the descending Ao where it crosses the upper portion of the main PA, i.e., the aortic opacity does not pass through the upper part of the PA. This has been termed the run-off sign.

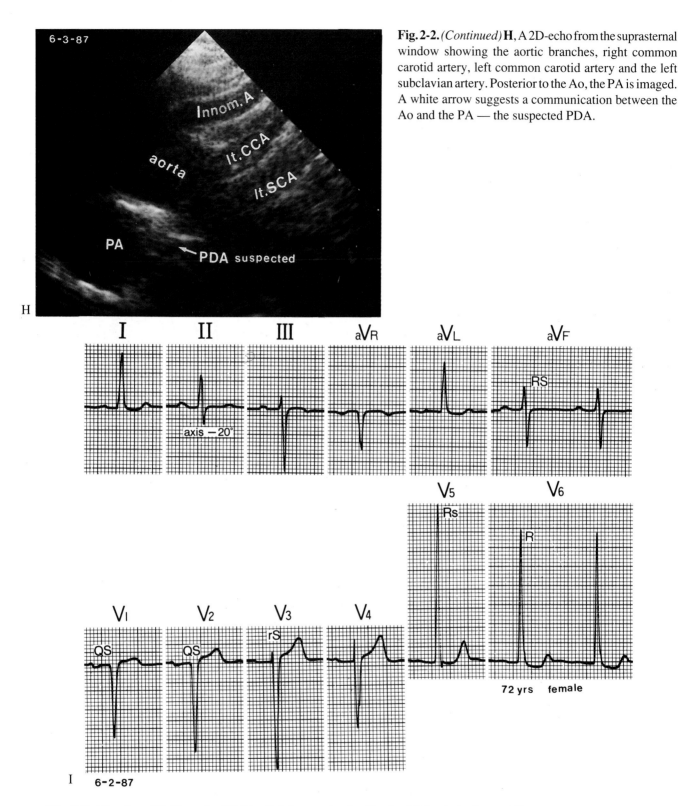

Fig. 2-2. *(Continued)* **H,** A 2D-echo from the suprasternal window showing the aortic branches, right common carotid artery, left common carotid artery and the left subclavian artery. Posterior to the Ao, the PA is imaged. A white arrow suggests a communication between the Ao and the PA — the suspected PDA.

Fig. 2-2. *(Continued)* **I,** Since the QRS is slightly negative in aVF, the QRS axis is about –20°; i.e., there is slight left-axis deviation. A prolonged PR interval of 0.24 seconds is present (first degree A-V block). The precordial leads V_1 and V_2 show QS waves and there is no septal q wave in V_5 and V_6 suggesting an abnormal simultaneous bidirectional or dominant right-to-left conduction in the septum, not necessarily due to myocardial infarction. Therefore, the initial negativity in V_1 and V_2 should not be interpreted as caused by myocardial necrosis but probably secondary to an incomplete LBBB pattern.[*] The tall R wave in leads V_5 and V_6 together with the deep S wave in lead V_1 satisfies the Sokolow voltage criteria for LV overload in diagnosing. The sagging ST depression in V_5 and V_6 suggests digitalis effect.

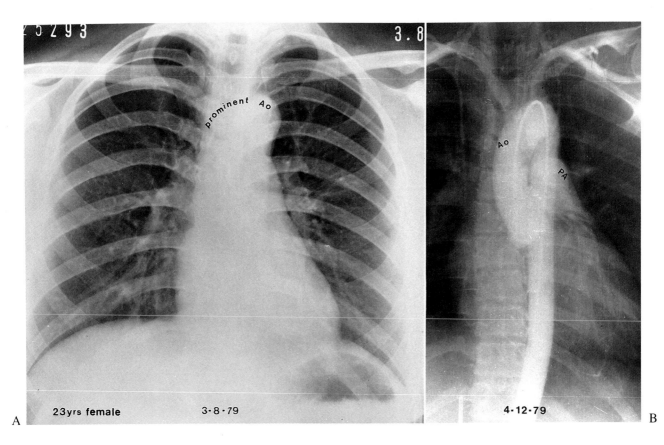

Fig. 2-3. Chest x-rays from a 23-year-old asymptomatic woman who intermittently has a continuous murmur at the base of her heart. **A** shows an aortic arch (Ao) that is prominent for her age, but her main PA is within normal limits. The pulmonary vascularity is unremarkable and does not suggest the presence of a left to right shunt. **B**, an aortogram demonstrates the main PA to be filled from the Ao and indicates the presence of a PDA.

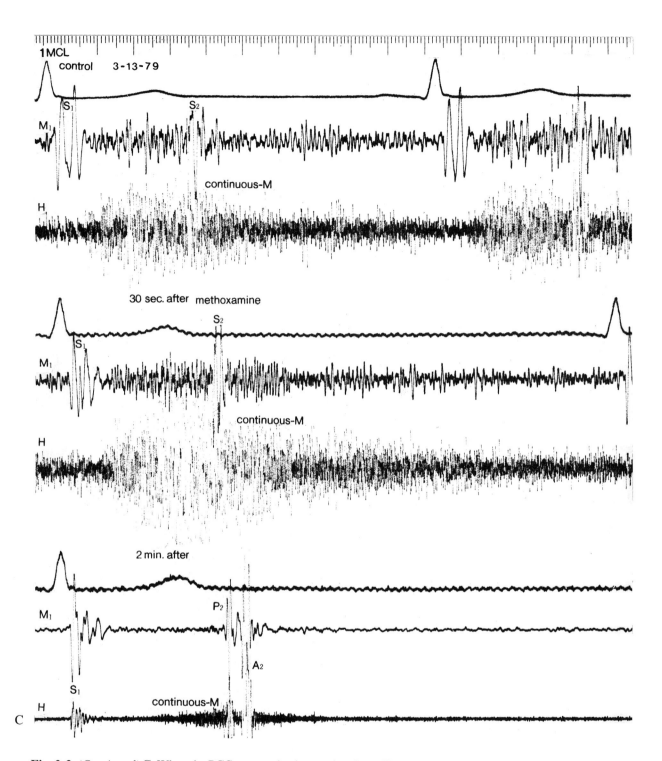

Fig. 2-3. *(Continued)* C, When the PCG was made, the previously audible continuous murmur was not heard. In order to reproduce the murmur, the vasopressor methoxamine was administered (0.09 mg/Kg). Her systolic blood pressure rose from 110 to 130 mm Hg; however, it failed to produce the murmur. Amyl nitrite was then given which produced the murmur maximal at the first left intercostal space, mid-clavicular line (1MCL) with radiation to the 3LSB in spite of a blood pressure drop from 110 to 94 mm Hg. The murmur became loudest 90 seconds after the administration of amyl nitrite and was still a continuous murmur after 1 hour. Methoxamine was given repeatedly. A coarse continuous murmur heard best at 1MCL became louder for a few seconds following the administration of methoxamine, then diminished rapidly, followed by a residual soft continuous murmur which lasted about 90 minutes. During this period, a soft splitting of the S_2 with A_2 and P_2 appeared, in that order, then became single and finally showed sharp paradoxical splitting of S_2 with an accentuated P_2. The markedly delayed A_2 from the terminal portion of the T wave of the ECG is due to methoxamine effect. After 90 minutes, amyl nitrite again produced a loud continuous murmur.

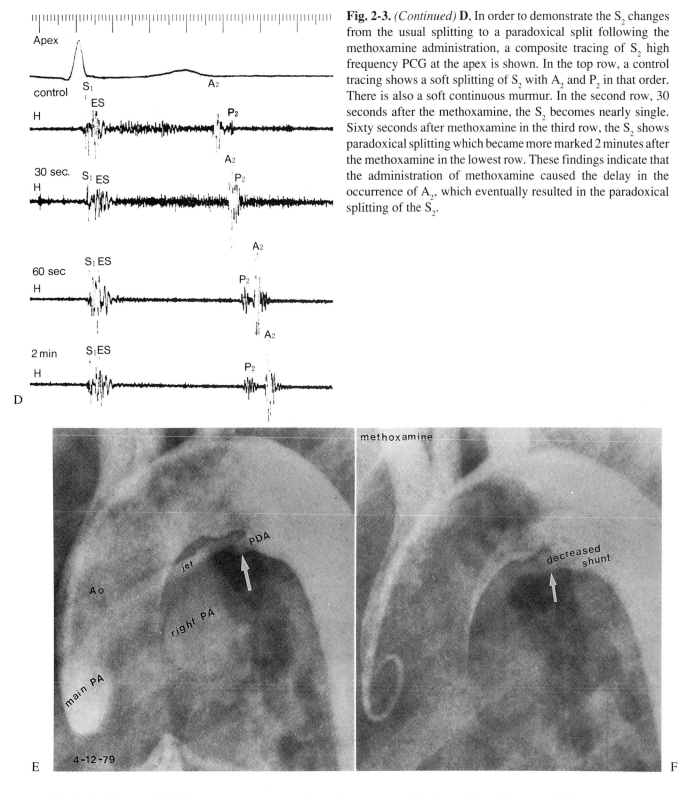

Fig. 2-3. *(Continued)* **D,** In order to demonstrate the S_2 changes from the usual splitting to a paradoxical split following the methoxamine administration, a composite tracing of S_2 high frequency PCG at the apex is shown. In the top row, a control tracing shows a soft splitting of S_2 with A_2 and P_2 in that order. There is also a soft continuous murmur. In the second row, 30 seconds after the methoxamine, the S_2 becomes nearly single. Sixty seconds after methoxamine in the third row, the S_2 shows paradoxical splitting which became more marked 2 minutes after the methoxamine in the lowest row. These findings indicate that the administration of methoxamine caused the delay in the occurrence of A_2, which eventually resulted in the paradoxical splitting of the S_2.

Fig. 2-3. *(Continued)* **E,** The control aortogram shows the presence of the shunt. The white arrow indicates a jet stream from the Ao to the main PA via a PDA. **F,** After administration of methoxamine, the murmur spontaneously resolved simultaneously with a decrease in the aortopulmonary shunt through the PDA. At catheterization, pressures were 22/8 in the RV and 36/23mm Hg in the main PA, with an oxygen step-up of only 2 vol/% indicating a very small shunt.

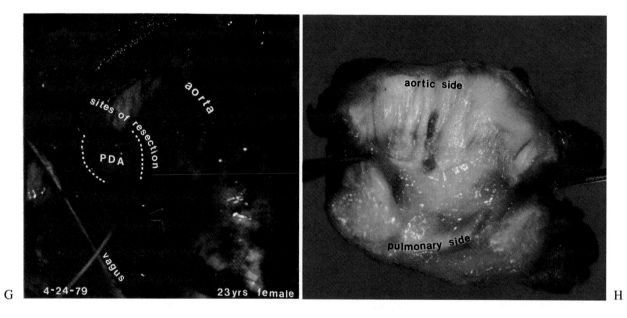

G 4-24-79   23yrs female   H

Fig. 2-3. *(Continued)* **G** and **H**, At surgery, a 1 × 2 cm PDA was resected. Ordinarily the peripheral vaso-constrictive action of methoxamine will increase the intensity of the PDA murmur and the peripheral vasodilating action of amyl nitrite causing a fall in aortic pressure will decrease the murmur. In the present case, these drugs acted paradoxically due to the presence of excessive smooth muscle in the media of the wall of the PDA: i.e., methoxamine induced spasm of the ductus muscle, nearly closing it off. There are several case reports of this reverse-action effect with methoxamine, but the author believes that this is the first histologically documented case.

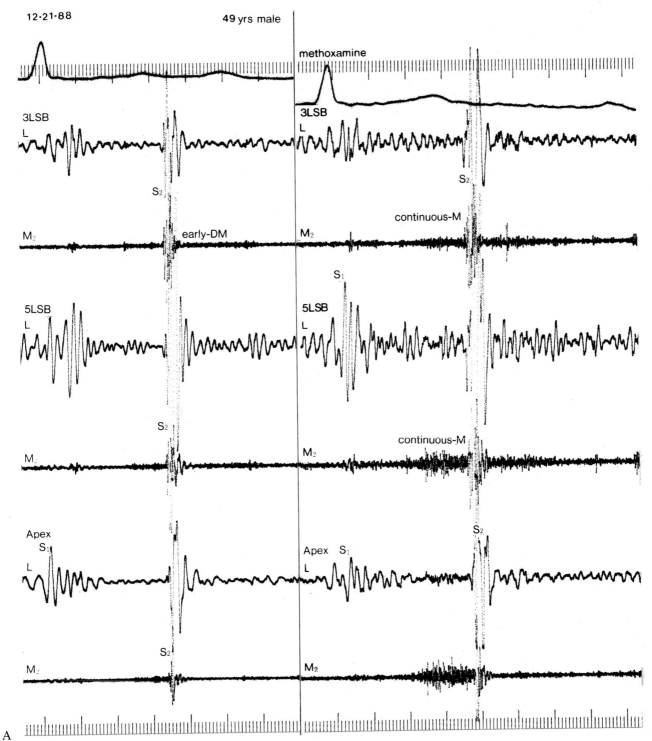

Fig. 2-4. PCG from a 49-year-old man with cerebral AV fistula. Preoperative chest x-rays, ECG, and echo were unremarkable. On auscultation a soft, early diastolic murmur (early DM) of AR was audible, **A**, but PCG showed a soft murmur enveloping the S₂ suggesting a continuous murmur, **B**. After methoxamine, the murmur became continuous in type with maximum intensity at the 5LSB. This rules out PDA, but the cause of the disease has not been established.

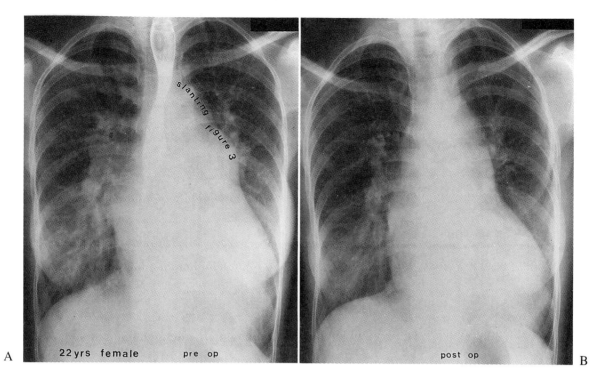

A   22 yrs female   pre op

post op   B

Fig. 2-5. This 22-year-old woman with a PDA had a preoperative chest x-ray, **A**, which showed a prominent aortic arch and a main PA resembling a slanting figure 3. The PA segment is enlarged, and the pulmonary vascularity is markedly increased indicating a left to right shunt. The postoperative chest x-ray, **B**, shows a marked reduction of the pulmonary blood flow as indicated by a smaller PA at the right hilum, reduction of vascular markings in the lungs, and resolution of the slanting figure 3. The haziness of the left lung may be due to pleural thickening as a result of surgery.

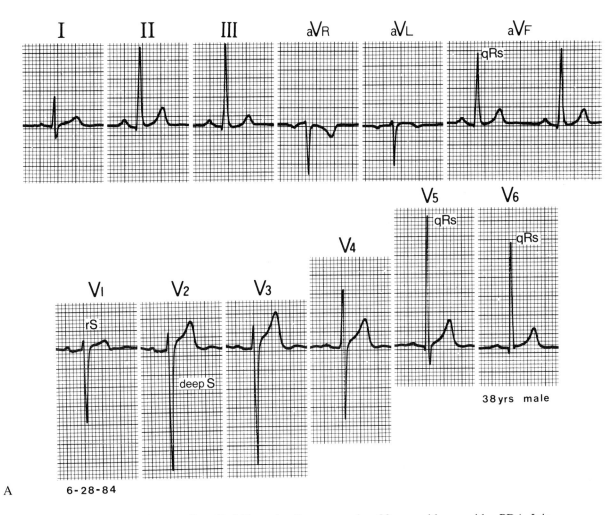

I II III aVR aVL aVF

qRs

V4 V5 V6

qRs qRs

VI V2 V3

rS

deep S

38yrs male

A   6-28-84

Fig. 2-6. A, This ECG shows a diastolic LV overloading pattern in a 38-year-old man with a PDA. It is indicated by the tall qR waves and the upright T waves in leads V_5 and V_6.

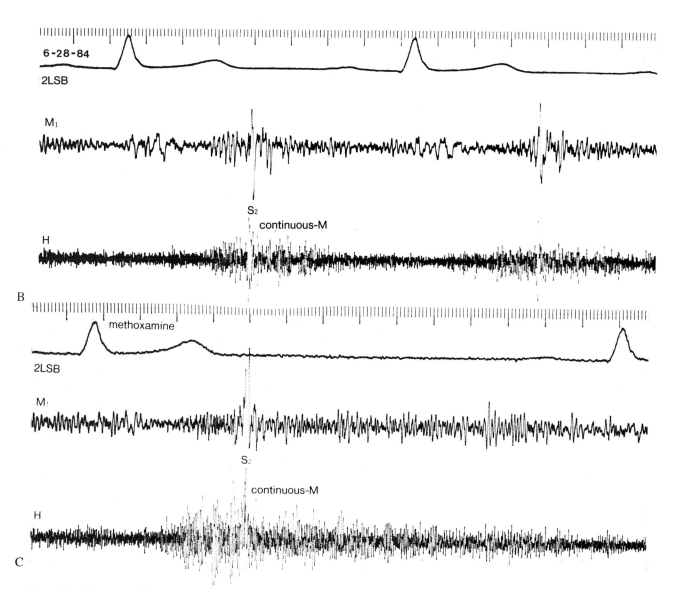

Fig. 2-6. *(Continued)* **B**, The patient's PCG shows a continuous murmur loudest at the 2LSB without transmission to the apex. **C**, After methoxamine, the murmur intensified. This and Figure 2-4 show that the peripheral vasoconstrictive action of methoxamine, which increases the blood pressure, will intensify the murmur.

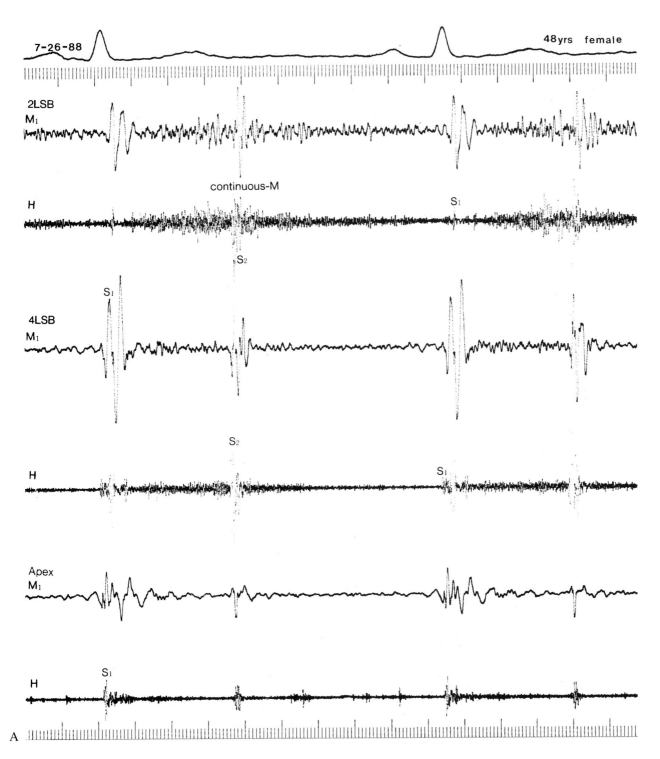

Fig. 2-7. A, PCG from a 48-year-old asymptomatic woman. During her youth, she was told she had a heart murmur but never sought medical care. A continuous murmur was loudest near the 2LSB and radiated to the 4LSB but not to the apex.

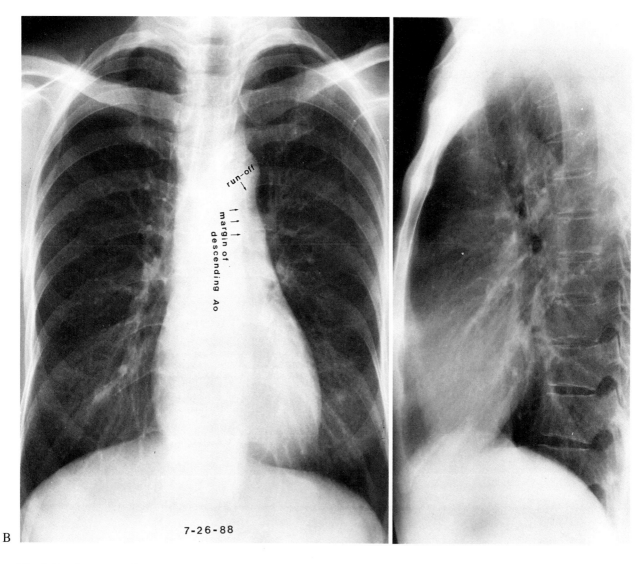

B   7-26-88   C

run-off

margin of descending Ao

Fig. 2-7. *(Continued)* **B**, The patient's chest x-rays show a prominent aortic arch without an enlarged main PA. The distal margin of the descending Ao is shifted medially, and the upper portion at the junction of the PA is not imaged. This is the run-off sign. There is no increment of peripheral PA vascularity to suggest a left to right shunt. In **C**, the anterior portion of her heart is against more than one third of the sternum suggesting some RA and RV enlargement.

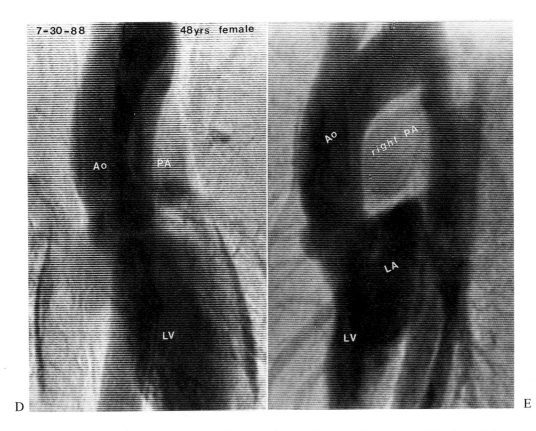

Fig. 2-7. *(Continued)* **D** and **E**, The patient's digital subtraction angiogram shows reopacification of the pulmonary arteries by a faint aortopulmonary shunt via a PDA.

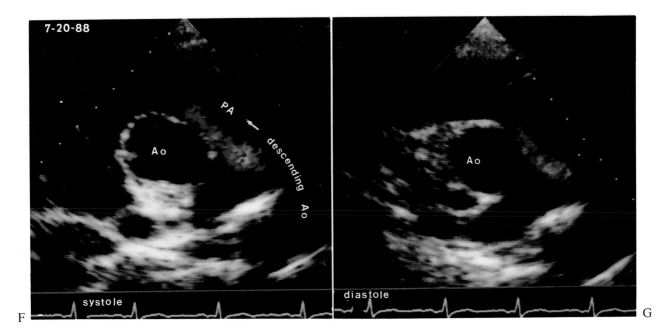

Fig. 2-7. *(Continued)* **F** and **G**, Short-axis 2D-color Doppler echoes of the Ao reveal a descending Ao to PA shunt during both systole and diastole, indicating the presence of a PDA.

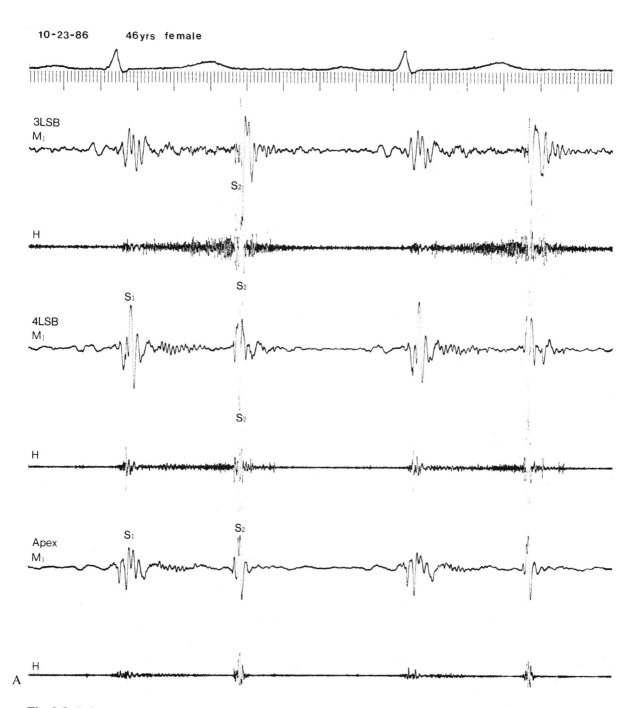

Fig. 2-8. A, In the presence of a continuous murmur, one must be alert to the possibility of a coronary artery-pulmonary artery fistula in which the murmur is usually maximal in the 3LSB or is louder in the 3LSB than in the 1LSB. This 46-year-old women had a continuous murmur loudest at the 3LSB. Since coronary flow occurs mainly in diastole, the diagnosis of a coronary artery-PA shunt is easier when the continuous murmur is louder in diastole. This is not seen in the present case.

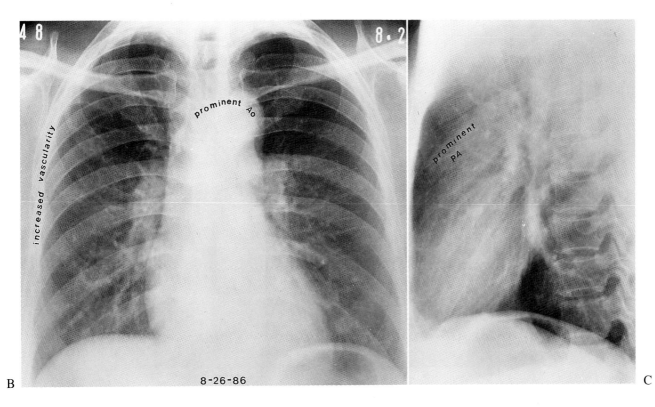

B   8-26-86   C

Fig. 2-8 *(Continued)* **B**, Patient's frontal chest x-ray shows a prominent aortic arch with increased peripheral pulmonary vascularity. **C**, Her lateral film shows a prominent main PA.

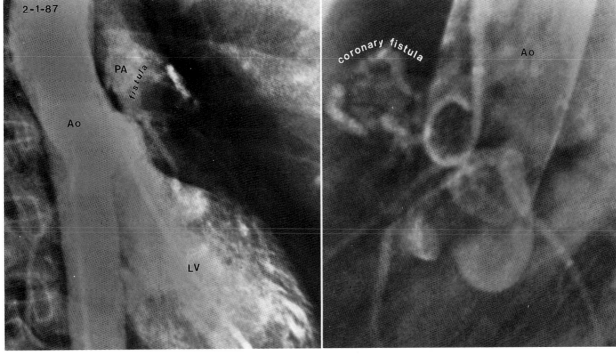

D   E

Fig. 2-8 *(Continued)* **D**, Patient's angiogram shows a dilated and tortuous left coronary artery to pulmonary artery fistula. **E**, through the fistula the contrast medium enters the PA.

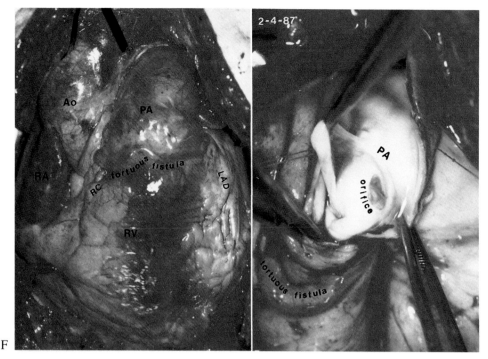

Fig. 2-8 *(Continued)* F, At surgery a dilated and tortuous coronary artery fistula traversed the root of the PA. G, The fistula communicated with the PA just below the pulmonary valve, via 2 orifices. The fistula was divided and the PA orifices were closed.

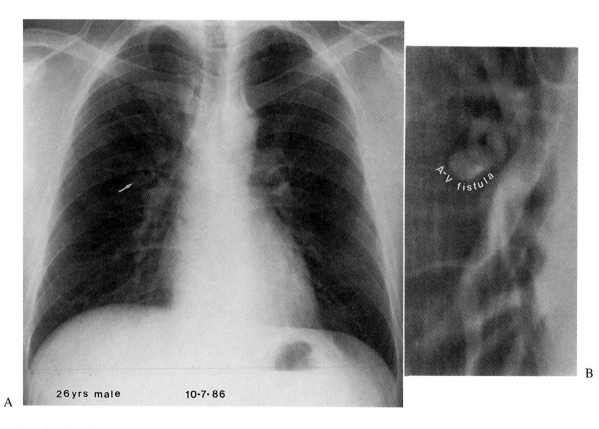

Fig. 2-9. **A,** Chest x-ray from a 26-year-old man with a pulmonary coin lesion (white arrow) detected at an annual physical examination. On auscultation, a continuous murmur was audible over the entire right side of the chest. When a continuous murmur is heard over a large area of the chest, one must suspect a pulmonary arteriovenous (AV) fistula. **B,** A tomogram of the lesion clearly demonstrates an AV fistula.

Chapter 3   Aortic Regurgitation

Pathophysiology and Clinical Clues

The major cause of aortic regurgitation (AR) is rheumatic fever; it is also often associated with aortic stenosis and mitral valve abnormalities. Another common cause of AR is a bicuspid aortic valve. Syphilis, formerly a common cause of AR, is now rare. Other causes of AR are hypertension of more than 110 mm Hg diastolic pressure, aortic dissection, Marfan's syndrome, aortitis syndrome, annulo-aortic ectasia and a high ventricular septal defect complicated by a prolapsed aortic cusp. Ankylosing spondylitis and rheumatoid arthritis are very rare causes of AR.

An approach to the diagnosis of AR is as follows:

★★★★ On auscultation, an early decrescendo diastolic murmur is heard along left sternal border (best heard during held expiration with the patient leaning forward). The early diastolic murmur is often associated with an ejection murmur due to increased forward flow or distortion of the valve. When the ejection murmur is soft, annulo-aortic ectasia, aortitis and/or a prolapsed aortic cusp is suspected.

★★★★ Chest x-ray usually shows an enlarged aortic arch and LV.

★★★★ Echo shows dilatation of the LV and often fluttering of the anterior leaflet of the mitral valve in the M-mode.

★★★★ On ECG, diastolic LV overloading or if severe and of long duration, a systolic overloading[*] pattern is observed.

[*] When low and/or negative T waves are associated with ST depressions in the LV leads, systolic overloading is suspected. In such cases, initial q waves may not be seen in the LV leads indicating the abnormal septal activation of an incomplete LBBB pattern.

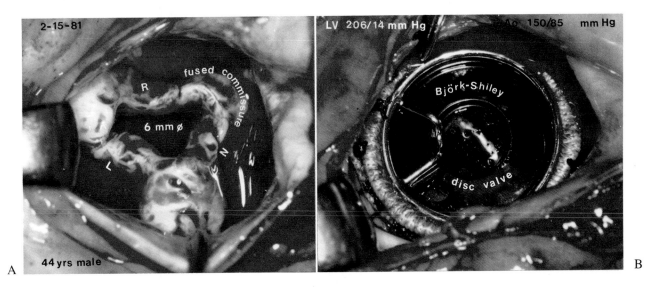

Fig. 3-1. A, Photographs from a 45-year-old man with rheumatic AR and aortic stenosis. At surgery, there was thickening of the left aortic cusp (L), the right cusp (R), and the noncoronary cusp (N), with fusion of the commissures. **B,** The patient's aortic valve was replaced with a Björk-Shiley disc valve.

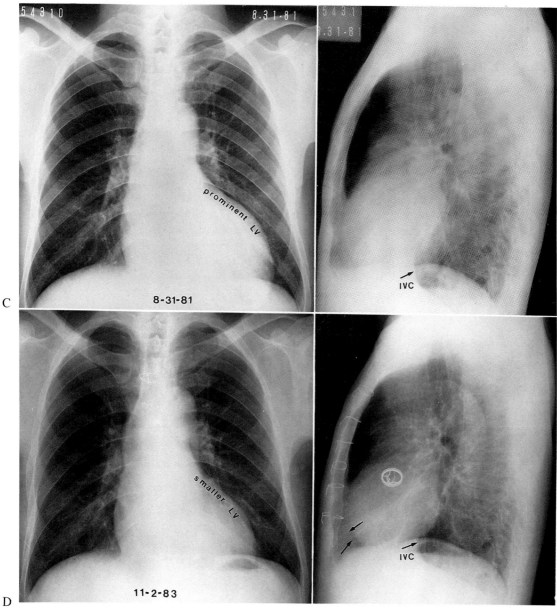

C

8-31-81

D

11-2-83

Fig. 3-1. *(Continued)* C, Patient's preoperative chest x-rays show an enlarged Ao and prominent LV. The lateral view shows that the inferior vena cava (IVC) intersects the posterior cardiac border below the level of the diaphragm, indicating LV enlargement. **D**, Postoperatively, although the size of the Ao remained unchanged, the LV became much smaller. This is also evident on the lateral view which now shows the junction of the IVC and LV above the level of the diaphragm. The disc valve is seen on the lateral view. The aortic valve is at the center of the longitudinal axis (a line from the bifurcation of the trachea to the sternophrenic angle) on the lateral projection.*

* In this chest x-ray, 2 black arrows pointing against each other at the sternophrenic angle designate a faint opaque white line representing an anterior pericardial stripe. Posterior to this line, a radiolucent (grey) area represents subepicardial fat; anterior to this line is pericardial fat. When a pericardial effusion develops, the anterior pericardial stripe becomes 5 mm or more thick.

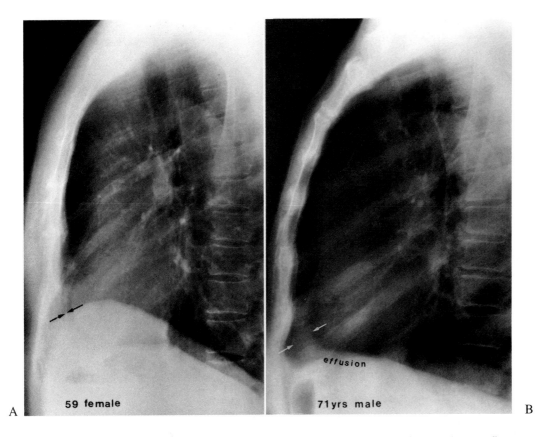

Fig 3-2. Two cases with an anterior pericardial stripe. **A,** A 59-year-old female shows a fine anterior pericardial stripe (black arrows) showing the absence of pericardial effusion. **B,** A 71-year-old man shows that his anterior pericardial stripe is wide (white arrows) suggesting a pericardial effusion.

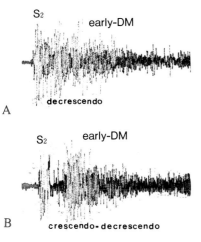

Fig. 3-3. A, Generally, the important clinical findings in AR are observation of high amplitude rapidly rising pulsations in the neck or suprasternal area and a diastolic high-pitched decrescendo murmur, which usually begins at the S_2 and ends at the S_1 (pandiastolic). **B,** shows that the murmur may begin shortly after the S_2 and produce an early crescendo-decrescendo beginning. It will have a very early peak, giving the impression of a short pause or hesitation after the S_2, and may imply mild to moderate AR.[*]

[*] Conventionally the systolic and diastolic murmurs over the femoral artery described by Duroziez, head-nodding of de Musset, and pulsating flushing of slightly compressed fingernails (Quincke's sign) are interesting but unimportant because they only occur with severe AR.

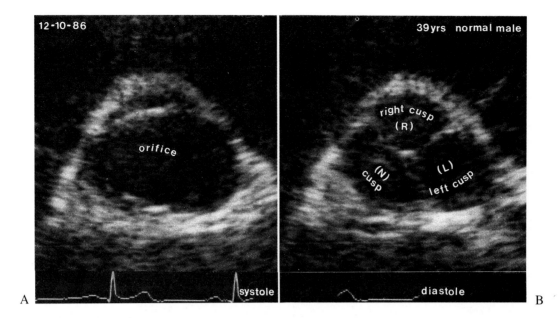

Fig. 3-4. Short-axis echoes of the aortic valve from a 39-year-old male noncardiac patient. **A**, During systole, there is complete opening of the valve. **B**, In diastole, the three cusps coapt in the center of the Ao.

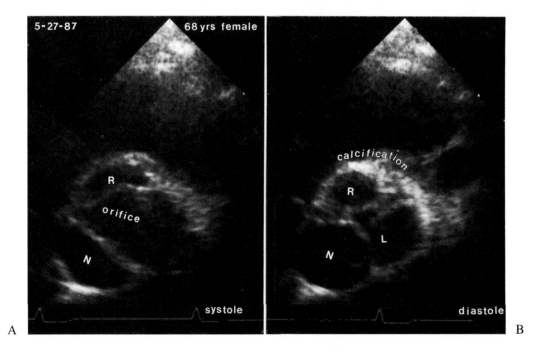

Fig. 3-5. Short-axis echoes of the Ao from a 68-year-old woman with rheumatic AR and aortic stenosis (AS). **A**, During systole, incomplete opening of the aortic valve is seen, especially of the right (R) and noncoronary (N) cusps. **B**, In diastole, the three cusps do not coapt in the center of the Ao and there are spaces between each cusp. The calcification of the aortic root is imaged along the right (R) and left (L) cusp. Each cusp is a bowl-like structure and the echo beam may project across the bottom of the bowl and show a space between the cusps in spite of their complete coaptation. For this reason the diagnosis of AR by short-axis view is hazardous.

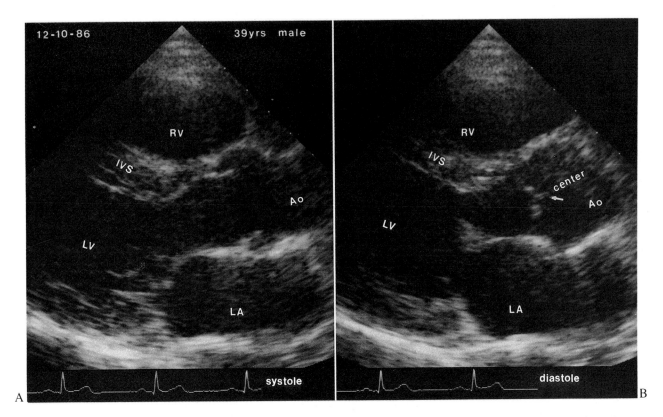

Fig. 3-6. Long-axis echoes from a 39-year-old noncardiac patient. **A,** During systole the aortic cusps are widely open and they are nearly touching the aortic wall. **B,** In diastole, the aortic cusps coapt in the center of the Ao indicating complete closure.

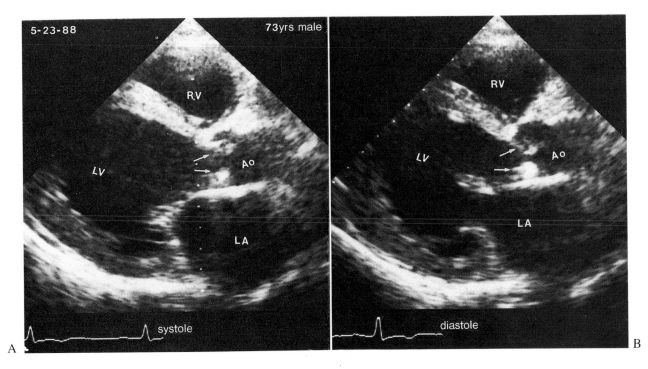

Fig. 3-7. Long-axis echoes from a 73-year-old man with rheumatic valvular heart disease. **A,** During systole, limited opening of the aortic valve with heavy calcification can be seen. **B,** During diastole, the aortic valve remains open (white arrows) suggesting the presence of AR.

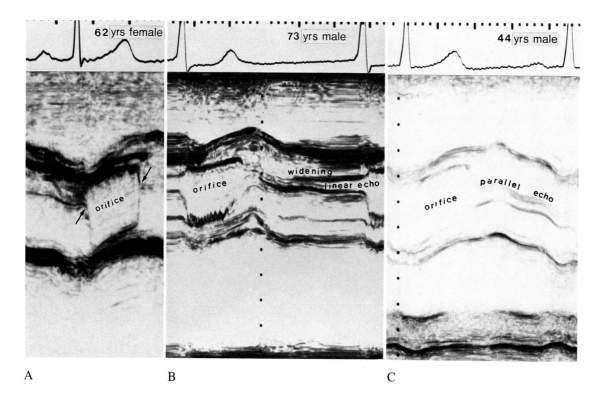

A   B   C

Fig. 3-8. As mentioned before, a definitive diagnosis of AR is rather difficult to establish by echo except by Doppler. In some cases, however, a finding that is strongly suggestive may be observed. **A,** An M-mode echo of a 62-year-old noncardiac patient shows normal opening and closing of the aortic valve with a box-like configuration. Closure appears to be a single line during diastole. **B,** A 73-year-old man with AR and incomplete opening of the aortic valve during systole. In contrast to a single linear valvular echo during diastole as in normal subjects, there are multiple layered echoes. However, they are rather thin linear echoes and they have a tendency to widen toward the beginning of systole. This differs from an ordinary multiple-layered echo and strongly suggests the presence of AR. **C,** An M-mode echo from a 44-year-old man with rheumatic AR. During diastole, the linear echoes are parallel. In the early days of echocardiography, this was suggestive of AR, but now is considered an inconclusive finding.

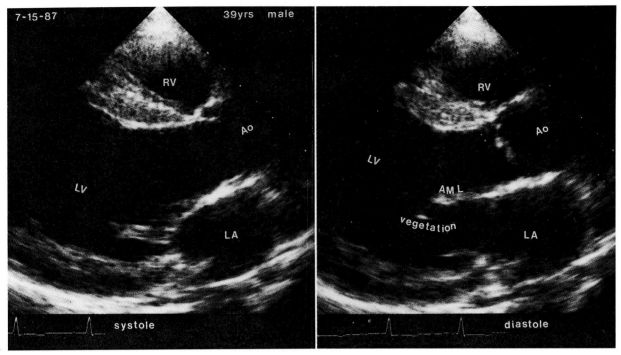

Fig. 3-9. A, Long-axis 2D-echoes from a 39-year-old man with combined valvular disease associated with infective endocarditis. Both the Ao and LV are enlarged. **B**, During diastole, the aortic valve does not seem to close completely. There is a strong echo in the LV between the mitral leaflets suggestive of a vegetation.

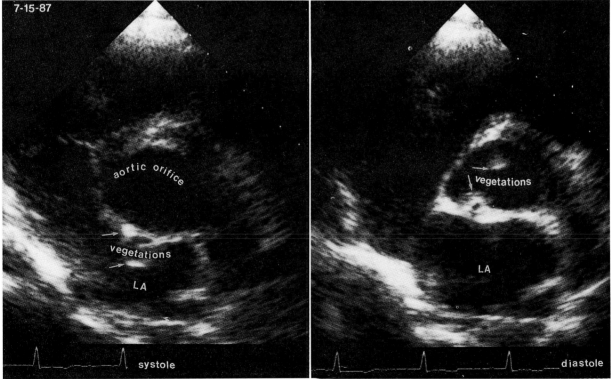

Fig. 3-9. *(Continued)* **C**, The short axis of the patient's Ao shows adequate opening of the aortic valve. Posterior to the Ao, a normal-sized LA is imaged,* but there are strong echoes suggestive of vegetations. **D**, During diastole, these strong echoes shift upward toward the aortic area.

* A left atrial dimension is considered normal if it is the same as that of the aortic root.

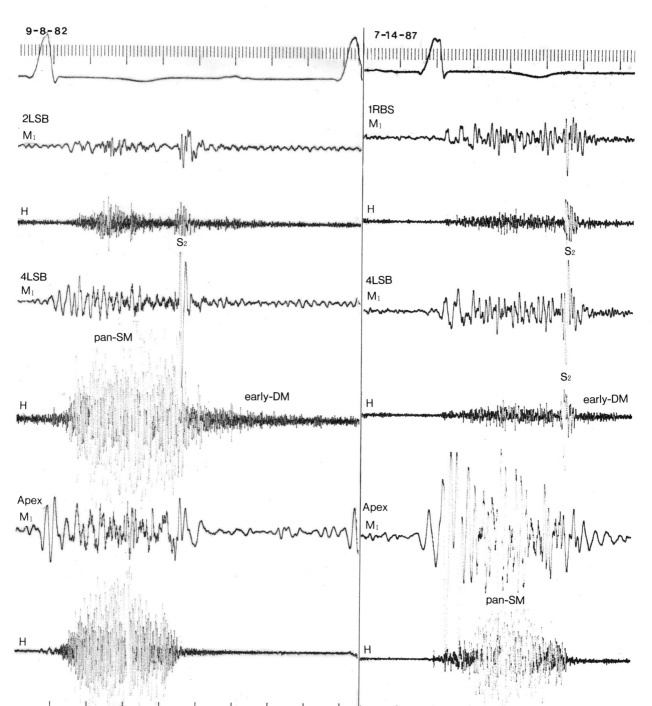

Fig. 3-9. *(Continued)* **E,** During the initial visit, PCG showed a pansystolic murmur (pan-SM) maximum at the fourth intercostal space (4LSB) and transmitted to the apex. An early diastolic murmur (early DM) is recorded from the base of his heart to the 4LSB suggesting the dominant lesions to be MR and AR. The patient was uncooperative and left the hospital after his recovery from congestive heart failure (CHF). **F,** A PCG on his readmission shows greatly reduced MR and AR murmurs, but he had a high fever, and the change in the murmurs was suggestive of infective endocarditis. Unfortunately, he again discharged himself from the hospital and no follow-up studies were possible.

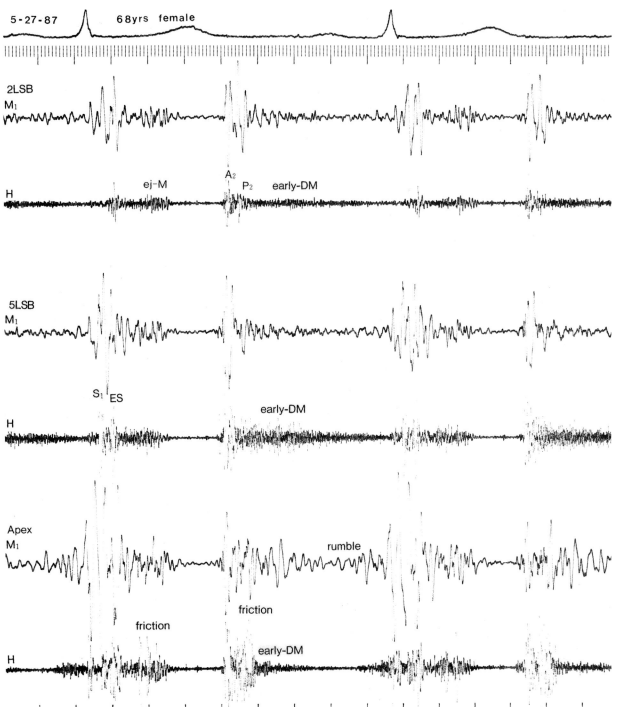

Fig. 3-10. A, PCG from a 68-year-old asymptomatic woman with a fusiform aneurysm of her ascending Ao. At the base of her heart, slight splitting of S_2 with an early diastolic murmur is present which is transmitted to 5LSB. A loud ejection sound (ES) is also seen. At the apex, there are high frequency presystolic, midsystolic, and early diastolic sounds which may be friction rubs. The presystolic component is also recorded at medium frequency (M_1) which may suggest that this is due to a rumble despite the absence of an opening snap (OS). In contrast to the early diastolic murmur, the ejection murmur (ej-M) is soft, which is unusual for AR of rheumatic origin.

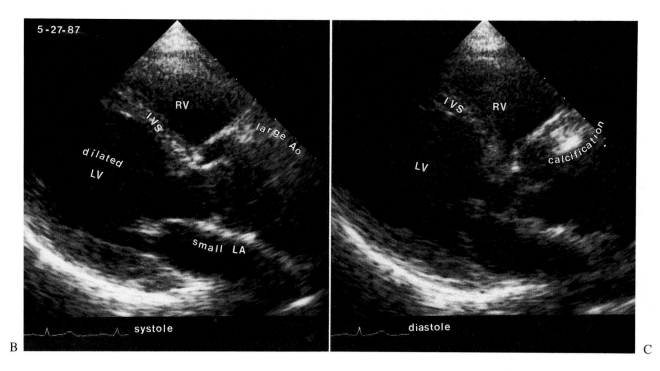

B

C

Fig. 3-10. *(Continued)* **B**, The patient's long axis shows a dilated LV and Ao. **C**, The markedly dilated and heavily calcified anterior and posterior aortic walls are seen compressing the LA. There is no evidence of concomitant mitral stenosis. The aortoseptal angle is sharp indicating a sigmoid septum. The presence of a rumble is probably an Austin Flint murmur.

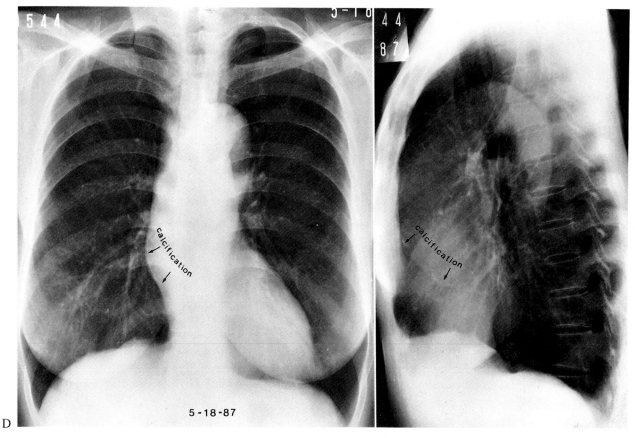

D

E

Fig. 3-10. *(Continued)* **D**, The patient's frontal chest x-ray shows a protrusion of the aortic root toward the right with a fine linear calcification. **E**, The lateral view shows the same linear calcification. The ascending Ao protrudes anteriorly and displaces the LV posteriorly.

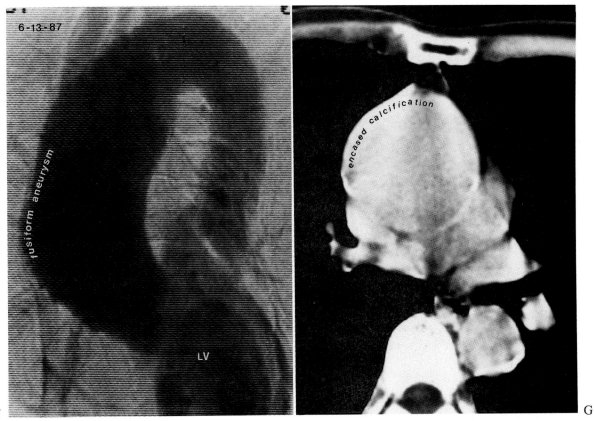

F

6-13-87

fusiform aneurysm

LV

encased calcification

G

Fig. 3-10. *(Continued)* **F**, A digital subtraction angiogram of the same patient shows a large fusiform aneurysm of the ascending Ao. **G**, A cardiac CT section at the level of the mid-ascending Ao shows marginal calcification also seen in the descending Ao.

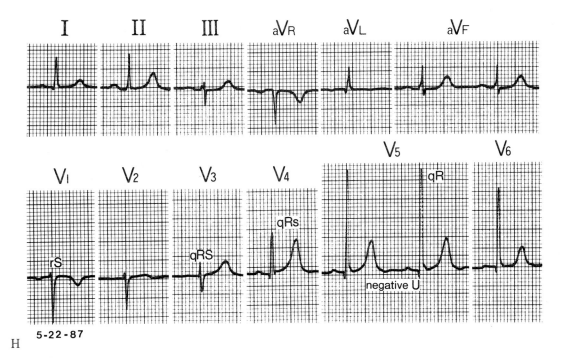

I   II   III   aVR   aVL   aVF

V5   V6

VI   V2   V3   V4

qR

rS   qRS   qRs

negative U

5-22-87

H

Fig. 3-10. *(Continued)* **H**, The same patient's ECG shows a qRS pattern in V$_3$ and a tall qR in V$_5$ associated with a negative U wave. The presence of a septal q wave as far to the right as V$_3$ often indicates either elongation or tortuosity of the Ao producing counterclockwise rotation of the heart. This correlates well with her chest x-ray.

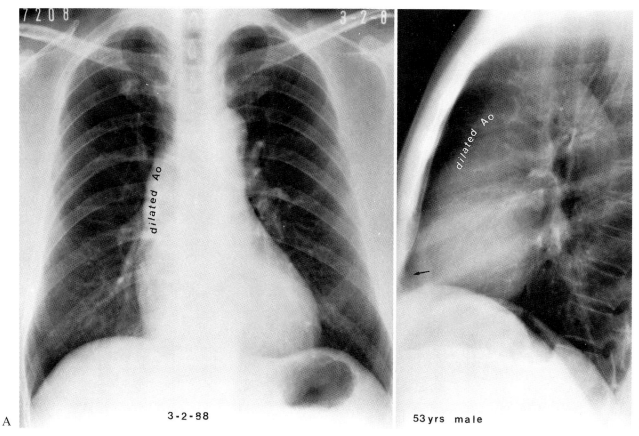

A

B

Fig. 3-11. A, Chest x-rays from 53-year-old man with AR showing dilated ascending Ao without LA enlargement. **B**, The lateral view shows a dilated ascending Ao without either LV or LA enlargement. An anterior pericardial stripe is clearly observable as indicated by the arrow.

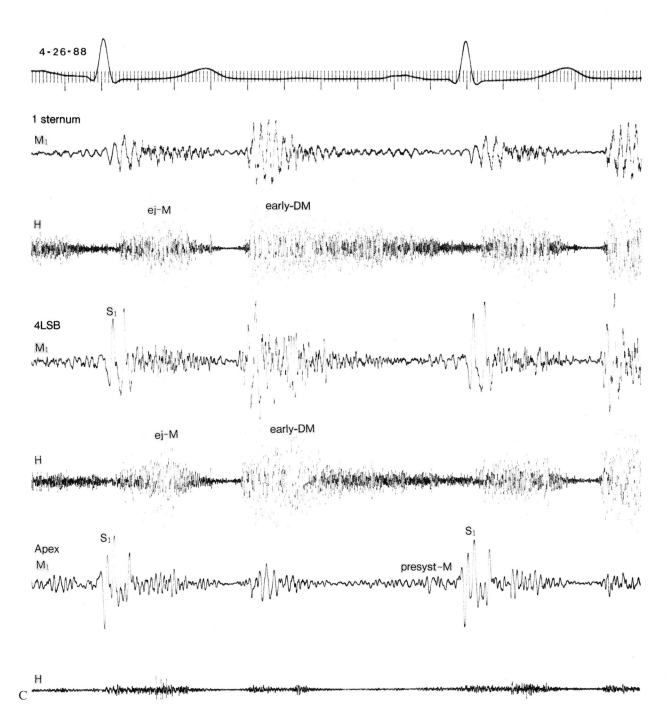

Fig. 3-11. *(Continued)* **C**, A PCG of the same patient shows an ejection murmur (ej-M) and an early diastolic murmur from the first intercostal space on the sternum (1 sternum) to the fourth intercostal space. At the apex, a medium frequency PCG shows a soft presystolic murmur. The S$_2$ is not clearly visible at any site.

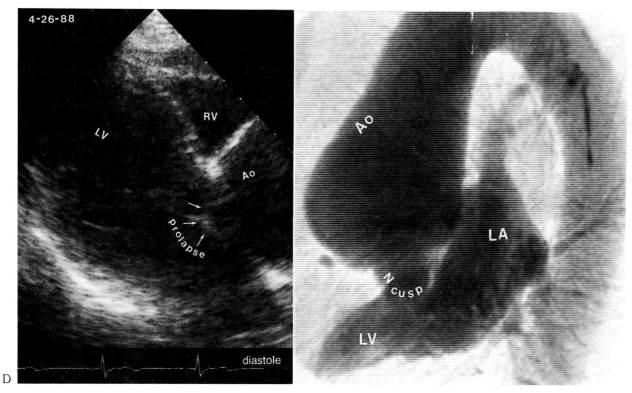

D

E

Fig. 3-11. *(Continued)* **D,** Patient's echoes show that one of the aortic cusps was prolapsed. **E,** A digital subtraction angiogram of the same patient shows a relatively small noncoronary cusp prolapsed. The aortic root is markedly dilated, which is suggestive of annulo-aortic ectasia.

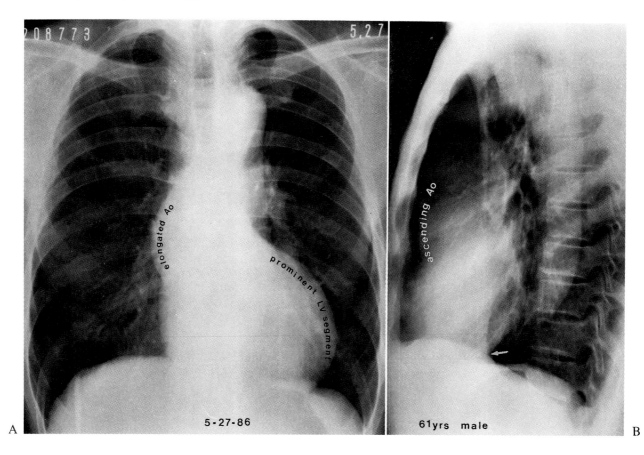

A

B

Fig. 3-12. See legend on facing page.

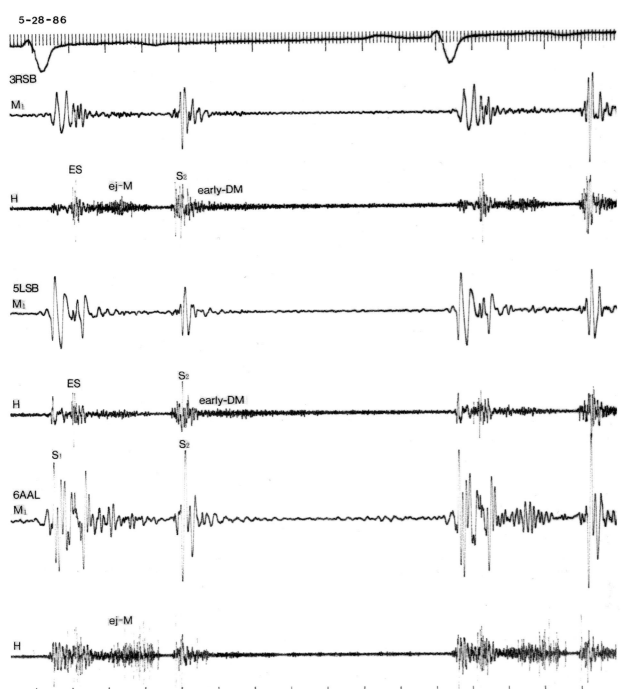

5-28-86

3RSB
M₁

ES   ej-M   S₂   early-DM
H

5LSB
M₁

ES   S₂   early-DM
H

S₁   S₂
6AAL
M₁

ej-M
H

C

Fig. 3-12. *(Continued)* **C,** His PCG shows a soft ejection murmur (ej-M) which begins with an ejection sound (ES) and ends before the S₂. An early diastolic murmur (early DM) is best heard at the third right intercostal space (3RSB) and is transmitted to the 5LSB.

←—

Fig. 3-12. Chest x-rays from a 61-year-old man with AR. A prominent ascending Ao is seen in both frontal, **A,** and lateral, **B,** projections. The junction of the IVC and posterior margin of the heart is above the level of the diaphragm suggesting that there is no LV enlargement. However, the LV segment is prominent as a slight bulge of the upper portion of the LV segment, **A,** suggesting concentric hypertrophy.

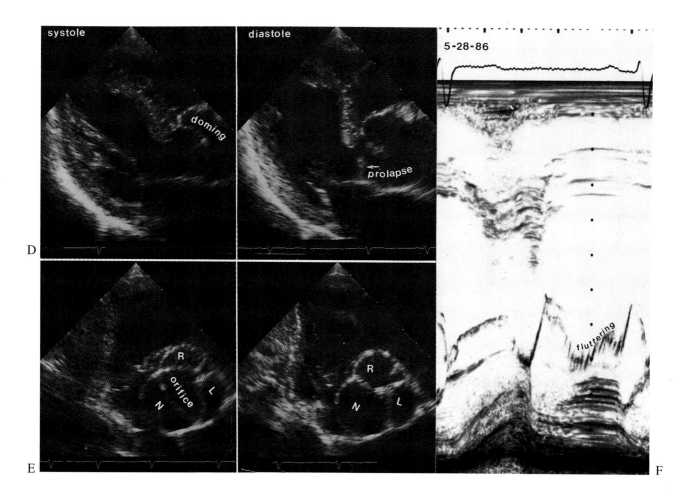

Fig. 3-12. *(Continued)* Long- and short-axis 2D-echoes show a deformed opening of the aortic valve during systole. **D,** During systole, the long-axis view shows doming of the aortic valve and, **E,** the short-axis view demonstrates an unusual shape and incomplete opening. During diastole, the long-axis view shows a prolapsed cusp. In the short-axis view, the noncoronary cusp is relatively larger than other cusps. An M-mode echo, **F,** shows fluttering of the anterior mitral leaflet. The E wave (mitral valve opening movement) is relatively low which suggests the presence of AR. There is no evidence of LV enlargement.

*Fluttering of the anterior leaflet of the mitral valve can be caused by AR or ruptured anterior chordae allowing a flail anterior leaflet to flutter.

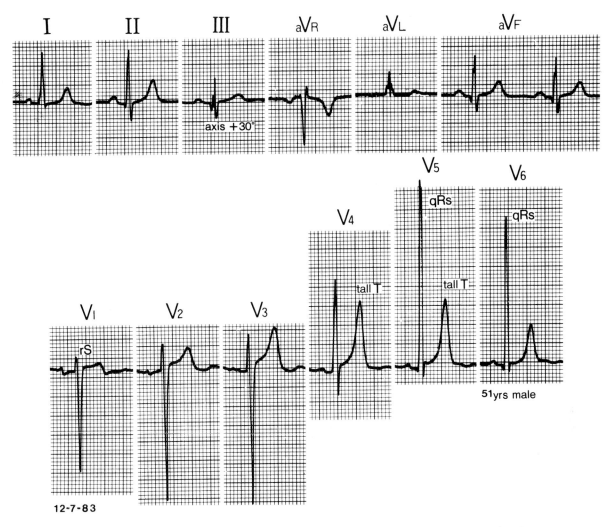

A

12-7-83

Fig. 3-13. A, ECG of 51-year-old man with rheumatic AR. ECG findings of diastolic LV overloading* which are frequently observed in AR include

1. A tall qR wave and T wave in the LV leads V_5 and V_6 with an upward concave ST elevation.
2. S waves equally deep (or deeper) over the right precordium than the amplitude of the R waves in the left precordium.
3. Usually no QT prolongation unlike what may be seen in systolic LV overloading.
4. In some cases, short PQ intervals may be observed.

* When diastolic LV overloading with right axis deviation is found, biventricular overload is likely.

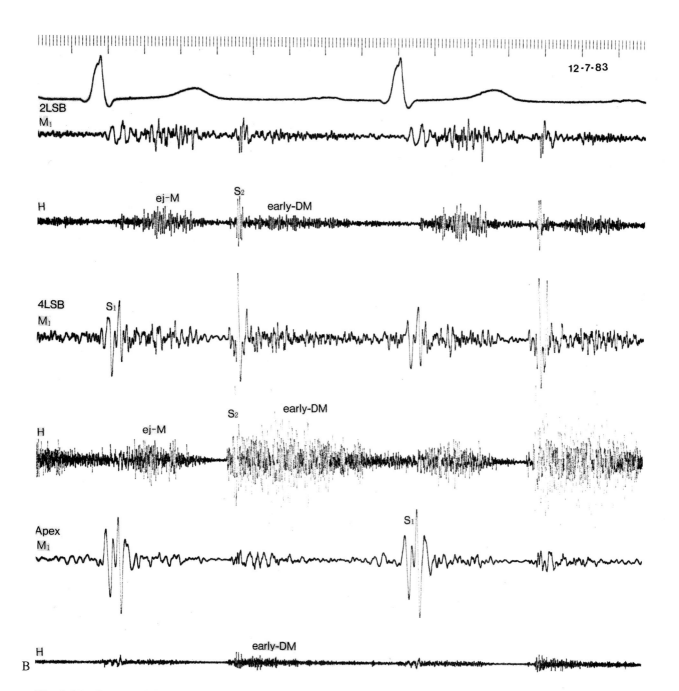

Fig. 3-13. *(Continued)* **B**, PCG of the same patient shows a soft ejection murmur (ej-M) at the 2LSB transmitted to the 4LSB. There is a crescendo-decrescendo type early diastolic murmur (early DM) indicating AR. The ejection murmur does not necessarily indicate the presence of AS.

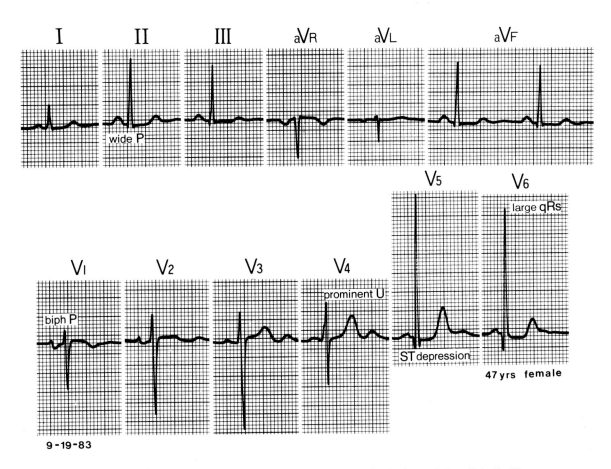

I II III aVR aVL aVF

wide P

V5 V6

large qRs

V1 V2 V3 V4

biph P

prominent U

ST depression

47 yrs female

A 9-19-83

Fig. 3-14. A, ECG from a 47-year-old woman with rheumatic AR and MS who is receiving digitalis. There are tall R waves in leads V_5 and V_6 with positive T waves. Although the ST segment is depressed (probably due to digitalis), the overall pattern suggests diastolic LV overloading. The P wave in V_1 shows a large area of terminal P negativity suggesting LA overloading.*

* The left atrial P waves together with small QRS complex in lead I, in spite of diastolic LV overloading, suggest associated MS.

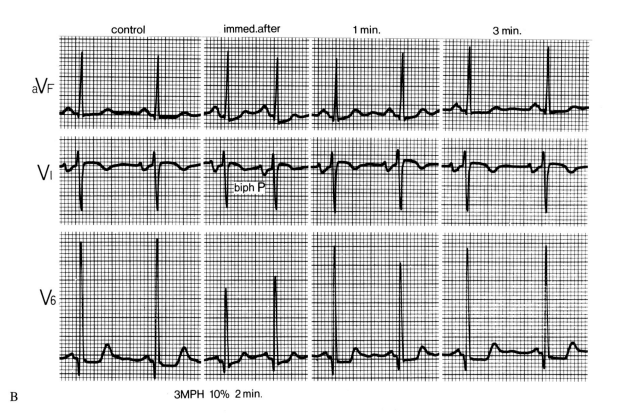

control immed.after 1 min. 3 min.

aVF

V1

biph P

V6

B   3MPH 10% 2 min.

Fig. 3-14. *(Continued)* **B,** In combined valvular heart disease which includes MS, the exercise ECG may or may not reveal ST depressions, but the P wave sign of LA overloading in V$_1$ may be the only change and often precedes ST changes. This patient with AR and MS showed flat and slightly sagging ST depressions in V$_6$ both in the control phase and after exercise. However, after exercise the P wave became biphasic (biph P) in V$_1$ and its terminal negative area became markedly enlarged indicating a greater degree of LA overloading.

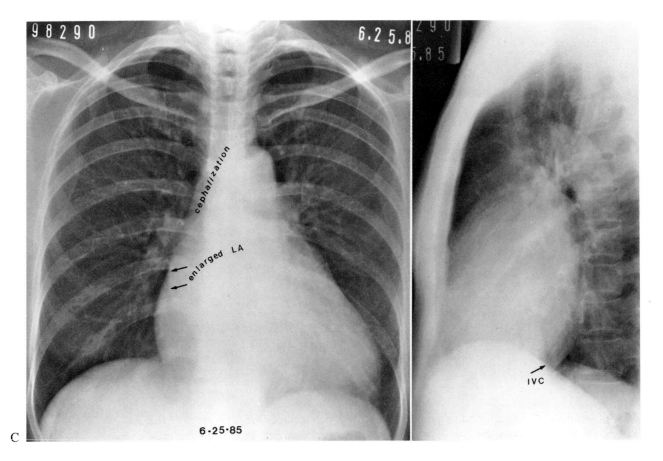

Fig. 3-14. *(Continued)* **C,** Chest x-rays of the same patient show right-sided heart enlargement. An enlarged LA is seen as a double density (arrow). There is some relative increase of the pulmonary vascularity in the upper lung fields suggesting elevation of LA pressure. **D,** The LV is also dilated and in the lateral view the junction of the IVC and the LV is below the level of the diaphragm.

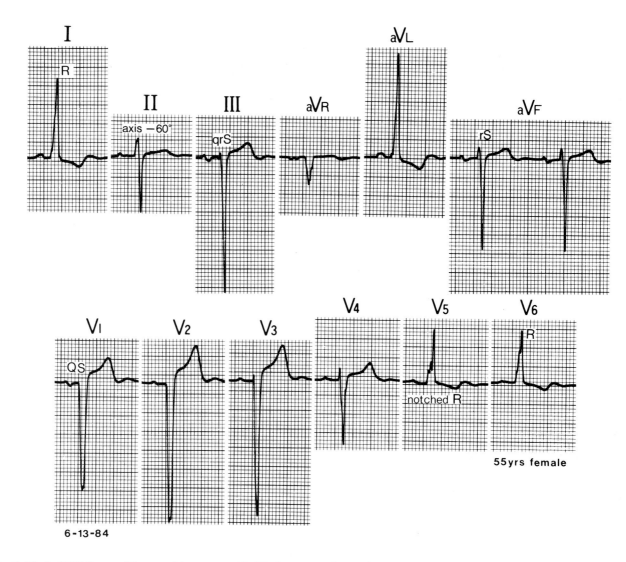

Fig. 3-15. A, ECG from a 55-year-old woman with AR due to annulo-aortic ectasia. Since the QRS complex in lead II is predominantly negative, there is a marked left axis deviation of nearly -60°. Furthermore, there is no initial septal q wave in the LV leads or a septal r wave in the right chest leads. The R wave is notched in leads V_5 and V_6. These initial QRS changes strongly suggest fibrosis in the IVS producing an incomplete LBBB pattern. Care must be taken to avoid an erroneous diagnosis of myocardial infarction in the presence of QS waves in the right precordial leads when there is an LBBB pattern. The heart was enlarged both radiographically and echocardiographically, with increased echoes from the IVS probably due to fibrosis.

Fig. 3-15. *(Continued)* **B**, The patient's chest x-ray shows cardiomegaly with marked dilatation of her ascending Ao. Since the main PA is not imaged, a counterclockwise rotation of the heart is suspected.

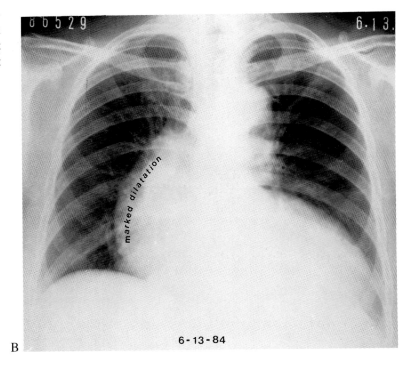

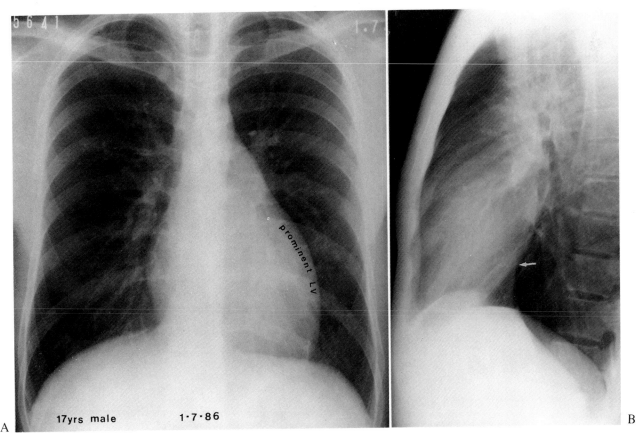

Fig. 3-16. A, Chest x-rays from a 17-year-old healthy, male high school student, show a prominent LV in the frontal view although the IVC crosses the posterior cardiac border well above the level of the diaphragm in the lateral view, **B**. There may be some increase in pulmonary vascularity, but there is no LA enlargement. The patient is an active basketball player and is asymptomatic. Because of a third heart sound (S$_3$) at the apex, a thorough examination was requested.

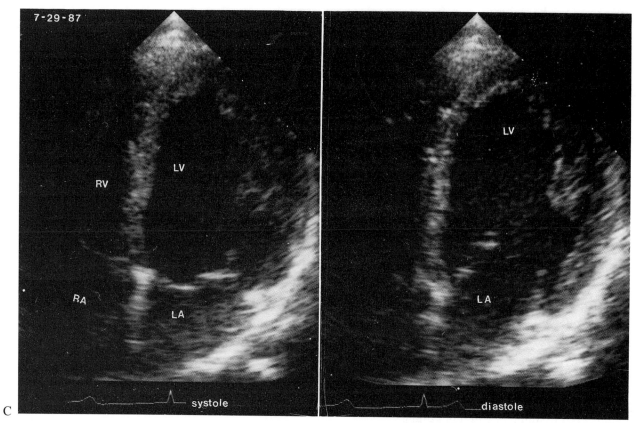

C

D

Fig. 3-16. *(Continued)* **C,** The 2D-echoes in the apical four-chamber view of the same patient show a large LV which becomes more marked during diastole, **D,** with clearly diminished LV movement. This suggests supressed LV contraction which was also observable in the short axis echoes. The LA and RA are normal.

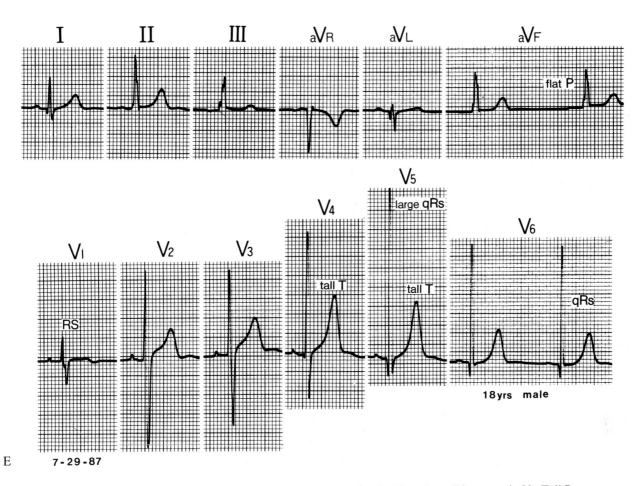

E   7-29-87

Fig. 3-16. *(Continued)* **E,** ECG of the same patient shows a normal axis. There is an RS pattern in V_1. Tall R waves associated with tall T waves in the LV leads suggest diastolic LV overloading.

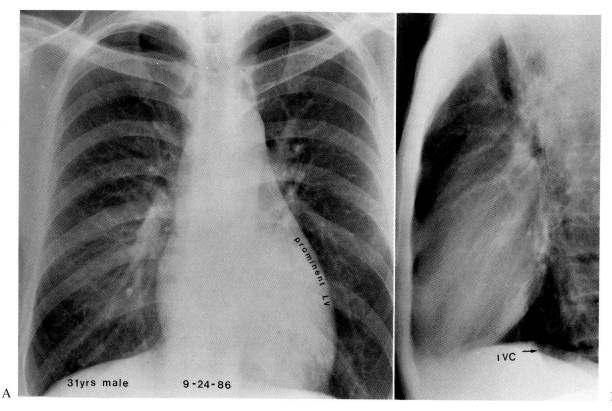

A

B

Fig. 3-17. Occasionally it is difficult to determine whether an individual who is active in sports is normal or abnormal. These chest x-rays are from a 31-year-old asymptomatic man who was thought to have an abnormal ECG. **A,** His chest x-rays show some prominence of the LV segment in the frontal view. **B,** The lateral view does not confirm LV enlargement, since the junction of the IVC and the LV is well above the level of the diaphragm.

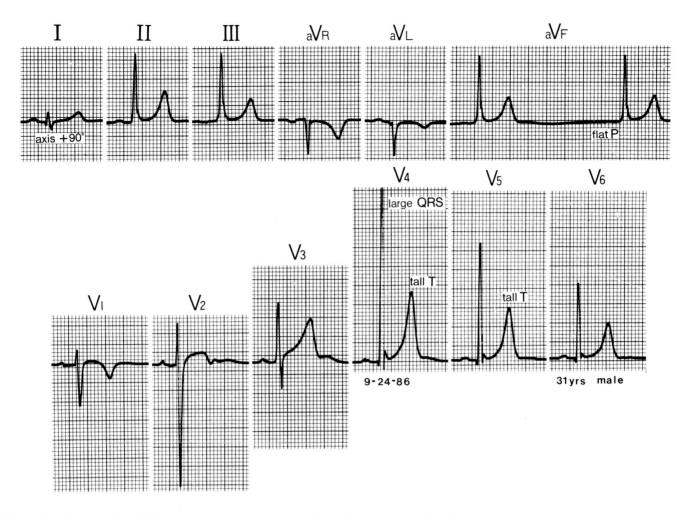

Fig. 3-17. *(Continued)* **C,** ECG shows a tall R wave in leads V₄ to V₆ associated with tall T waves resembling diastolic LV overloading. The QRS axis is about +90° since there is an equiphasic QRS in lead I. Many normal athletes may have findings suggestive of cardiac enlargement. This is because they have physiological LV overloading. Auscultation as well as an echo study disclosed no abnormality.

Chapter 4 Aortic Stenosis

Pathophysiology and Clinical Clues

Although the most common cause of aortic stenosis (AS) is valvular damage from rheumatic carditis, AS is almost as often caused by arteriosclerotic changes in very elderly patients, especially on a congenital bicuspid valve. These conditions result in calcification of the aortic valve or fusion of the commissures. Other causes of AS include hypertrophic subaortic stenosis (HSS) also known as hypertrophic obstructive cardiomyopathy (HOCM), discrete subvalvular stenosis, and supravalvular AS.[*] When the AS is significant, there will be a pressure gradient between the Ao and the LV of more than 50 mm Hg. Hypertrophy of the LV compensates for the obstruction to outflow. Diminished blood flow to the aortic arch from exertion or arrhythmias may cause presyncope or syncope. If the AS is severe or there is also concomitant coronary artery disease, angina and/or congestive heart failure will eventually occur. If the stenosis is at or very near the valve, a coarse ejection murmur is heard, loudest at the second right interspace, and is often transmitted to the neck where it coincides with a shudder or thrill over the carotid pulse. Diminution of the second heart sound is usually due to a calcified valve or the presence of cardiac dysfunction.

The clinical features of AS are as follows:

★★★★ On auscultation there is a prominent ejection murmur often associated with an ejection sound. There is usually a coexistent early diastolic murmur of AR. Occasionally, there may be paradoxical splitting of the second heart sound (S_2) i.e., it will split on expiration and become single on inspiration.

★★★★ In the ECG, systolic LV overloading may be manifested by systolic LV overloading pattern (LVH strain pattern) and/or an incomplete LBBB pattern.

★★★★ Chest x-rays may show an enlarged ascending Ao due to poststenotic dilatation. Calcification of the valve may be observed in the center of the cardiac silhouette in the lateral projection. Concentric LV hypertrophy without dilatation is present unless there is cardiac decompensation or an associated aortic regurgitation (AR).

★★★★ In the echo, besides thick walls, a thickened or calcified aortic valve with limited movement is expected.

[*] Either sub- or supravalvular AS is due to obstruction by membranous or fibrous tissue.

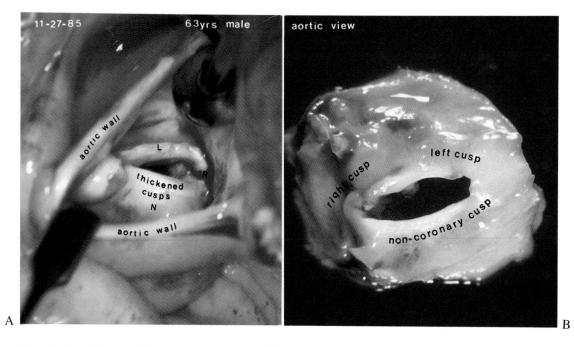

Fig. 4-1. This 63-year-old man with rheumatic AS had valvular replacement due to repeated congestive heart failure. **A**, At surgery all cusps were hypertrophied and the commissures were fused. **B**, The surgical specimen viewed from the aortic side shows a hypertrophied left (L) and noncoronary cusp (N). The right cusp (R) was atrophied so that the valve appeared to be bicuspid.

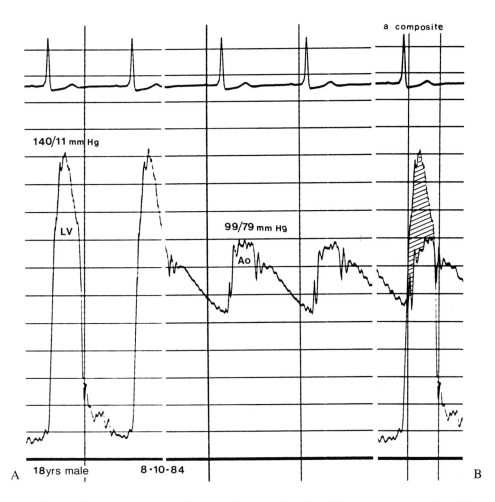

Fig. 4-2. A, LV and Ao pressure tracing from an 18-year-old male high school student who had a systolic murmur since childhood. His LV pressure was 140/11 and his Ao pressure 99/79 mm Hg. This 40 mm Hg pressure gradient across his aortic valve caused an ejection murmur. **B**, On the right is a composite tracing showing a slight delay in the onset of the upstroke of the Ao from that of the LV. This is caused by the isovolumic contraction period during which the mitral and aortic valves remain closed. A sharp notch on the descending limb of the aortic pressure curve is the incisura, which coincides with closure of the aortic valve and the A$_2$.

*The dicrotic notch of the external carotid artery pulse tracing is delayed after the incisura because of the distance from the Ao; therefore, the A$_2$ occurs slightly before the dicrotic notch. The external carotid dicrotic notch is due to the same phenomenon as the aortic incisura, i.e., they mark closure of aortic valve.

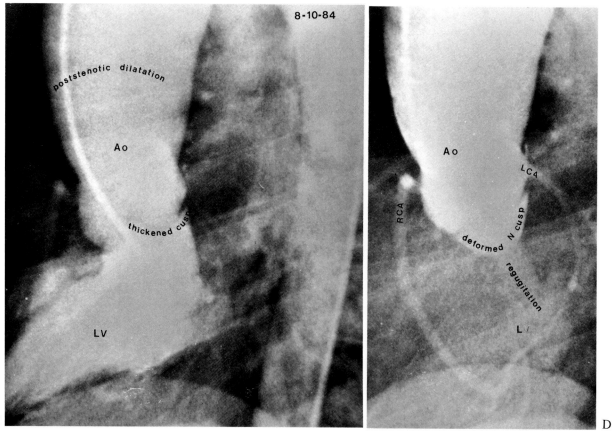

C

D

Fig. 4-2. *(Continued)* C, An aortogram of the same patient shows poststenotic dilatation of the ascending Ao. Both the left (LCA) and right coronary artery (RCA) are visualized. D, A faint aortic regurgitant jet is also visible.

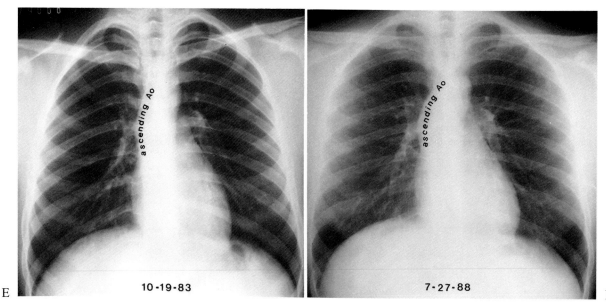

E

F

Fig. 4-2. *(Continued)* E, Initial frontal chest x-ray of the same patient shows a normal cardiac silhouette except that the ascending Ao is slightly prominent due to the poststenotic dilatation. If one were to overlook the abnormal ascending Ao, the diagnosis of AS would not be suspected. In F, 5 years later, the protrusion of the ascending Ao is more marked indicating greater poststenotic dilatation.

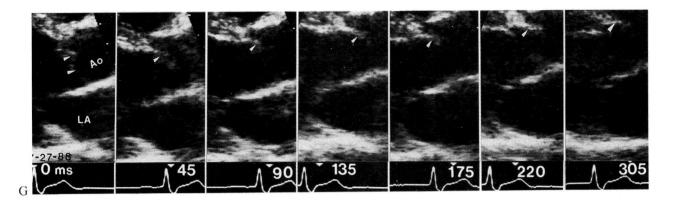

Fig. 4-2. *(Continued)* **G,** Serial tracing of his long-axis 2D-echoes of the aortic valve shows very limited opening throughout systole. The numbers in milliseconds indicate the delay from the peak of the R wave in the ECG.

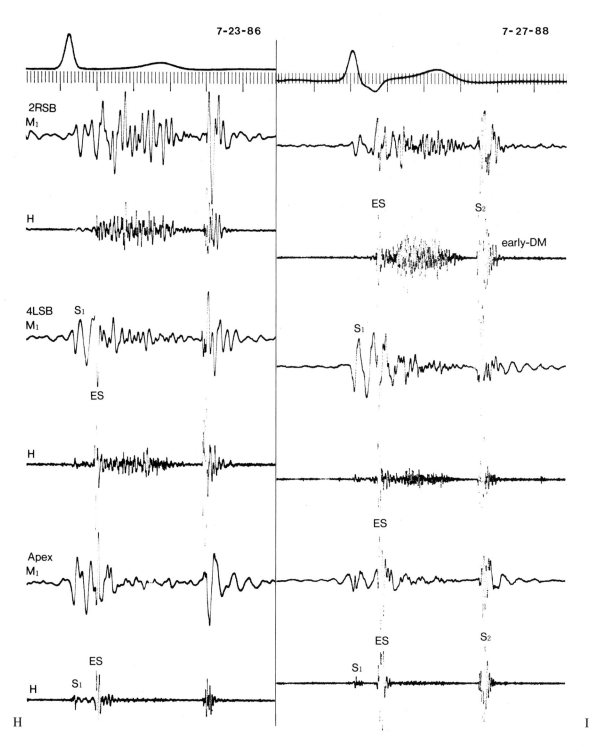

Fig. 4-2. *(Continued)* **H,** The patient's PCG showed a relatively soft ejection murmur at the base with a sharp ejection sound (ES). **I,** Two years later the ejection murmur is more high-pitched and a soft early diastolic murmur (early DM) follows the S$_2$ which is also more prominent.

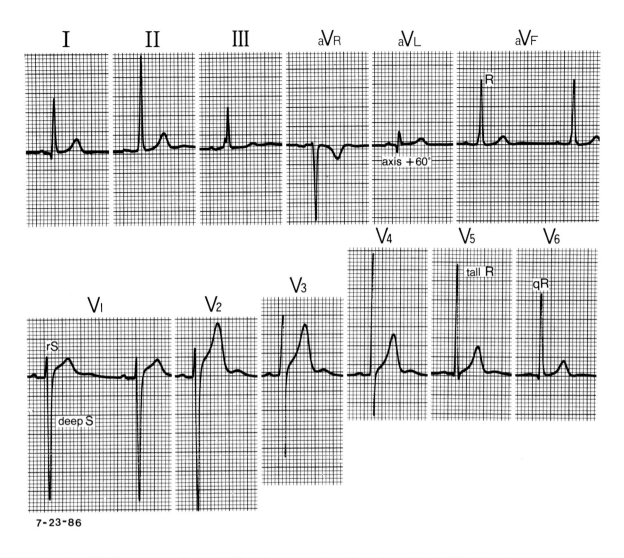

I II III aVR aVL aVF

V1 V2 V3 V4 V5 V6

7-23-86

J

Fig. 4-2. *(Continued)* **J**, Two years earlier, an ECG of the same patient showed an axis of +60°. A deep S wave in V_1 and V_2 and tall R wave in V_5 and V_6 satisfies the Sokolow voltage criteria for left ventricular hypertrophy.* However, there are no ST·T changes of a strain pattern.

*Sokolow criteria: $SV_1 + RV_5$ or $_6 \geq 35$ mm.
  Modified Sokolow criteria: $SV_2 + RV_6 \geq 35$ mm.

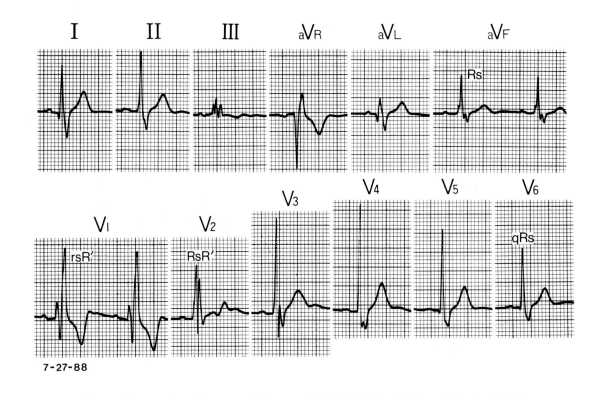

K   7-27-88

Fig. 4-2 *(Continued)* **K**, ECG 2 years later shows an rsR′ pattern in V₁ of right bundle-branch block (RBBB). There is no inferior or right-axis change or peaked P waves to indicate that this RBBB is due to diastolic RV overloading. This suggests that an increased Ao and LV pressure gradient caused interventricular septal ischemia or fibrosis which produced the RBBB. The patient is being evaluated for possible surgical treatment.

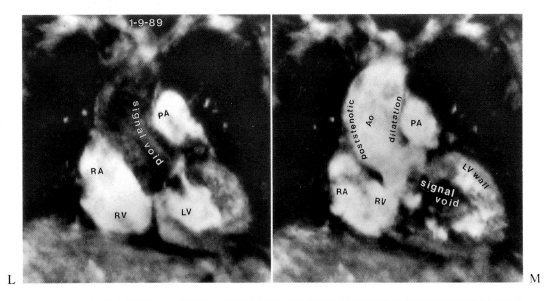

Fig. 4-2 *(Continued)* **L**, The patient's cine magnetic resonance image (MRI) in the coronal section shows marked poststenotic dilatation of his ascending Ao. There is signal void in the entire ascending Ao indicating the AS. **M**, Dilatation of the sinuses of Valsalva and the hypertrophy of the LV wall can be seen. Below the aortic valve a signal void indicates inflow from the mitral valve and the regurgitant flow of AR.

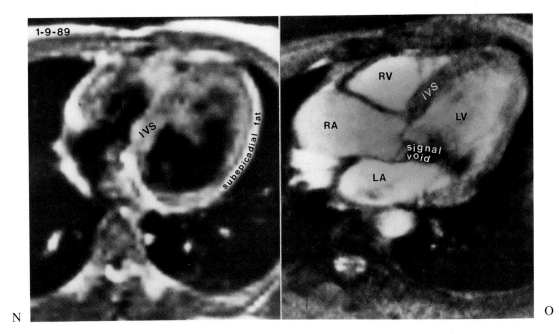

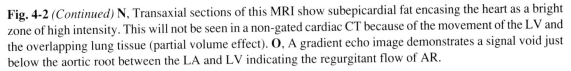

Fig. 4-2 *(Continued)* **N**, Transaxial sections of this MRI show subepicardial fat encasing the heart as a bright zone of high intensity. This will not be seen in a non-gated cardiac CT because of the movement of the LV and the overlapping lung tissue (partial volume effect). **O**, A gradient echo image demonstrates a signal void just below the aortic root between the LA and LV indicating the regurgitant flow of AR.

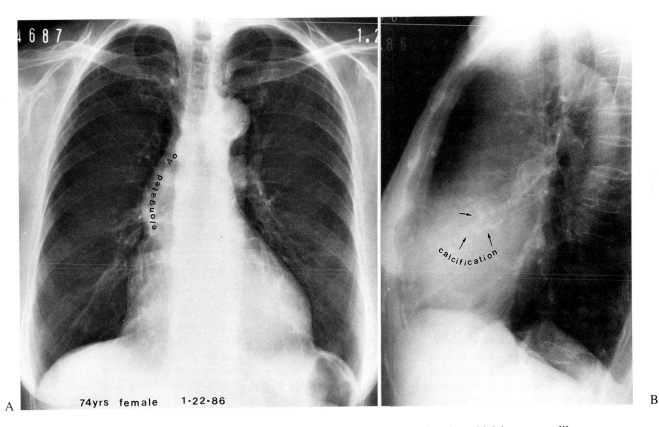

Fig. 4-3. **A**, X-rays of 74-year-old woman with AS show calcification of her aortic valve which is more readily observed on the lateral film, **B**. In this view, the valve is almost in the center of the cardiac silhouette on a line between the tracheal bifurcation and the sternophrenic angle. The calcification of a bicuspid aortic valve often appears as an almost circular calcification, unlike irregular ordinary aortic valve calcification of rheumatic heart disease and/or arteriosclerosis.

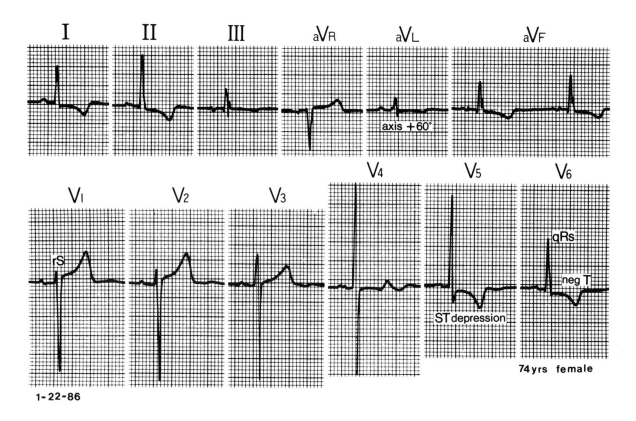

Fig. 4-3. *(Continued)* **C**, ECG of the same patient demonstrates systolic LV overloading as manifested by LV leads with J point depressions and downsloping upward convex ST segments to negative T waves. The QRS axis is normal at about +60°.*

* Left-axis deviation (LAD) of above 0° is not expected in LV overloading unless there is associated myocardial damage.

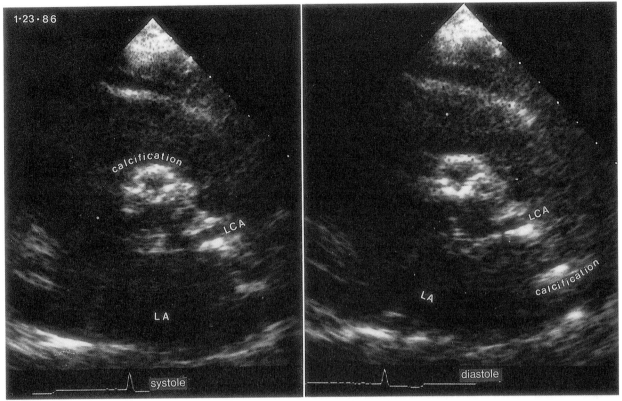

D   E

Fig. 4-3. *(Continued)* **D,** The short axis echoes of the Ao of the same patient show a calcified valve, and severely limited opening and closing. **E,** There is a strong echo at the inlet of the left main coronary artery (LCA) which may also indicate calcification.

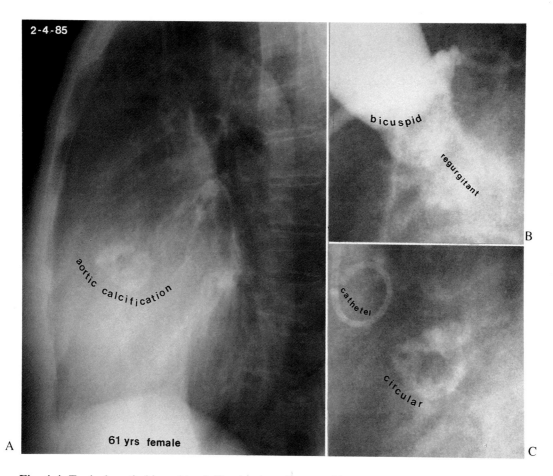

Fig. 4-4. Typical aortic bicuspid calcification in a 61-year-old woman. **A,** Lateral chest x-ray shows a circular calcification in the center of her cardiac silhouette. **B,** Aortogram shows a bicuspid aortic valve with mild AR. **C,** A magnified view of calcification reveals a circular configuration with dots in the center. This is typical of bicuspid aortic valvular calcification. (Courtesy of S. Matsuyama, M.D.)

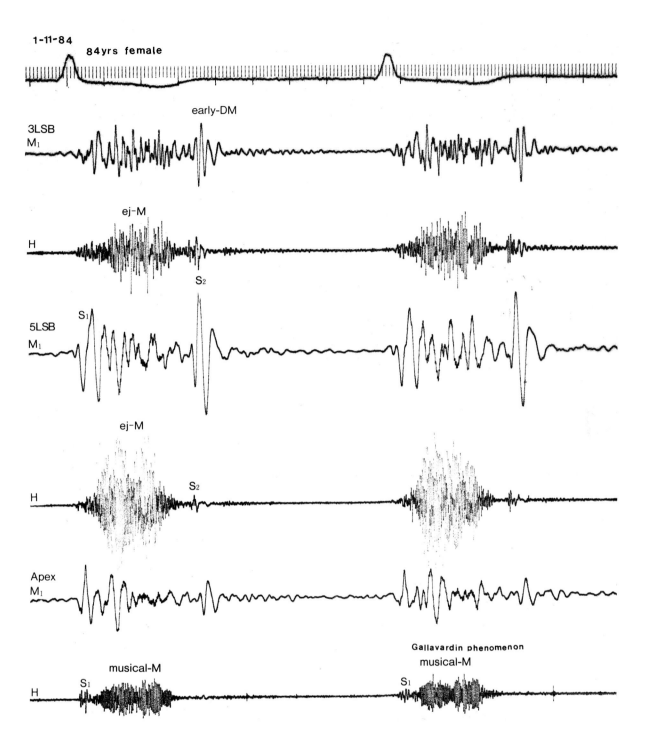

Fig. 4-5. PCG of an 84-year-old woman with a calcified aortic valve demonstrates the Gallavardin phenomenon. A coarse ejection murmur (ej-M) is audible from the 3LSB to the 5LSB with a trivial early diastolic murmur (early DM) of AR. The ejection murmur then changed to a high pitched murmur at the apex. The Gallavardin phenomenon refers to the transmission of the high frequency components of the AS murmur to the apex which simulates MR.

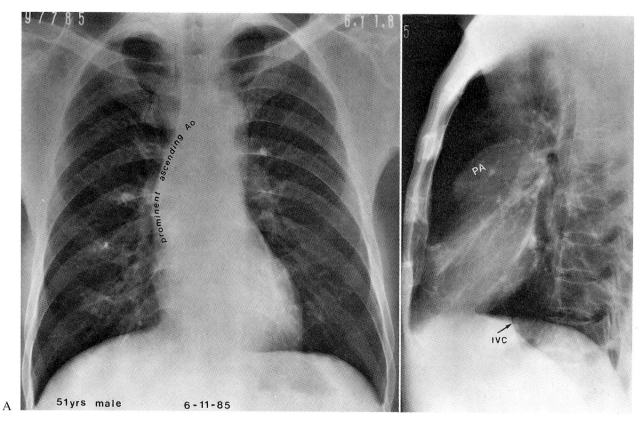

Fig. 4-6. A and B, Chest x-rays from a 51-year-old man whose bicuspid aortic valve was complicated by infective endocarditis. They are unremarkable except for a prominent ascending Ao. There is no evidence of LV enlargement.

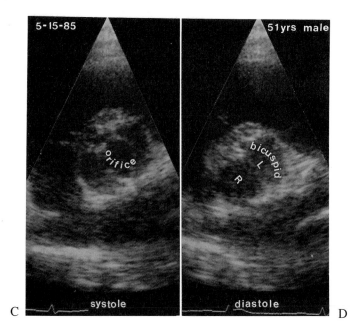

Fig. 4-6. *(Continued)* Short-axis 2D-echoes of the Ao show a vertical-type bicuspid valve and absence of the noncoronary cusp. **C**, During systole the aortic orifice is vaguely seen. **D**, In diastole, closure of the bicuspid valve is observed.

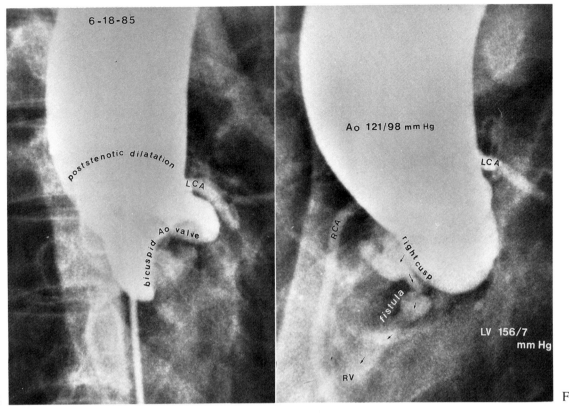

E

F

Fig. 4-6. *(Continued)* **E**, Angiogram of the same patient shows the bicuspid valve with poststenotic dilatation of the ascending Ao. **F**, Besides the bicuspid valve, there is a fistula immediately below the right coronary artery (RCA) communicating with the RV. Aortic pressure was 121/98 and he had a 35 mm Hg pressure gradient between the Ao and LV. Thus his AS is relatively mild.

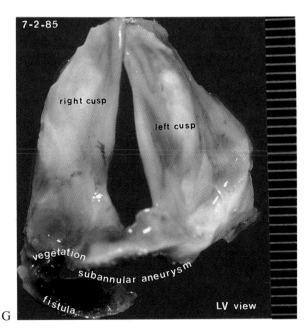

G

Fig. 4-6. *(Continued)* **G**, Because of infective endocarditis manifested by the appearance of AR, the aortic valve was replaced. The resected specimen in the LV view shows a vertical bicuspid valve and a subannular aneurysm with a fistula originating behind the right coronary cusp and communicating with the RV.

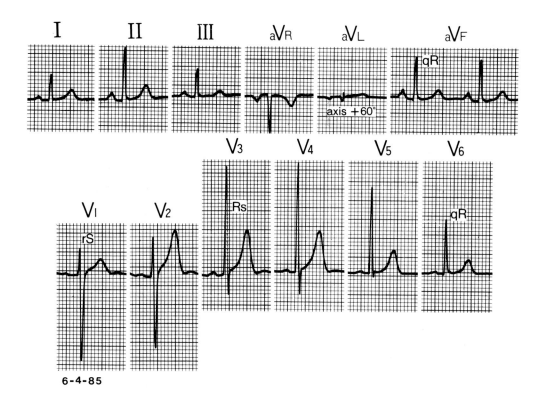

H   6-4-85

Fig. 4-6. *(Continued)* **H**, Preoperative ECG shows no remarkable changes other than a high voltage QRS in the LV leads and an anterior QRS indicated by an equiphasic area between V_2 and V_3. The anterior QRS may be due to counterclockwise rotation of the heart as a result of Ao elongation. The tall R wave in V_3 and V_4 supports the hypothesis that the LV comes closer to the anterior chest wall as a result of the twisting effect of the elongated Ao.

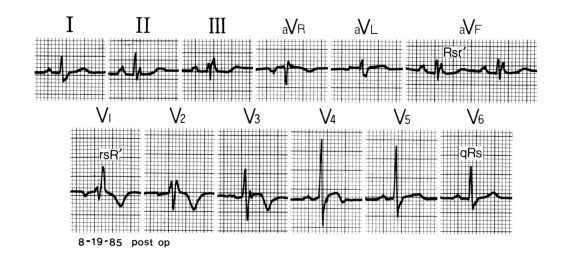

I   8-19-85 post op

Fig. 4-6. *(Continued)* **I**, Six weeks postoperatively, patient's ECG shows an rsR′ pattern in V_1 and inverted T waves in V_1 to V_3 caused by the surgical intervention.

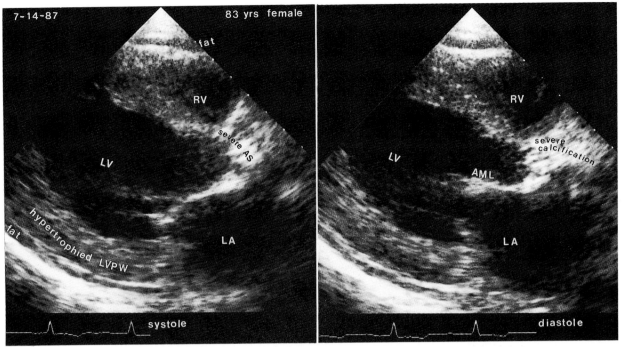

Fig. 4-7. Long-axis echoes from an 83-year-old man with severe AS caused by a calcified aortic valve. **A** and **B**, During both systole and diastole, a severely calcified aortic valve is seen but its movement is not clear. Posterior to the hypertrophied left ventricular posterior wall (LVPW) and anterior to the RV, there are extra echo spaces suggesting the presence of subepicardial fat.

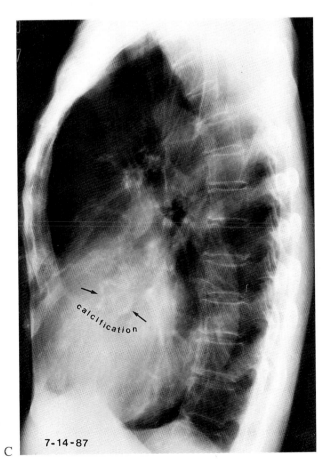

Fig. 4-7. *(Continued)* **C**, Lateral chest x-ray shows an irregular calcification of the aortic valve, or annulus, in the center of his cardiac silhouette indicated by arrows.

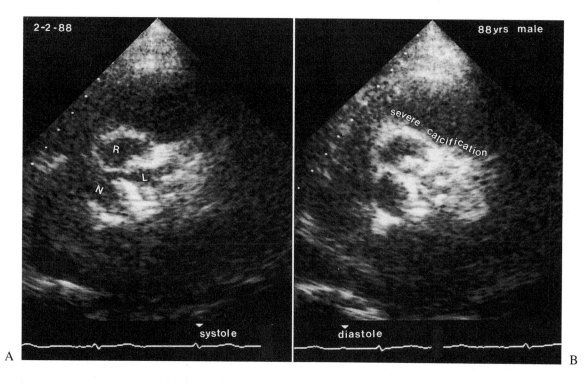

Fig. 4-8. Short-axis 2D-echoes of the Ao from an 88-year-old man with severe diabetes and hypertension. Heavy calcification of the left coronary cusp (L) adjacent to the right (R) and noncoronary cusps (N) shows clearly. **A,** The aortic orifice during systole is severely limited, and its closure appears to be incomplete during diastole, **B.** The patient had both AR and AS murmurs.

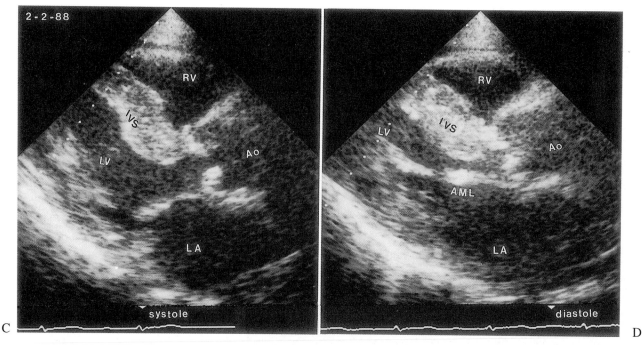

Fig. 4-8. *(Continued)* **C,** Long-axis 2D-echoes show a heavily calcified aortic valve whose movement is very limited both in systole and diastole, **D.** Calcification of the anterior mitral leaflet (AML) is also seen during diastole. Both the left ventricular posterior wall and septum (IVS) have very strong echoes with a granular appearance which are suggestive of deposits of metabolic products or degenerative changes of the myocardium.

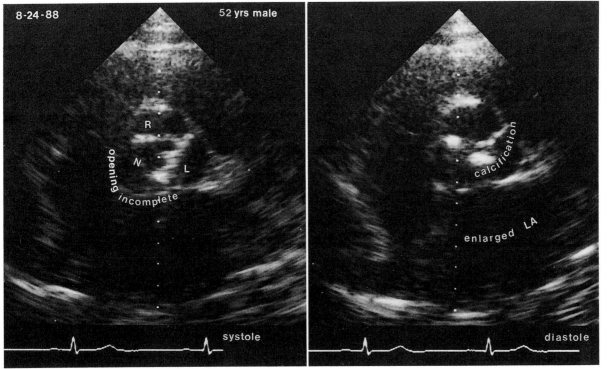

Fig. 4-9. A, The short-axis 2D-echoes of a 52-year-old man who has combined valvular disease show limited opening of the Ao during systole. The calcified cusps are seen in the center of the Ao but their coaptation is not clear. **B,** Behind the Ao, an enlarged LA is seen.

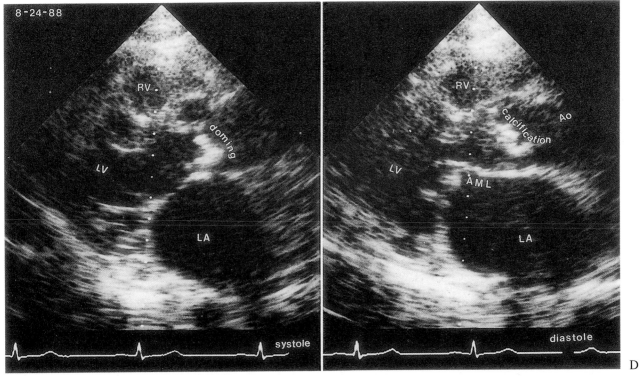

Fig. 4-9. *(Continued)* Long axis 2D-echoes show a heavily calcified aortic valve both in systole and diastole. **C,** Doming of the aortic valve during systole indicates the presence of AS. **D,** An enlarged LA with limited opening of the anterior mitral leaflet (AML) indicates the presence of MS.

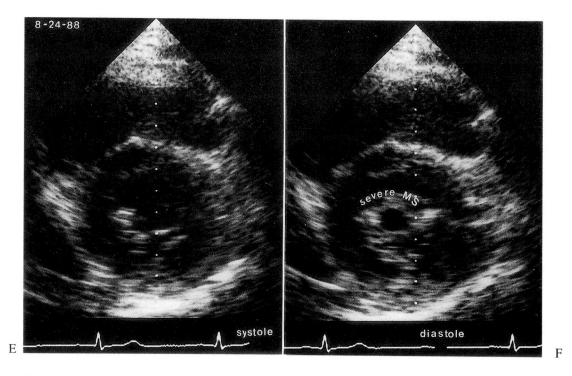

Fig. 4-9. *(Continued)* **E,** The presence of MS is confirmed by the short-axis 2D-echoes. **F,** During diastole, the mitral valve opening is very limited showing an approximately 10 × 10 mm orifice.

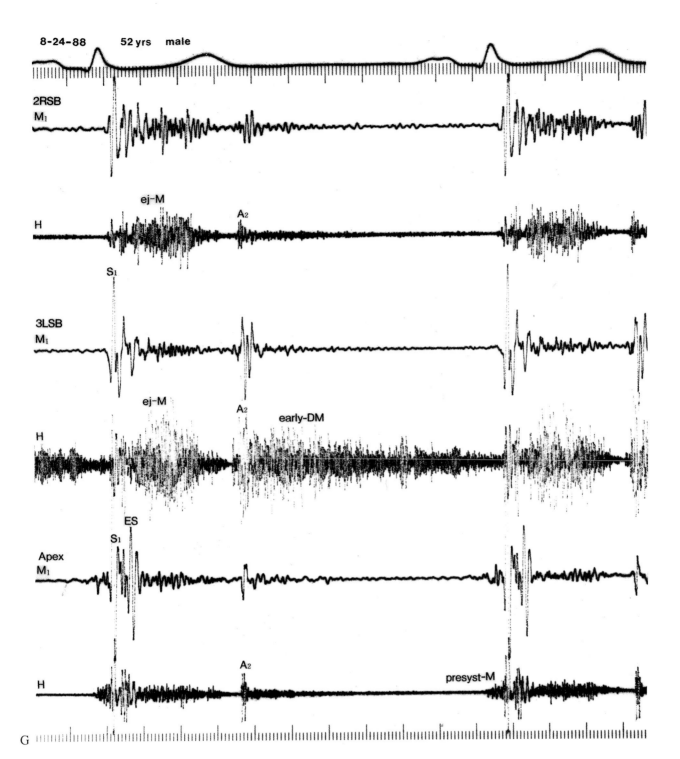

Fig. 4-9. *(Continued)* **G**, PCG shows a coarse ejection murmur (ej-M) with an early diastolic murmur (early DM) of AR best heard at the 3LSB. An ejection sound (ES) is recorded at the apex along with a soft presystolic murmur (presyst-M).

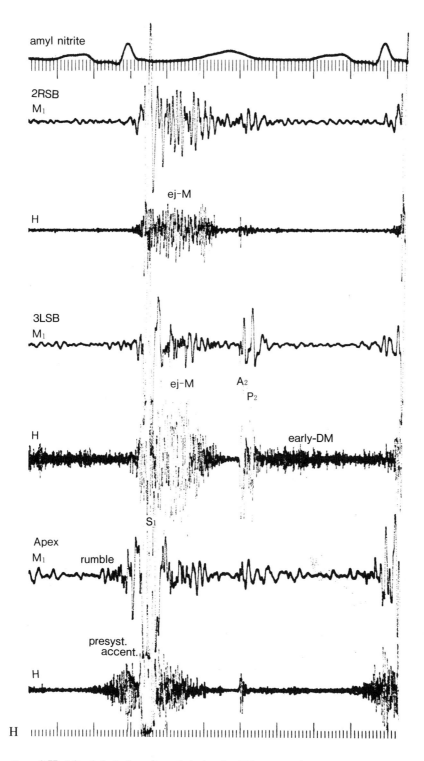

Fig. 4-9. *(Continued)* **H,** After inhalation of amyl nitrite, the AR murmur became softer and the ejection murmur (ej-M) increased at the apex. A diastolic rumble with presystolic accentuation occurred at apex. The decrease of the AR murmur after inhaling amyl nitrite is caused by a reduction of the peripheral resistance; the increase of the diastolic rumble is due to an increased flow through the mitral orifice.

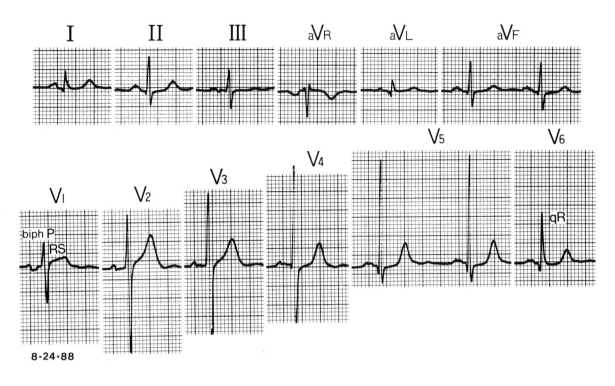

8-24-88

I

Fig. 4-9. *(Continued)* **I**, ECG shows LA overloading by a slightly increased width of the P wave, and in V₁ as a large area of terminal negativity (biph P). The QRS axis is somewhere between 0° and +30°. In spite of receiving digitalis, the T waves in the LV leads are upright, which suggests the presence of diastolic LV overloading. The overall appearance of this ECG is compatible with MS and AR.

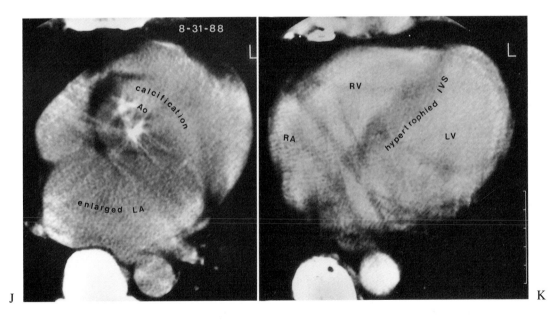

J   K

Fig. 4-9. *(Continued)* **J**, His combined MS and AR are also shown in his cardiac CT findings. His CT section at the level of the LA shows calcification as a "star sapphire" in the center of the cardiac silhouette indicating calcification of the aortic valve or its ring. In **K**, a slightly hypertrophied IVS is observed with a moderately enlarged LV cavity, and an enlarged LA.

Chapter 5　Aortitis Syndrome

Pathophysiology and Clinical Clues

The cause of aortitis is uncertain, but past histories of syphilis, tuberculosis, collagen disease, and septicemia have been implicated. Another suspected cause of aortitis is based on autoimmunity (often called Takayasu's disease) and involves mainly the aortic arch producing narrowing or occlusion of the brachiocephalic trunk and subclavian arteries which results in reduced pulses in the upper extremities. Therefore Takayasu's disease has been called pulseless disease, or the aortic arch syndrome. In the acute stages, night sweats, general malaise, arthralgia, anorexia, weight loss, gastrointestinal symptoms, and a striking elevation in sedimentation rate occur. The diagnosis of the aortitis syndrome is usually made retrospectively based on differences in the blood pressures of the extremities, or on finding cardiac murmurs. It occurs mostly in young women but is also common in middle-aged women. It occurs only rarely in men. In some cases, faintness may be the initial symptom, occurring when the patient raises her head to look upward.*

The clinical findings of the aortitis syndrome include:
★★★★　On auscultation, there may be an early diastolic murmur of AR with or without an ejection murmur at the base of the heart. A continuous murmur in the neck is also common.
★★★★　On the chest x-ray, linear calcifications along the Ao and scalloping of the descending Ao are common. An abnormal decrease in peripheral pulmonary vascularity and/or rib notching may be observed.
★★★★　On echo, dilatation of the Ao with or without an aneurysm may be seen.
★★★★　On ECG, hypertension results in systolic LV overloading.†

---

*　The blood pressure of the right upper extremity may normally exceed that of the left by about 10 mm Hg. When this becomes reversed, narrowing of or occlusion near the innominate artery is suspected. Routine examinations of pulses and blood pressures bilaterally are indicated.

†　Occasionally there is unexplained prolongation of the QT interval. There also occurs prolongation of the interval between the first and the second heart sound which would tend to produce a tic-tac rhythm in which systole tends to equal diastole in duration.

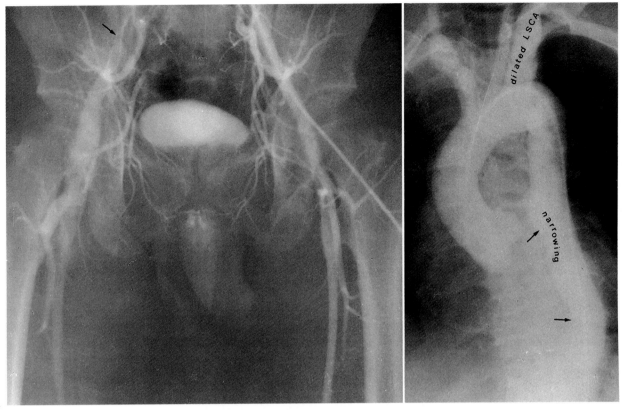

Fig. 5-1. A, Preoperative angiogram of a 21-year-old man with right femoral artery occlusion shows narrowing of the proximal portion of the right femoral artery (arrow) with dilatation of its distal portion. A successful embolectomy was performed. **B**, His aortogram shows narrowings of the descending Ao (arrows). The left subclavian artery (LSCA) and the innominate artery are dilated but the right subclavian artery is not imaged.

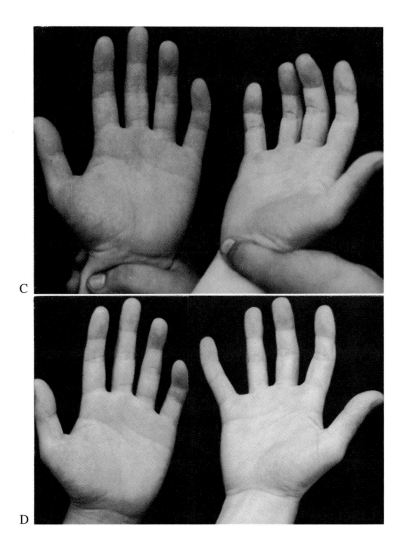

Fig. 5-1. *(Continued)* **C**, Right radial pulse was weak and ulnar artery compression by simultaneous pressure on both wrists by a firm grip produced pallor of the right hand. **D**, With release of the occlusions, a delayed flushing occurred only on the right.

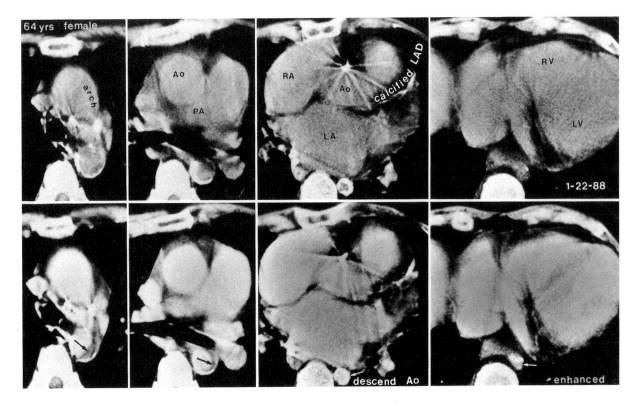

Fig. 5-2 Cardiac CT sections from a 64-year-old woman with aortitis syndrome. In the upper row, the plain sections show calcifications in the aortic arch which extend to the markedly narrowed lower thoracic aorta. In the lower row, the contrast-enhanced sections show a mural thrombus and/or thickening of the wall in the descending Ao (black arrows). The white arrows indicate the markedly narrowed lower thoracic Ao. This is an example of the aortitis syndrome which involves the Ao extensively. Calcifications may be seen from the ascending to the abdominal Ao.

Fig. 5-3. X-ray of a 52-year-old woman with the aortitis syndrome. Her right lateral oblique projection shows fine linear calcifications which begin at the aortic root and continue to the abdominal Ao. Characteristically the calcification in aortitis is fine and linear in contrast to the thick calcifications in atherosclerosis.

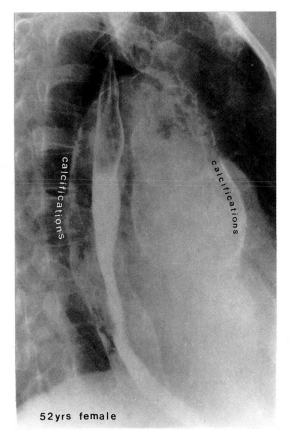

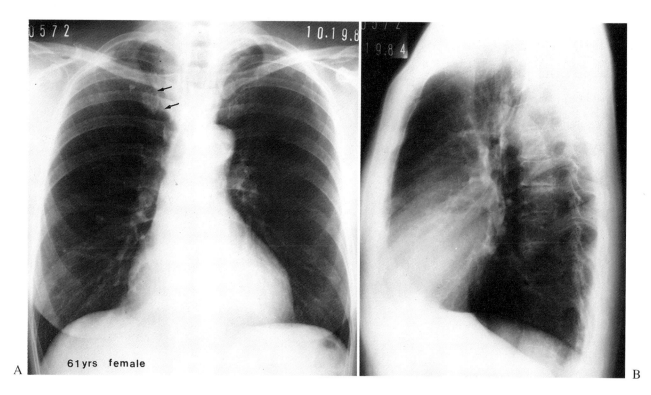

A   61yrs female   B

Fig. 5-4. Chest x-rays are from a 61-year-old woman with the aortitis syndrome. **A,** The frontal view shows slight cardiomegaly with a prominent aortic arch containing calcification. The right innominate artery (arrows) is prominent above the aortic arch. The descending thoracic Ao is not imaged and its scalloping is not clearly outlined. **B,** Lateral view, there is no obvious deformity of the descending Ao.

Fig. 5-4. *(Continued)* **C,** Since the patient's left radial pulse was not palpable, the aortitis syndrome was suspected. Her digital subtraction angiogram (DSA) shows a prominent ascending Ao with a dilated right innominate artery. Her left subclavian artery (SCA) is completely occluded at its origin and there is narrowing of the mid-portion of her thoracic Ao with scalloping.

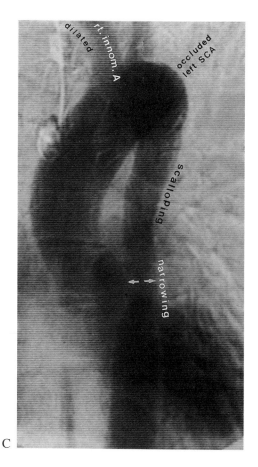

C

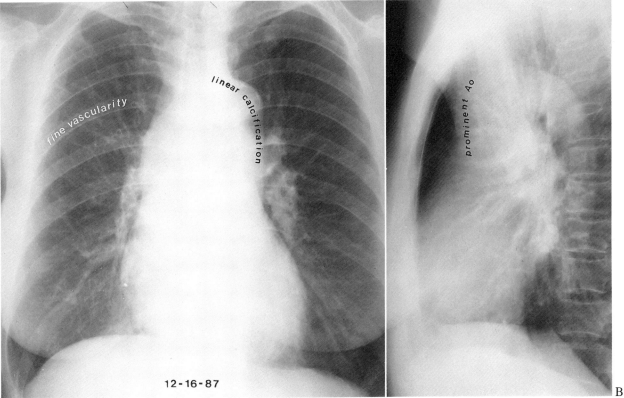

Fig. 5-5. Chest x-rays from a 39-year-old woman with the aortitis syndrome. **A**, Her ascending Ao is prominent but it contains no visible calcification. The aortic arch is also prominent and has linear calcifications. There is reduced peripheral pulmonary vascularity in the right upper lung field. **B**, The ascending Ao is prominent but the narrowing of the descending Ao is not definite.

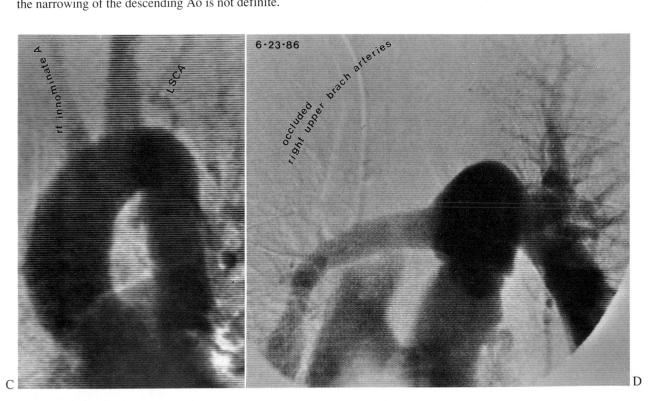

Fig. 5-5. *(Continued)* **C**, DSA of same patient shows narrowing of right innominate and left subclavian arteries (LSCA). **D**, The right pulmonary artery is diffusely narrowed with marked reduction in filling of its branches.

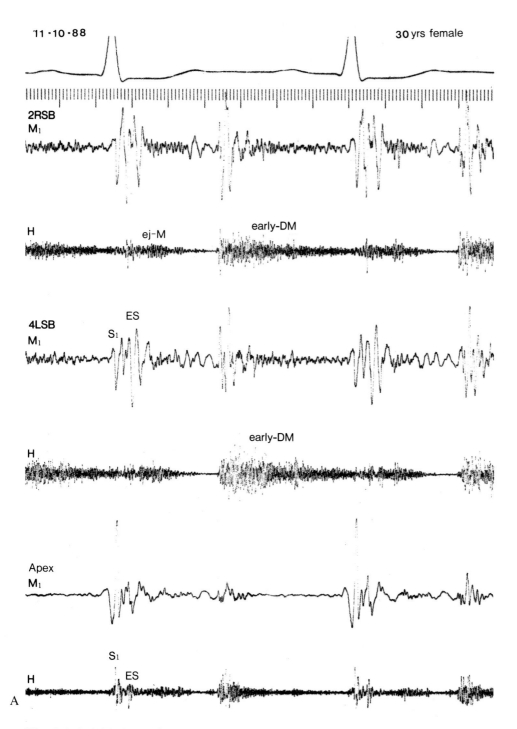

Fig. 5-6. A, PCG from a 30-year-old woman with the aortitis syndrome. There is an early diastolic murmur (early DM) of AR at the second right intercostal space which is transmitted to the apex. There is also a very soft ejection murmur (ej-M) which is common either in aortitis, annulo-aortic ectasia, or a prolapse of the aortic cusp.

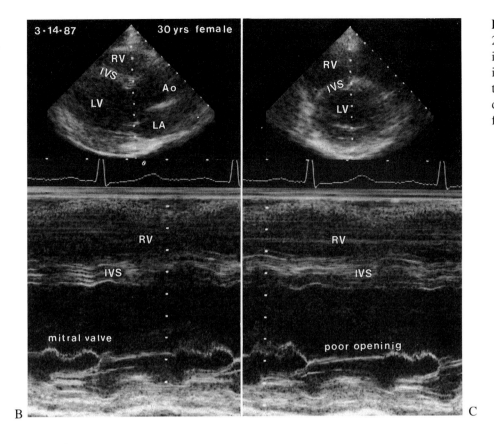

Fig. 5-6. *(Continued)* **B and C,** Her 2D and M-mode echoes show a limited opening of the mitral valve during diastole which is so low in amplitude that it resembles that seen in dilated cardiomyopathy with heart failure.

B

C

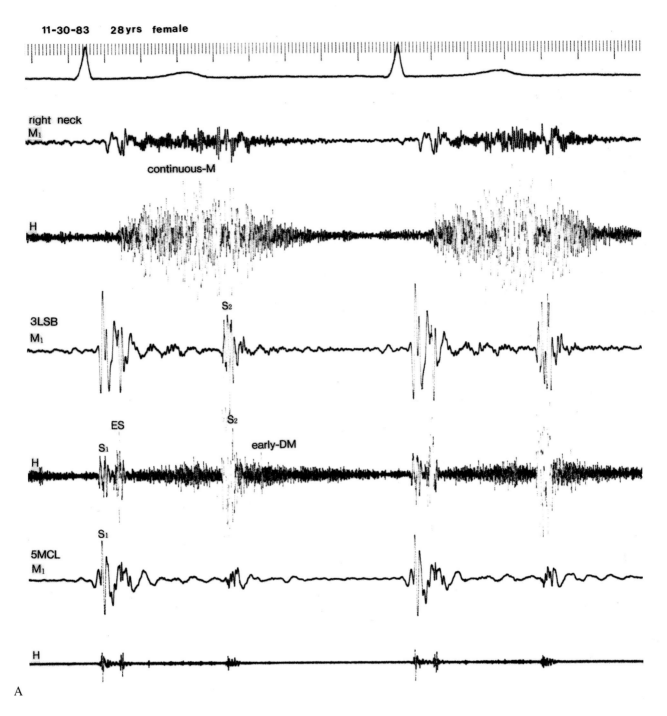

Fig. 5-7. A, PCG from a 28-year-old woman with the aortitis syndrome. A continuous murmur is present at the right side of her neck. A systolic murmur begins with ejection sound (ES) and lasts until the S_2. An early diastolic murmur (early DM) at the 3LSB may represent transmission of the continuous murmur.

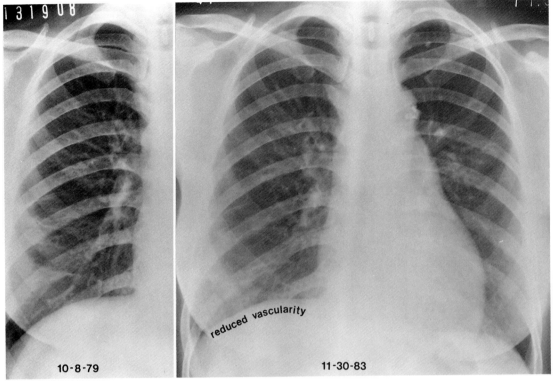

B, 10-8-79   C, 11-30-83   reduced vascularity

Fig. 5-7. *(Continued)* **B,** Chest x-ray shows normal distribution of the peripheral pulmonary arteries in her right lung. **C,** There is decreased pulmonary vascularity in the right lower lung region 4 years later. Since the reduction of the caliber of the right descending pulmonary artery is also visible, an obstruction of this artery is suspected. Reduction of vascularity is also noted in the left lower lung field.

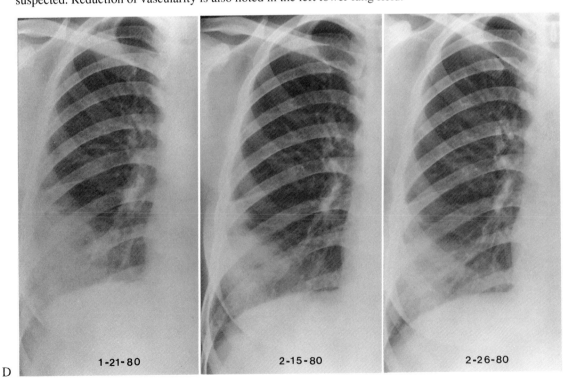

D, 1-21-80   2-15-80   2-26-80

Fig. 5-7. *(Continued)* **D,** Chest x-rays from the same patient when she was admitted for an upper respiratory infection. Because of cough and fever, pneumonitis was suspected. Consolidation in the right lower lung field that extended centrally from the periphery possibly was caused by pulmonary infarction. The opacification did not resolve after one month, and reduced size of the descending pulmonary artery is noted.

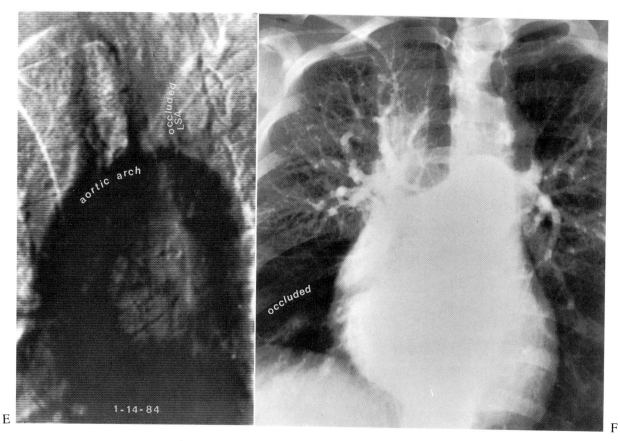

Fig. 5-7. *(Continued)* **E**, DSA of the thoracic Ao and a pulmonary angiogram 6 weeks later showed occlusion of her left subclavian artery (LSA). **F**, The peripheral pulmonary arteries show multiple narrowing and obstruction of the segmental branches in both lower lung regions. Pulmonary thromboembolism is quite common in the aortitis syndrome.

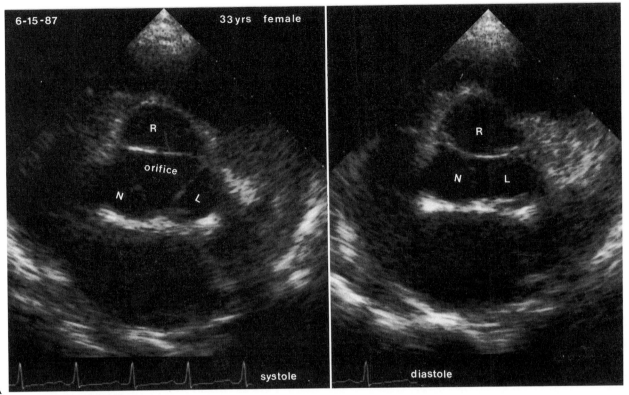

A

B

Fig. 5-8. A 33-year-old unmarried woman entered the hospital for an upper respiratory infection. She was engaged to be married in 1 week and did not wish to be hospitalized. Her temperature was 38°C and she was in acute heart failure. She had sinus tachycardia of 110, a short ejection murmur, and a diastolic murmur of AR. Blood pressure was 130/30 mm Hg bilaterally. Sedimentation rate was 110 mm per hour. Six years prior to the present illness, she experienced high fever of unknown etiology and was admitted to a local hospital for 6 weeks. No cardiac murmur was noted. During the present admission, the patient responded rapidly to digitalis and diuretics. **A** and **B**, The 2D-echoes of the Ao made during her recent admission showed incomplete opening of her aortic valve.

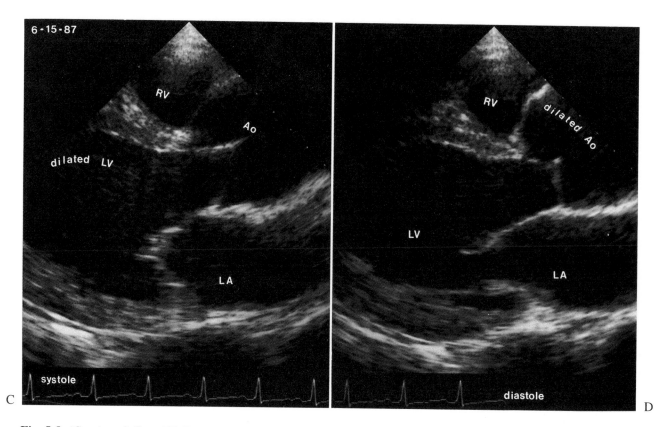

Fig. 5-8. *(Continued)* **C and D**, Long-axis 2D-echoes show dilatation of her LV as well as of her aortic root.

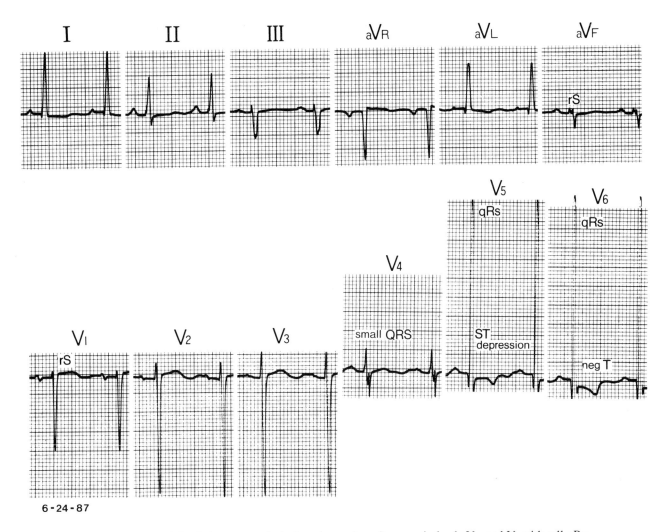

I II III aVR aVL aVF

rS

V1 V2 V3 V4 V5 V6

rS small QRS qRs qRs

ST depression

neg T

6-24-87

Fig. 5-8. *(Continued)* **E**, ECG 10 days post-admission shows deep S waves in leads V$_2$ and V$_3$ with tall qRs complexes in V$_5$ and V$_6$, associated with ST depressions and negative T waves, indicating systolic LV overloading.

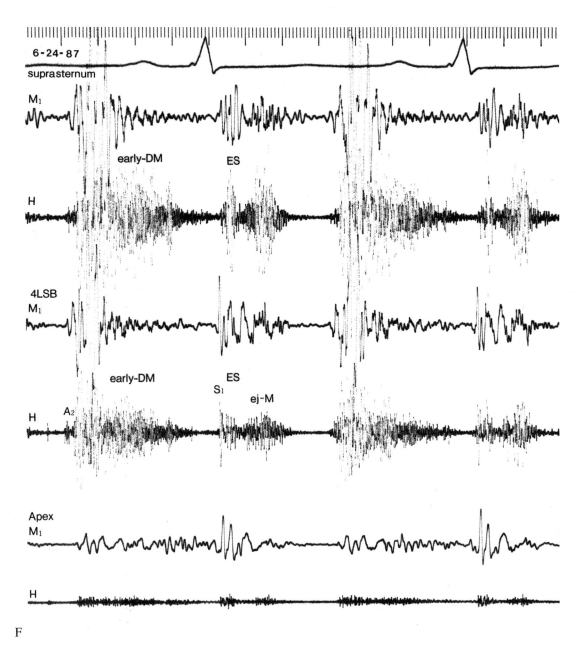

Fig. 5-8. *(Continued)* **F**, The patient experienced forceful suprasternal pulsations. Her PCG shows a loud ejection sound (ES) with a short ejection murmur (ej-M). S₂ is followed by an early diastolic murmur (early DM) of AR with a rapid decrescendo.

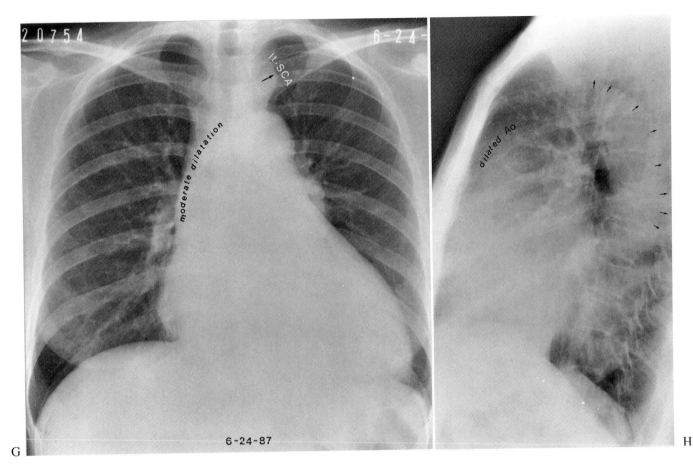

G

H

Fig. 5-8. *(Continued)* **G**, Her chest x-rays show moderate dilatation of the ascending Ao and aortic arch, with generalized cardiomegaly. Aneurysmal dilatation of the left subclavian artery (SCA) is suspected above the aortic arch (arrow). **H**, The ascending Ao occupies the anterosuperior portion of the cardiac silhouette. The descending Ao has an uneven surface (arrows). There is no calcification of the aortic wall.

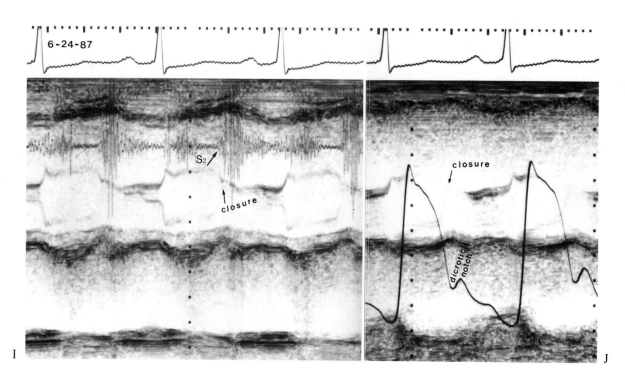

Fig. 5-8. *(Continued)* **I**, Simultaneous recording of the PCG and M-mode echo of the Ao shows a very soft S$_2$ that coincides with aortic closure. **J**, Carotid artery tracing shows a low dicrotic notch following aortic valvular closure.

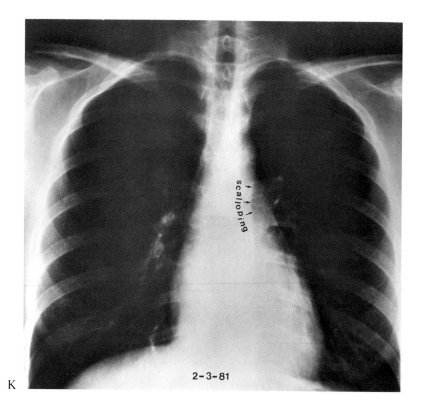

Fig. 5-8. *(Continued)* **K**, Fortunately a chest x-ray taken 6 years before was available showing her heart to be a normal size. But the descending Ao shows scalloping of its lateral margin, indicating that she had aortitis before this hospitalization.

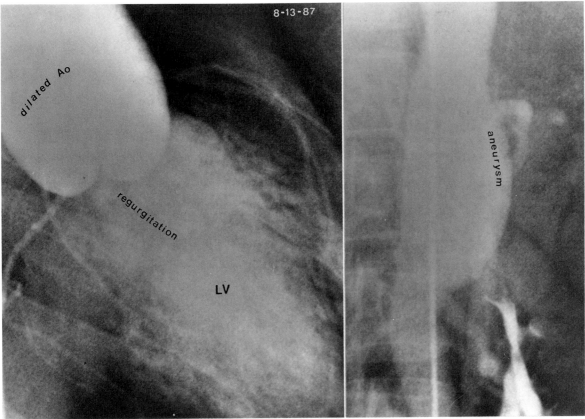

Fig. 5-8. *(Continued)* **L,** Aortogram shows a dilated aortic root with marked AR. **M,** The patient had an aneurysm in her aortic arch and another in her descending Ao. Multiple aneurysms are a rather uncommon finding in the aortitis syndrome.

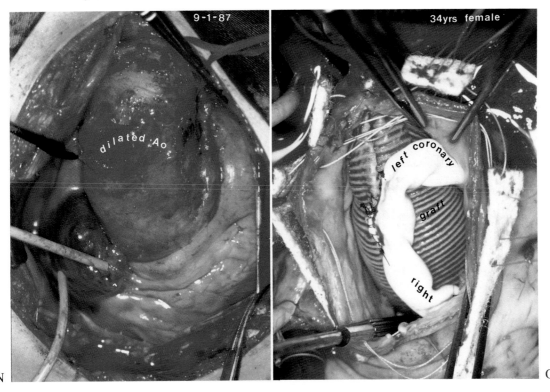

Fig. 5-8. *(Continued)* **N,** At surgery, a large aneurysmal dilatation of the ascending Ao was resected and a dacron graft, **O,** containing a disc valve was implanted.

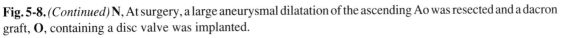

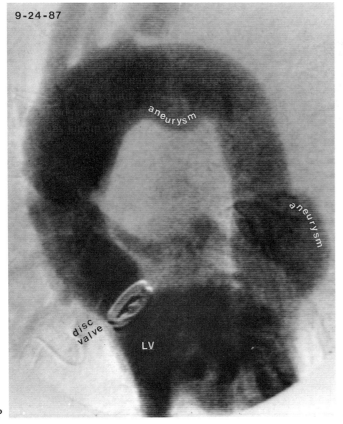

9-24-87

aneurysm

aneurysm

disc valve

LV

P

Fig. 5-8. *(Continued)* **P**, Three weeks postoperatively a digital subtraction angiogram demonstrates a well functioning disc valve and aortic graft. The aneurysms of the left subclavian artery, aortic arch, and descending Ao were unchanged.

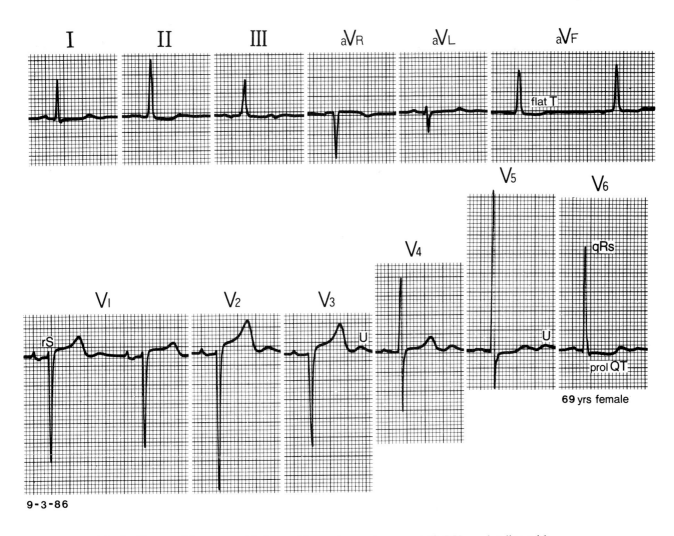

I   II   III   aVR   aVL   aVF

V5   V6

V4

V1   V2   V3

qRs

rS   U   U

prol QT

69 yrs female

9-3-86

Fig. 5-9. A, ECG of a 69-year-old woman with the aortitis syndrome shows systolic LV overloading with a marked QT prolongation of about 0.48 seconds. The T waves in the extremity leads and in V_5 and V_6 are low with associated relatively high U waves. These findings are rather common in the aortitis syndrome. The patient has not received any diuretics.

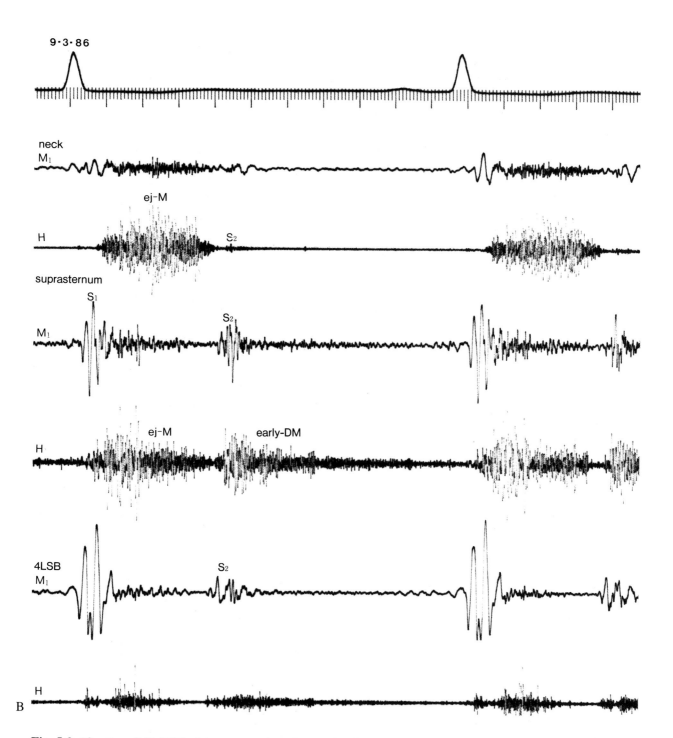

Fig. 5-9. *(Continued)* **B**, PCG of the same patient shows a harsh vascular murmur over her neck. There is a different shaped ejection murmur (ej-M) over the sternum above the sternal angle originating at the Ao. An early diastolic murmur (early DM) characteristic of AR is present. This is a typical "to and fro" murmur, and it is transmitted to the 4LSB.

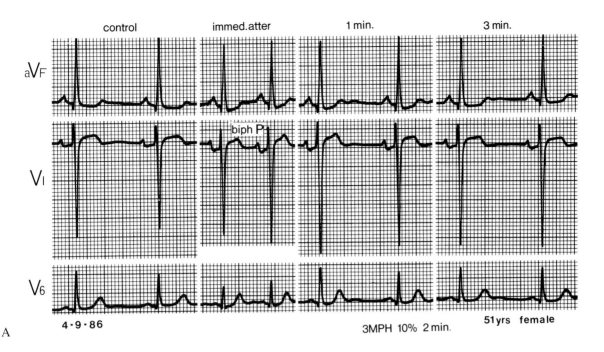

Fig. 5-10. A, This exercise ECG is from a 51-year-old woman with the aortitis syndrome as described in Figure 5-5. In the control phase, there is a slightly sagging ST depression. After exercise (3 miles per hour with a 10% slope change in 2 minutes), there is no significant ST depression. However, the P wave in V_1 developed a more marked terminal negativity (biph P), suggesting LA overloading that lasted until 3 minutes after completion of the exercise.

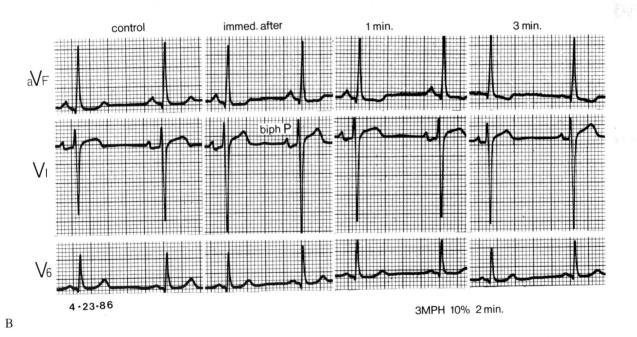

B

Fig. 5-10. *(Continued)* **B,** After digitalis and a vasodilator, an exercise ECG made 16 days later shows a lesser degree of the terminal negativity of the P wave in V_1. This indicates improvement of the LA overloading. The T wave negativity in aVF after 3 minutes of exercise may have been due to a digitalis effect.

Chapter 6   Coarctation of the Aorta

Pathophysiology and Clinical Clues

Coarctation occurs in the descending Ao immediately at or distal to the bifurcation of the left subclavian artery where the ligamentum arteriosum is located. It is frequently associated with a bicuspid aortic valve, ventricular septal defect, or persistent ductus arteriosus. The most striking clinical finding is hypertension in the upper extremities with poor circulation in the lower extremities. This may produce headache, epistaxis, and cold lower extremities with or without intermittent claudication. One must never omit an examination of the lower extremities of hypertensive patients, particularly young people.

The clinical findings are as follows:

★★★★ Chest x-rays may show an enlarged poststenotic dilatation of the descending Ao. There is dilatation of the left subclavian artery above the aortic arch, and rib notching. Contrast medium in the esophagus (barium swallow) shows a reversed figure 3 due to pressure on the esophagus by the aortic arch and the poststenotic dilatated segment of the Ao.

★★★★ Auscultation of the heart may reveal an accentuated S_2 and the murmurs of AS and AR. Continuous murmurs are heard over the tortuous and dilated posterior intercostal arteries as well as over the site of the coarctation.

★★★ The electrocardiograph may be unremarkable in spite of the hypertension which may be due to congenital hypoplasia of the LV.

★★ A diagnosis of coarctation is difficult by echocardiography unless the descending Ao is recorded.

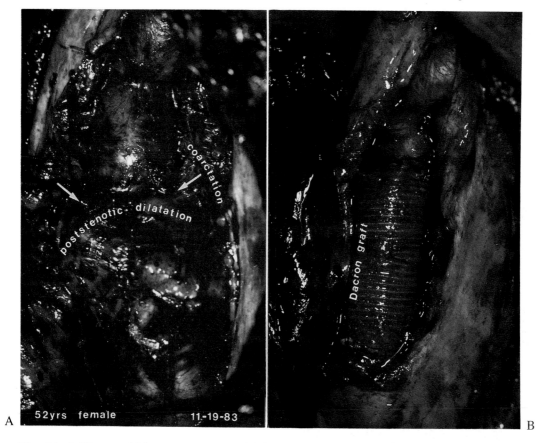

Fig. 6-1. A 53-year-old former nurse was told during childhood that she had a heart murmur. After she became a nurse, hypertension was detected with no known cause and she had to quit her job at age 40 because she was easily fatigued and had coldness in her feet. At age 52, a consultant cardiologist found that blood pressure in both her arms was 220/120 mm Hg, and her lower extremities were cold with no pulse. A grade 2 to 3 ejection murmur was found at the base of her heart. After angiography she was referred for surgery. **A,** At surgery, there was a coarctation with aneurysmal dilatation of the descending Ao immediately below the left subclavian artery. **B,** The coarctation was resected and replaced with a dacron graft.

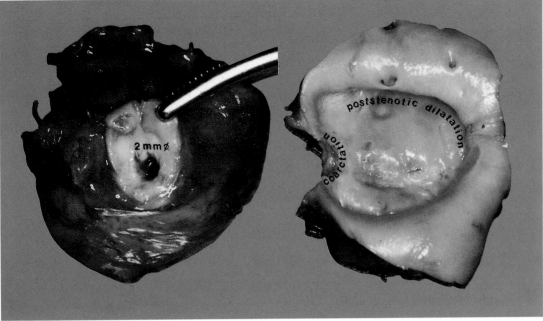

Fig. 6-1. *(Continued)* **C**, The resected specimen at the coarctation had an orifice only 2 mm in diameter, with poststenotic dilatation.

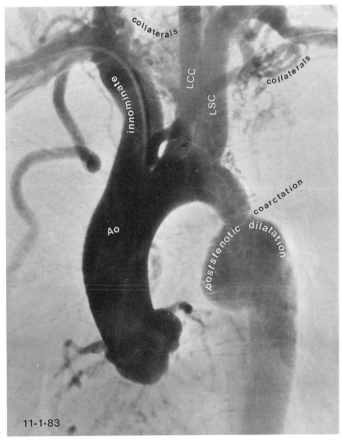

Fig. 6-1. *(Continued)* **D**, Preoperative digital subtraction angiogram (DSA) shows marked aneurysmal poststenotic dilatation 5 cm in diameter immediately below the coarctation. Both internal mammary arteries are dilated and there are numerous collateral networks in the lower neck and upper mediastinum.

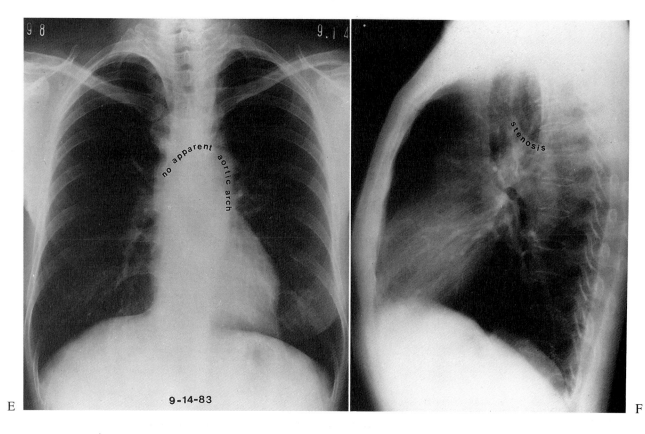

Fig. 6-1. *(Continued)* **E**, Chest x-rays of the same patient show a protrusion resembling the aortic arch, though it is somewhat lower than the usual site. This protrusion is due to the aneurysmal poststenostic dilatation of the descending Ao. **F**, The lateral view shows a deformed Ao at the beginning of the descending portion. This deformity is caused by the coarctation.

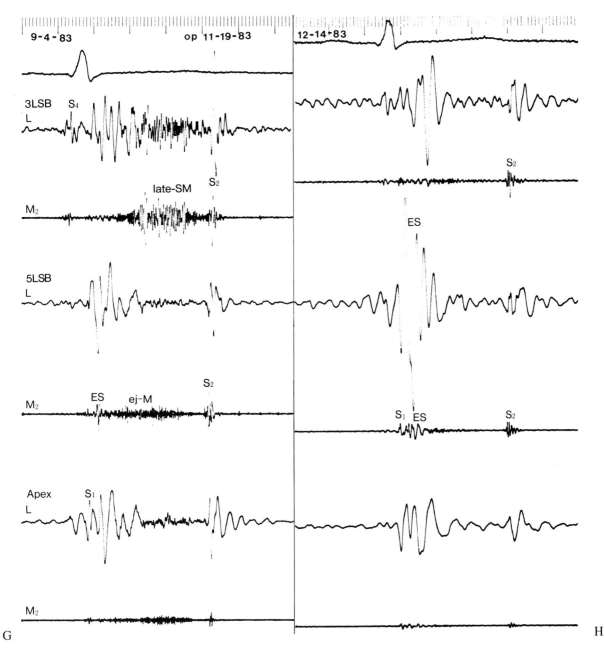

Fig. 6-1. *(Continued)* **G,** Preoperative PCG shows a systolic murmur which is delayed after the S_1 and enhanced toward the end of systole. This indicates that the murmur is vascular in origin rather than from the aortic valve. **H,** Postoperatively, the previously described murmur and the accentuated S_2 are no longer seen.

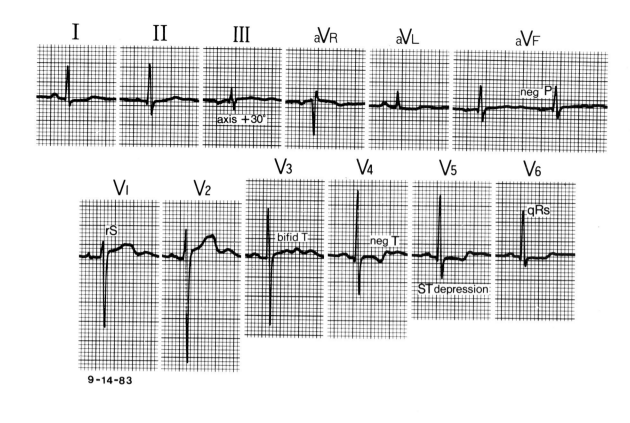

Fig. 6-1. *(Continued)* **I,** Preoperative ECG shows a negative P wave in aVF suggesting that the pacemaker is low atrial. Horizontal ST segment depressions are seen in leads I, aVL and V$_6$, and negative T waves in V$_4$ and V$_5$. This suggests LV myocardial damage or fibrosis.

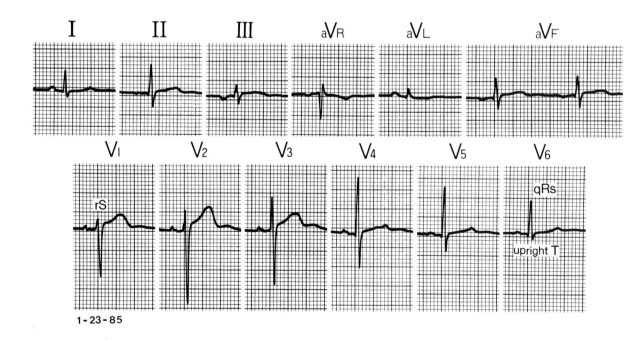

Fig. 6-1. *(Continued)* **J,** Postoperative ECG approximately 18 months after surgery shows a notched T wave in V$_4$ and the T in V$_1$ considerably taller than the T in V$_6$ as the only signs of any abnormality.

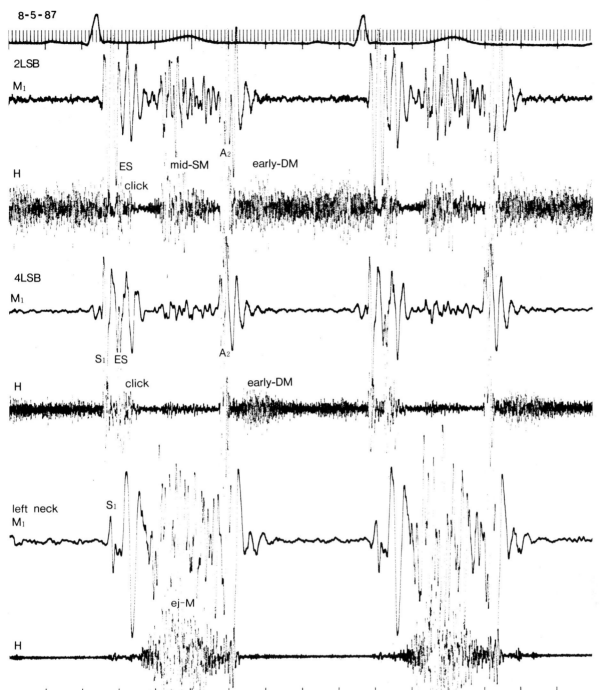

Fig. 6-2. This 25-year-old housewife was told that she had AR at the birth of her first child 3 years prior to her present examination for an upper respiratory infection. She had noted a strong pulsation at the left side of her neck when she was in her teens. She did not participate in any active sports during her school years, but she was not told she had a heart murmur. She is 150 cm tall and her arm span is 165 cm suggesting a Marfan stature. The blood pressure is 110/60 in her right arm and 120/70 mm Hg in her left. Despite palpable pulses in the lower extremities, blood pressures are 110/70 mm Hg bilaterally. **A,** Auscultation reveals a delayed mid-systolic murmur (mid SM) at the 2LSB, suggesting vascular origin. This murmur is associated with an early diastolic murmur (early DM) of AR. There is an ejection murmur (ej-M) on the left side of her neck, with a forceful systolic pulsation and a thrill. This murmur radiates to the upper region of her back. An early diastolic murmur of AR is heard in the second right interspace and across the sternum to the 4LSB. There is an ejection sound (ES) followed by a click, simulating a double ejection click.

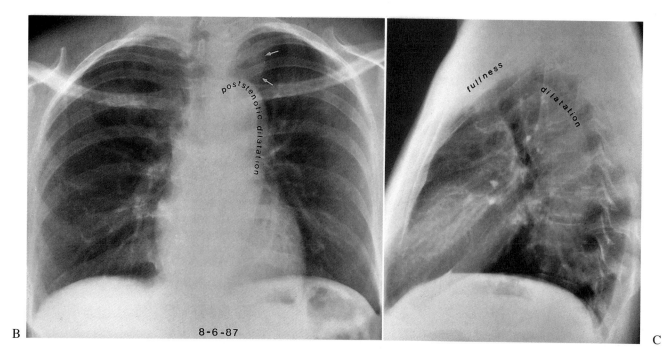

Fig. 6-2. *(Continued)* **B,** Frontal chest x-ray shows a protruding opacity along the left sternal border suggesting an aortic arch. However, this is above the level of the clavicle, and there is a faint opacity above it (white arrows). **C,** Lateral view shows no cardiac enlargement but a dilatation of the ascending Ao which occupies the anterosuperior portion of the cardiac silhouette. The character of the murmurs, her stature and the x-ray findings suggest a coarctation with a possible bicuspid aortic valve. However, the normal leg blood pressures rule out a significant coarctation.

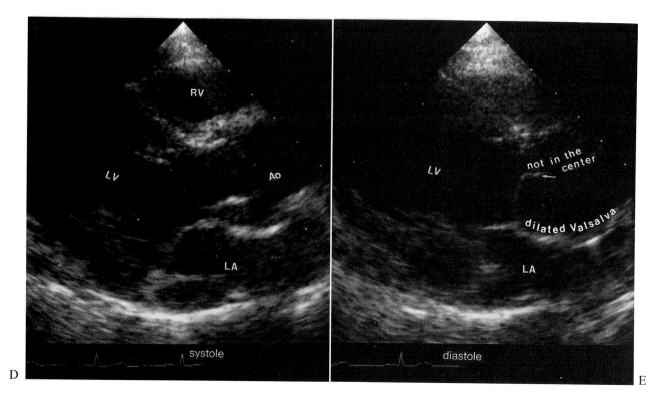

Fig. 6-2. *(Continued)* **D and E,** Long-axis 2D-echoes of the same patient show enlargement of the sinuses of Valsalva and the cusps are closed slightly above the center of the Ao, suggesting a bicuspid aortic valve.

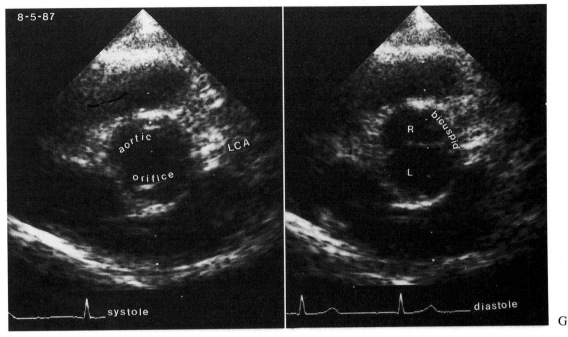

F   G

Fig. 6-2. *(Continued)* **F and G**, Short-axis 2D-echoes of the Ao reveal a horizontal-type bicuspid valve with a right cusp (R) and left cusp (L). There is no significant AS. The left coronary artery (LCA) may be somewhat larger than normal.

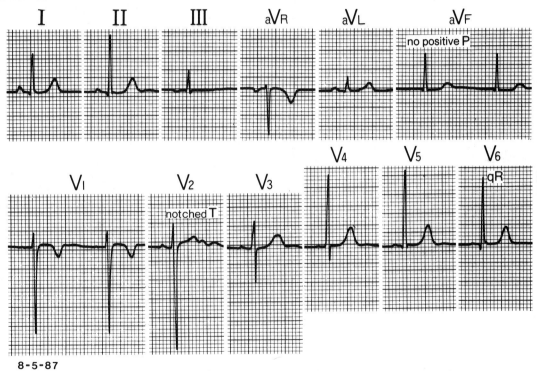

H

Fig. 6-2. *(Continued)* **H**, A notched T wave in V_2 demonstrates a normally notched T, i.e., between a negative T in V_1 and a positive T in V_3. There is a Sokolow index for left ventricular hypertrophy which could still be a variation of normal, especially in her age group.

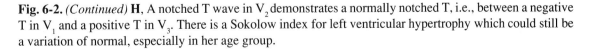

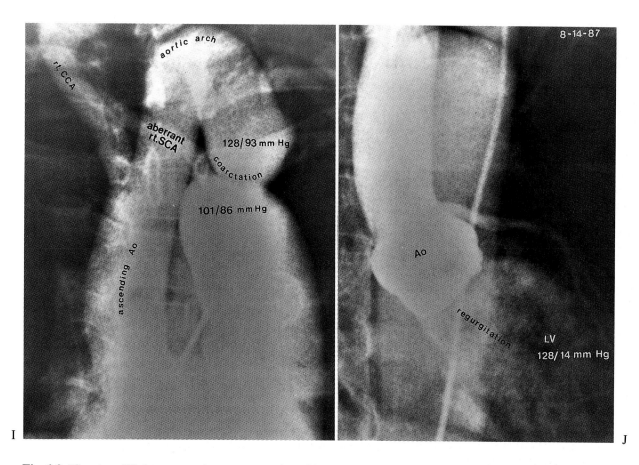

Fig. 6-2. *(Continued)* **I,** Aortogram shows a coarctation with marked poststenotic dilatation which was mistaken for the aortic arch in the plain chest x-ray. The ascending Ao is elongated; the true aortic arch is in the supraclavicular region on the left. This was seen as a faint opacity above the poststenotic dilatation on the plain chest x-ray. There is an aberrant right subclavian artery (rt.SCA) originating from the descending Ao just below the coarctation. The right common carotid artery (rt.CCA) originates from the ascending Ao at the same level as the coarctation. **J,** A mild degree of AR is also observed. The pressures across the coarctation show a 30 mm Hg gradient. Since the patient is asymptomatic, and there is only a slight pressure gradient at the site of the coarctation with no cardiac enlargement, no surgical procedure was performed. The patient is being followed every 6 months.

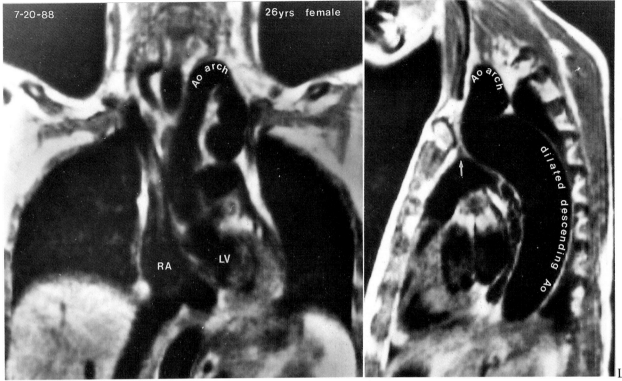

Fig. 6-2. *(Continued)* **K**, MRI shows her aortic arch to be well above the clavicle in the left side of the neck. The site of the coarctation and a markedly dilated descending Ao are clearly visualized. **L**, On the sagittal section, an arrow points to the site of the ligamentum arteriosum.

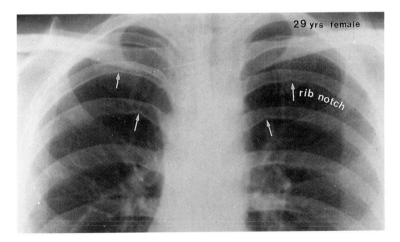

Fig. 6-3. This 29-year-old woman has rib notching bilaterally. Rib notchings occur in the aortitis syndrome, coarctation of the aorta, and in tetralogy of Fallot after a Blalock-Taussig operation. The cause of rib notching is dilatation and tortuosity of the intercostal arteries; it tends to occur in the posterior portions usually below the fourth ribs.

Chapter 7   Aortic Dissection

Pathophysiology and Clinical Clues

The term "dissecting aortic aneurysm" is generally used despite the common lack of associated aneurysmal dilatation of the Ao. Thus, the term "aortic dissection" is more appropriate. The real cause of aortic dissection is not known. Rupture of a vasa vasorum due to hypertension, tearing of an intimal atheroma, and cystic necrosis of the media (either of the congenital or acquired type) have all been postulated. Cystic medial necrosis is often found in Marfan's syndrome[*] or in annulo-aortic ectasia. A dissection may originate just above the aortic valve (proximal) or far from the aortic valve (distal). DeBakey has proposed four types:

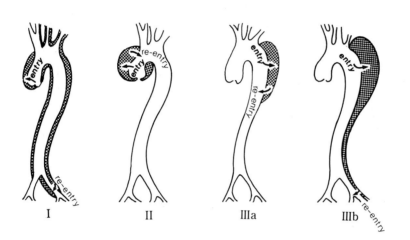

Fig. 7-1. Types of dissection: I. From the ascending Ao to the bifurcation of the abdominal Ao; II. Localized to the ascending Ao; IIIa. From a point distal to the left subclavian artery down to the descending Ao; IIIb. From distal to the left subclavian artery to the bifurcation of the abdominal Ao.

The dissection usually occurs in the lateral aspect of the Ao, but occasionally involves the medial side. There may be a high mortality in types I and II, with rupture proximally into the pericardial sac producing acute tamponade, or distally to produce acute renal failure. Major symptoms of the dissection are chest oppression, back pain, and/or abdominal pain. This is usually precipitated by the patient assuming an unusual posture, like lifting a heavy article onto a high shelf. Sometimes only ordinary activity precipitates dissection, i.e., putting on socks or lying in bed and reaching toward a side table. Dramatically, a drummer developed dissection during one of his performances. But, there may be neither precipitating factors nor symptoms. If an ECG made during or immediately after the onset of chest pain shows no ST changes in an elderly patient with hypertension, and the blood pressure remains high, an aortic dissection rather than a myocardial infarction should be suspected.

[*] The appearance of a person with the Marfan syndrome characteristically includes a tall body with long extremities. It is often associated with 1. pectus excavatum or pectus carinatum, 2. kyphoscoliosis, 3. arachnodactyly, 4. ectopia lentis, 5. high arched palate, and 6. hyper-extensibility of joints. It has been suggested that Abraham Lincoln may have had the Marfan syndrome because of his long arms, legs and fingers. Armspan is normally equal to the body height, and it may be more than this in the Marfan syndrome. Arachnodactyly is assessed by a plain radiograph of the hand. Ratios of more than 8.4 in the male and 9.2 in the female of the lengths to the widths of the metacarpal bones in an average of four fingers are considered abnormal.

The following features are found in aortic dissection:

★★★★ Chest x-ray shows a widened mediastinum due to an enlarged Ao. The thickness of the outer aortic wall is greater than 5 mm as measured from the calcification on the intimal surface. Often counterclockwise rotation of the heart is indicated by the absence of a main pulmonary artery segment.

★★★★ On auscultation, an accentuated S_2 and an early diastolic murmur of AR may be present.

★★★★ The M-mode echo reveals a double layered wall and the 2D-echo may show an intimal flap.

★★★ An ECG frequently shows systolic LV overloading.*

* There may be a septal q wave as far to the right as V_2 and/or V_3 due to counterclockwise rotation of the heart.

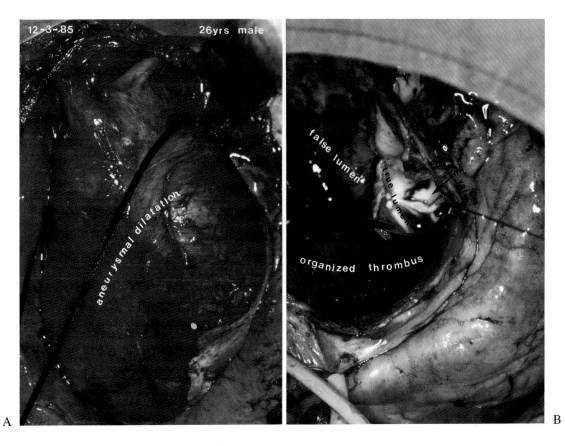

Fig. 7-2. A and B, A 26-year-old man was referred for a complete checkup and possible surgical treatment. At 17, while removing a book from the lowest shelf in a library, he experienced severe chest pain which radiated to his back. The pain eased in a few minutes. He did not see a physician until he had a physical examination for employment 9 years later. He was told he had an abnormal chest x-ray and a CT was done which revealed an aortic dissection. At surgery, he was found to have aneurysmal dilatation of the ascending Ao with an organized thrombus in the false lumen.

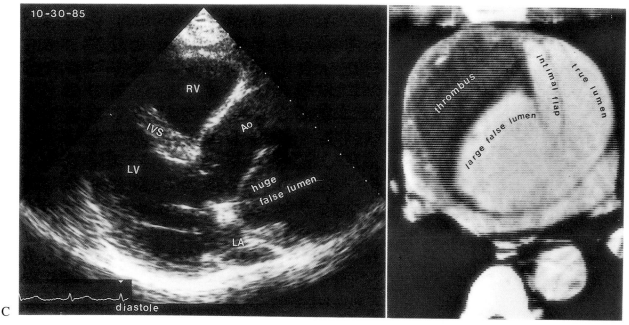

Fig. 7-2. *(Continued)* **C**, Preoperative long-axis 2D-echo during diastole shows an enlarged Ao with markedly sharp aortoseptal angulation. Closure of the aortic cusps is not clear. A large space behind the Ao usually occupied by the LA is now occupied by a false lumen of the aortic dissection which compresses the LA and displaces it toward the LV cavity. **D**, An enhanced CT section of the heart made above the aortic valvular level shows an intimal flap between the true lumen laterally and the false lumen medially with a large thrombus in the false lumen. The descending Ao is large but with no obvious dissection.

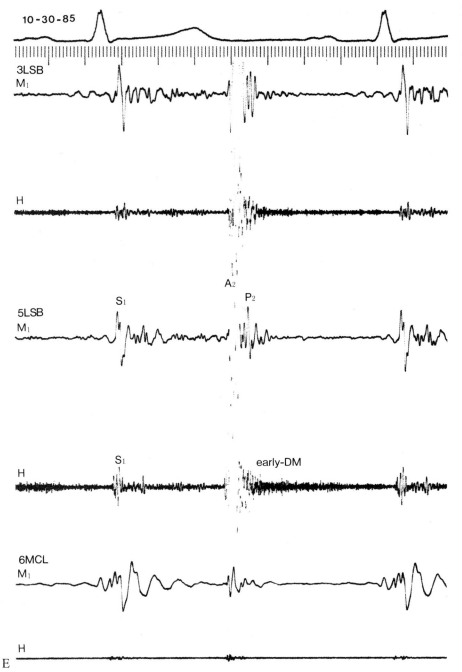

10-30-85

3LSB
M₁

H

A₂

S₁   P₂

5LSB
M₁

S₁   early-DM

H

6MCL
M₁

H

E

Fig. 7-2. *(Continued)* **E,** A PCG of the same patient shows an accentuated S_2 in the 3LSB to 5LSB followed by an early high-frequency diastolic murmur (early DM) of AR.

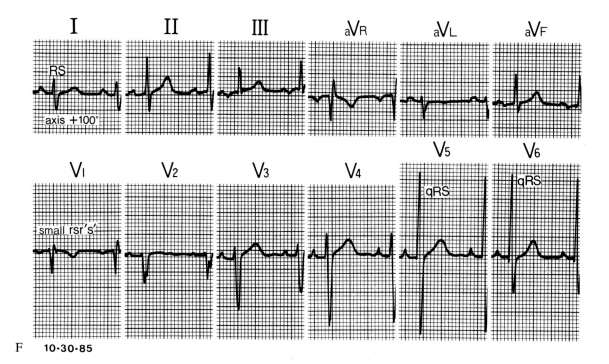

F   10·30·85

Fig. 7-2. *(Continued)* **F,** A slightly negative QRS is in lead I and a positive QRS in aVF indicates that the QRS axis is +100°. This slight right-axis deviation may be normal in a young person. The most prominent findings of this ECG are the tall QRS in the LV leads and small QRS in the right precordium. The transitional zone at V₅ suggests either a clockwise rotation or a posterior rotation of the QRS vector caused either by a conduction defect or by posterior tilting of the LV by the tortuous Ao. The small QRS in the right precordial leads suggests that there is an extra structure between the heart and the chest wall which correlates with the finding at surgery of a huge thrombus in the false lumen. The large amplitude of QRS in V₅ and V₆ may be the result of the heart being closer to the chest wall because of a leftward shift.

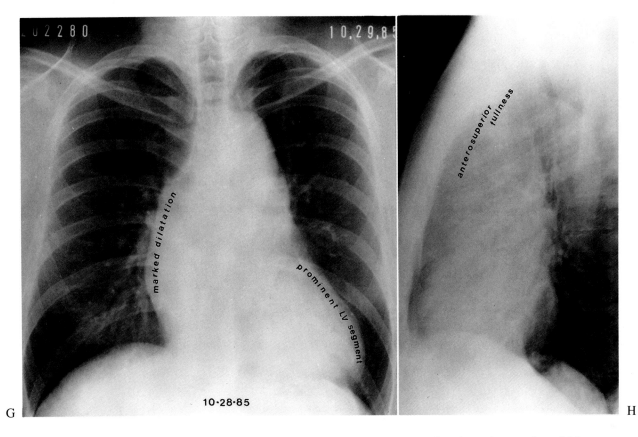

G

H

Fig. 7-2. *(Continued)* **G,** Chest x-rays demonstrate a dilated and tortuous ascending Ao and a prominent LV segment. The descending Ao is also elongated, its arch being at the level of the clavicle.* **H,** The lateral view shows the region anterosuperior to the heart occupied by an enlarged ascending Ao, and the posteriorly-shifted LV which appears dilated probably because the marked dilatation of the ascending Ao has displaced the heart posteriorly.

* The aortic arch is normally at least 1 to 2 cm below the sternoclavicular junction.

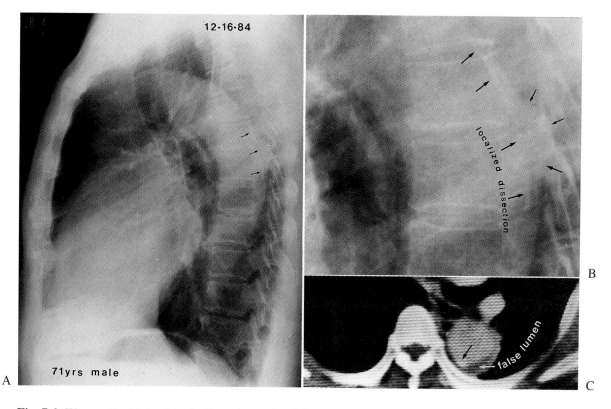

Fig. 7-3. We usually think of aortic dissection as involving a great length of Ao. This 71-year-old man with rheumatic MS and MR had atrial fibrillation (AF) and was taking digitalis. **A**, Chest x-rays during a routine checkup showed a small opacity protruding along the posterior margin of the descending Ao at the level of the tracheal bifurcation, arrows. **B**, A magnified view of the same region shows a linear calcification 3 mm inside the outer margin of the Ao (arrows) and an opacity 1 cm in height and 3 cm in length protruding from the descending Ao. **C**, Enhanced CT at the level of the protrusion shows an intimal calcification (black arrow) a few mm inside the outer margin of the descending Ao with a thrombus (white arrow) in a probable false lumen. It is debatable whether this is a localized aortic dissection or a saccular aneurysm with partially displaced intima. Because of the age of the patient, the fact that he was without symptoms, and the fact that the lesion was very small, surgery was not considered. This case underscores the fact that small, localized aortic disease can be overlooked on routine chest x-rays unless one cultivates a high degree of suspicion.

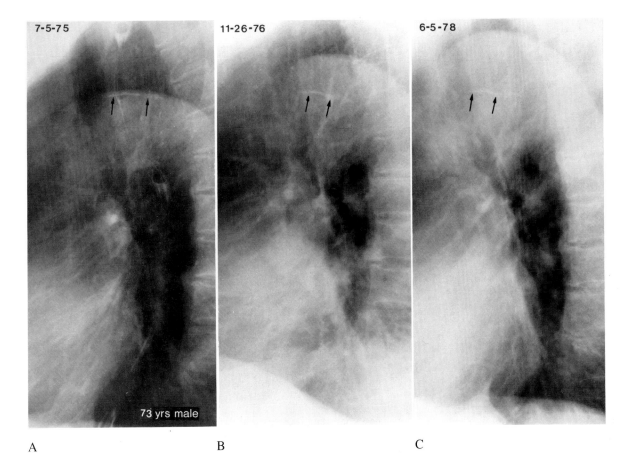

Fig. 7-4. A, This 73-year-old hypertensive executive experienced no symptoms but was referred for an abnormal chest x-ray that showed enlargement of the aortic arch with linear calcification at the top of the arch. He was told that he might have an aortic dissection and was advised to be aware of any chest discomfort. **B,** Although he was asymptomatic, his chest x-ray 17 months later showed that the previously noted linear calcification was now 15 mm from the aortic margin indicating interval development of an aortic dissection. He refused invasive studies. Eighteen months after that, he reached for an ash tray and felt an uneasy sensation in his chest. Because of earlier advice, he came to the hospital by ambulance. **C,** On admission he had already become asymptomatic, but his frontal x-ray showed further enlargement of his Ao which now reached the level of his left clavicle. The previously noted linear calcification in the lateral view is now 25 mm from the aortic margin, strongly indicating that he had further progression of an aortic dissection. An aortogram showed a type I dissection, and conservative treatment was unsuccessful. He died from acute cardiac tamponade and renal failure. This case emphasizes the importance of the location of the aortic calcification, particularly on the lateral view.

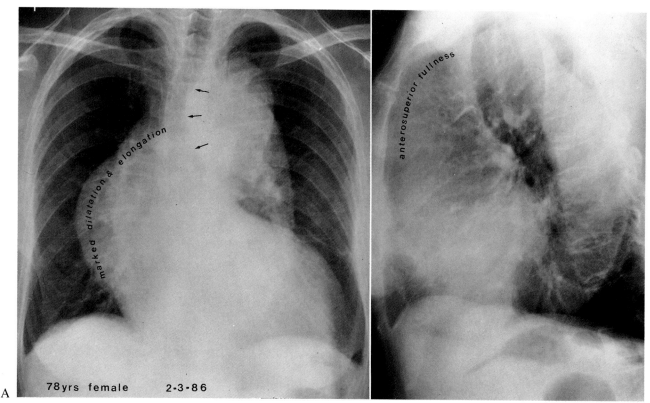

A 78 yrs female 2·3·86

B

Fig. 7-5. A 78-year-old woman was admitted because of an upper respiratory infection. **A,** Chest x-rays on admission reveal a huge ascending Ao with enlargement of the aortic arch that shifted the trachea to the right. **B,** Lateral view shows a tortuous aortic arch, and a huge ascending Ao which occupies the anterosuperior portion of the chest. She had no chest pain.

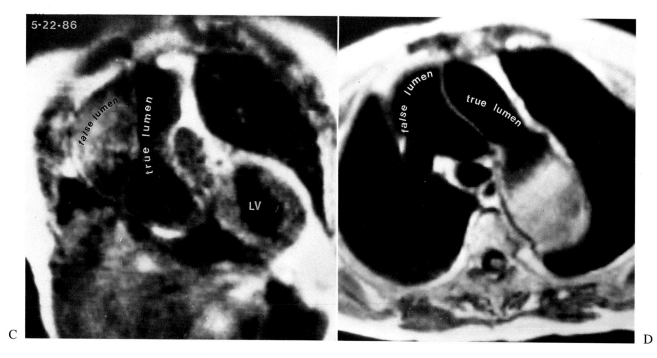

C

D

Fig. 7-5. *(Continued)* **C,** The coronal section of magnetic resonance imaging (MRI) shows a huge false lumen in the ascending Ao.* **D,** A transaxial section shows a large false lumen throughout the entire thoracic Ao.

* On the coronal section, the thrombus-like opacity in the false lumen may be due to blood stasis or slow blood flow.

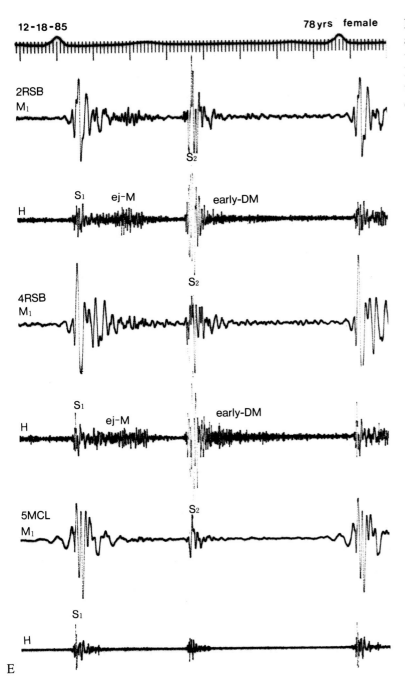

Fig. 7-5. *(Continued)* **E,** An ejection murmur (ej-M) and an early diastolic murmur (early DM) of AR were recorded best along the 2RSB to 3RSB correlating with x-ray evidence of a dilated ascending Ao to the right of the sternum. The patient was treated conservatively and had an uneventful recovery.

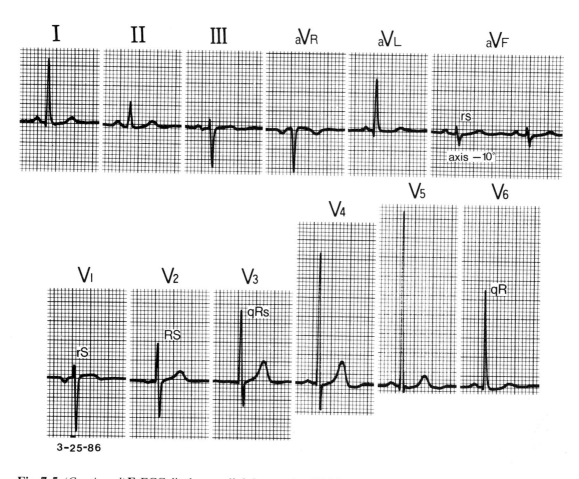

F

Fig. 7-5. *(Continued)* **F**, ECG discloses a slightly negative QRS in aVF, indicating a QRS axis of –10°. She has LVH by index of Sokolow with an anterior QRS (transitional zone at V_2) which may be due to a tortuous and elongated Ao causing counterclockwise rotation of the heart.

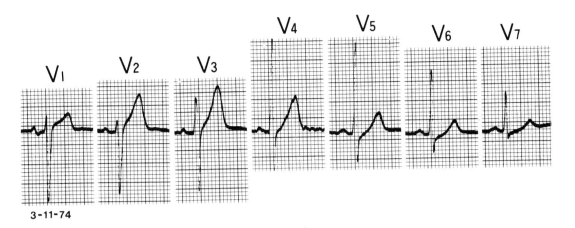

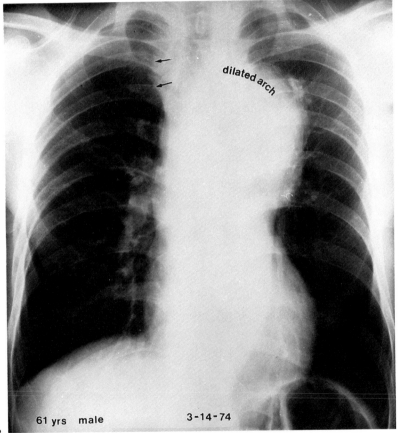

Fig. 7-6. A, A 63-year-old hypertensive man developed severe back pain and was admitted to our hospital. His ECG nearly 1 year before showed a transitional zone between V_3 and V_4 which is normal.

Fig. 7-6. *(Continued)* **B,** His chest x-ray 1 year before showed a markedly dilated aortic arch and prominence of the innominate artery (arrows). The patient may have had a dissecting Ao by this time.

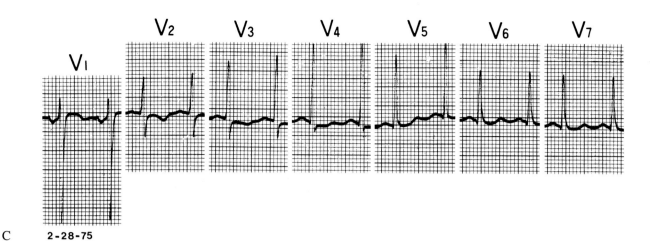

C   2-28-75

Fig. 7-6. *(Continued)* **C,** On admission his ECG shows a more anterior QRS than a year before as shown by a shift to the right of the transitional zone suggesting a possible counterclockwise rotation of the heart. The T waves are inverted in V₂ and V₃ and they are low in the LV leads indicating myocardial damage.

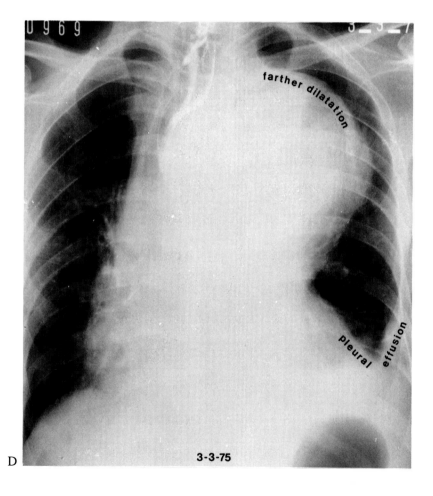

D   3-3-75

Fig. 7-6. *(Continued)* **D,** Despite conservative treatment for 4 days, his x-ray shows more marked dilatation of his aortic arch and a pleural effusion or extrapleural hemorrhage on the left suggesting a progression of the dissection or a rupture of the aneurysm. The patient died 6 days after admission. An autopsy showed an old organized dissection with thrombus throughout the entire thoracic Ao. There was a newly developed dissection distal to the left subclavian artery with a huge aneurysmal dilatation which could have caused the anterior shift of the QRS on the ECG by producing counterclockwise rotation of the heart. This case emphasizes the importance of a suddenly developed counterclockwise rotation which may indicate an aortic dissection.

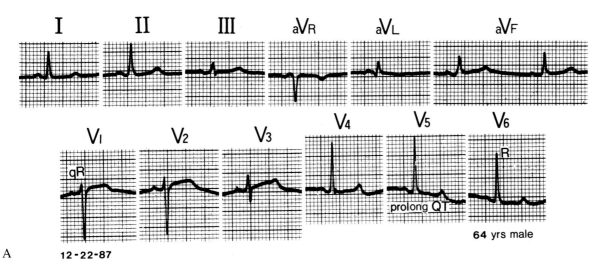

I   II   III   aVR   aVL   aVF

V₁   V₂   V₃   V₄   V₅   V₆

qR

prolong QT

R

64 yrs male

A   12-22-87

Fig. 7-7. A, A 64-year-old man was admitted to the hospital because of back pain. On admission, the patient was asymptomatic but his ECG shows generalized low voltage with some QT prolongation. There is no evidence of acute myocardial damage. An aortic dissection was then suspected.

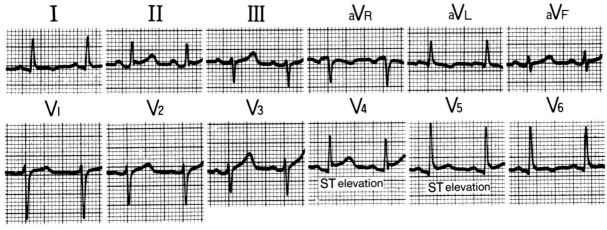

I   II   III   aVR   aVL   aVF

V₁   V₂   V₃   V₄   V₅   V₆

ST elevation   ST elevation

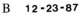

B   12-23-87

Fig. 7-7. *(Continued)* **B**, An ECG on the following day shows further reduction of QRS amplitudes with ST elevation in V₄ to V₆ suggesting pericardial effusion. The patient was transferred to another hospital for possible surgical treatment.

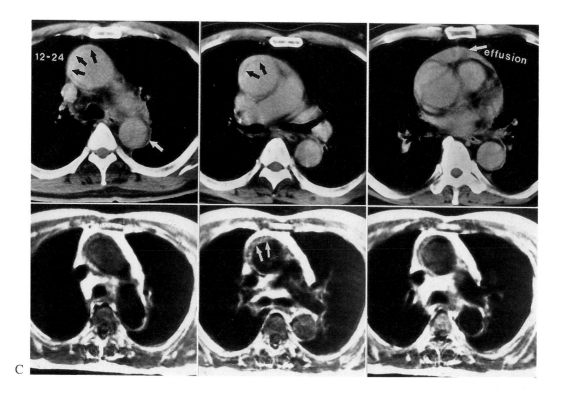

Fig. 7-7. *(Continued)* **C,** Transaxial cardiac CT and MRI showed the aortic dissection with a mural thrombus. CT sections in the upper row show a pericardial effusion anteriorly: the content is most likely blood.

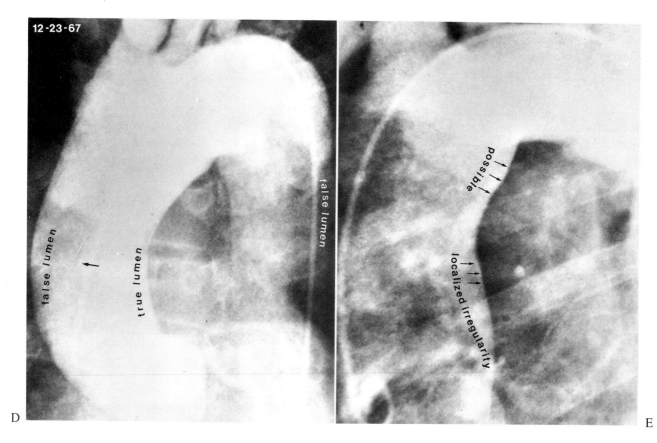

Fig. 7-7. *(Continued)* **D,** An aortogram confirmed a dissection which occurred a few cm above the aortic root (arrow). **E,** The medial margin of the ascending Ao shows an irregular margin which may indicate the sites of the lesions. The patient was conservatively treated but suddenly developed acute cardiac tamponade and died 1 week later.

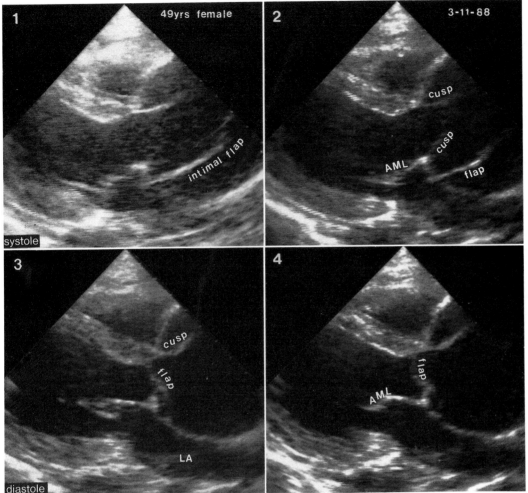

Fig. 7-8. A, A 49-year-old woman with the Marfan syndrome developed an aortic dissection. Her long-axis 2D-echoes show a markedly dilated aortic root with an intimal flap along the posterior aortic wall during systole. During diastole, this intimal flap covers the entire aortic orifice and prevents AR. The portion of the intimal flap over the aortic orifice prolapses into the LV outflow tract.

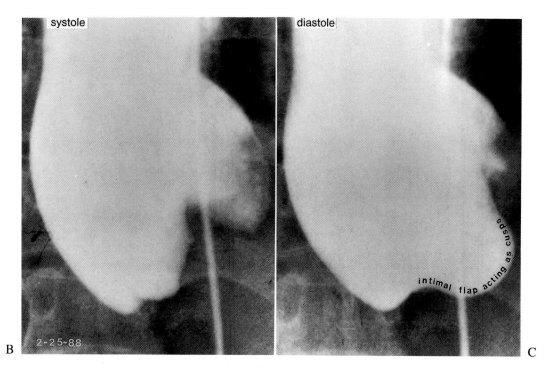

Fig. 7-8. (Continued) B, An aortogram of the same patient shows a markedly dilated aortic root. During systole, deformed cusps were observed. C, During diastole the intimal flap acts as an aortic cusp and overlays the aortic orifice to prevent regurgitation.

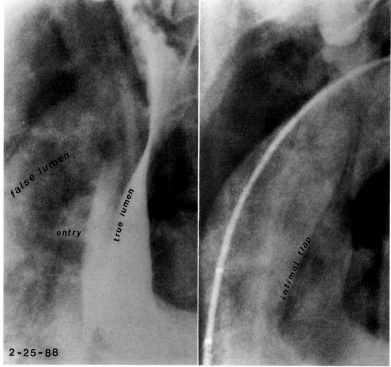

Fig. 7-8. (Continued) Another view of the aortogram above the aortic root shows the entry site of the dissection. D, A jet is imaged from the true lumen to the false lumen. E, A catheter is located in the false lumen and a long intimal flap is imaged. (Courtesy of S. Matsuyama, M.D., and S. Kawata, M.D.)

Chapter 8 Hypertrophic Cardiomyopathy

Pathophysiology and Clinical Clues

Hypertrophic cardiomyopathy (HCM) can be classified as symmetric or asymmetric, and as obstructive or nonobstructive in type. The obstructive type is termed hypertrophic obstructive cardiomyopathy (HOCM) or hypertrophic subaortic stenosis (HSS). Asymmetric hypertrophy (ASH) denotes either septal (IVS) or free wall hypertrophy. The obstructive form usually indicates the presence of an obstruction in the LV but occasionally in the RV outflow tract. Hypertrophy of the IVS with LV outflow tract (LVOT) obstruction is also described as idiopathic hypertrophic subaortic stenosis (IHSS), or simply HSS. Any exercise or drug that increases LV contractility and diminishes the end-systolic or end-diastolic volume (such as a Valsalva maneuver, tachycardia, digitalis, isoproterenol, or amyl nitrite) may increase the LVOT obstruction in HOCM. A decrease in afterload or blood pressure will also increase the obstruction by allowing the anterior mitral leaflet to move closer to the septum during systole.[*]

Clinical findings of HCM and HOCM are as follows:

★★★★ In the echo, isolated hypertrophy of the IVS and/or some portion of the LV, narrowing of the LV cavity, and systolic anterior movement (SAM) of the anterior mitral leaflet are the important findings. In some cases, mid-systolic semiclosure of the aortic valve may be found.

★★★★ In the ECG, there may be a deep septal Q wave associated with an upright T wave in LV leads and a reciprocally tall R wave in V_1. In many cases of HCM especially with apical hypertrophy there is a tall QRS complex with giant negative T waves in the LV leads. Often, especially with apical hypertrophy, there are no septal q waves in V_5 and V_6, and negativity of the T wave varies widely from day to day. A peaked P wave in V_1 and left axis deviation are common.

★★★ In patients with HCM, there is almost always an S_4. In HOCM, the loudest ejection murmur is at the 4LSB or apex. With severe obstruction there may be paradoxical splitting of the S_2.

★★★ In the chest x-ray, a normal or slightly prominent LV segment with a small aortic arch may be seen, unlike the prominent arch seen in hypertension.

[*] In either idiopathic or familial types of HCM and HOCM, a pertinent echo feature is an involvement of the RV which differs from the LV hypertrophy observed in hypertension.

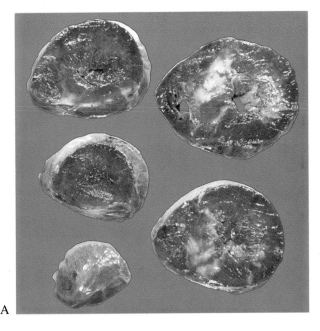

Fig. 8-1. A, These specimens of LV are from a 39-year-old woman who died of uterine cancer. At autopsy, the LV, RV and IVS were so markedly hypertrophied that there was nearly no ventricular cavity. This was the first autopsied case of apparent HCM encountered by the author (1969).

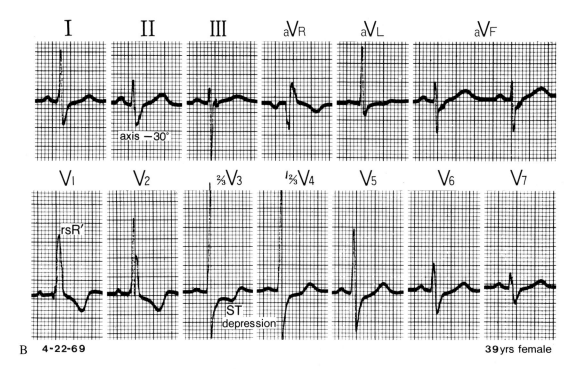

axis −30°

V_1 V_2 ⅔V_3 1⅔V_4 V_5 V_6 V_7

rsR′

ST depression

B 4-22-69

39 yrs female

Fig. 8-1. *(Continued)* **B**, Her ECG shows a right bundle-branch block (RBBB) with left-axis deviation of −30°. V_1 shows an rsR′ pattern with inverted T waves in V_1 to V_3. ST depressions are seen in V_3 to V_5. From these findings, LV overloading is not readily apparent.

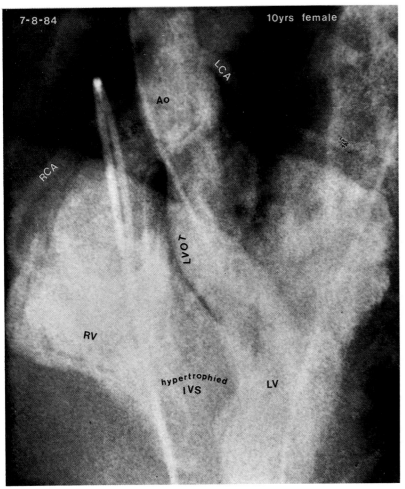

Fig. 8-2. A, This 10-year-old female student had an abnormal ECG during an annual physical examination. A biventriculogram revealed a hypertrophied IVS. There seems to be some protrusion of the upper segment of the IVS which compresses the left ventricular outflow tract (LVOT).

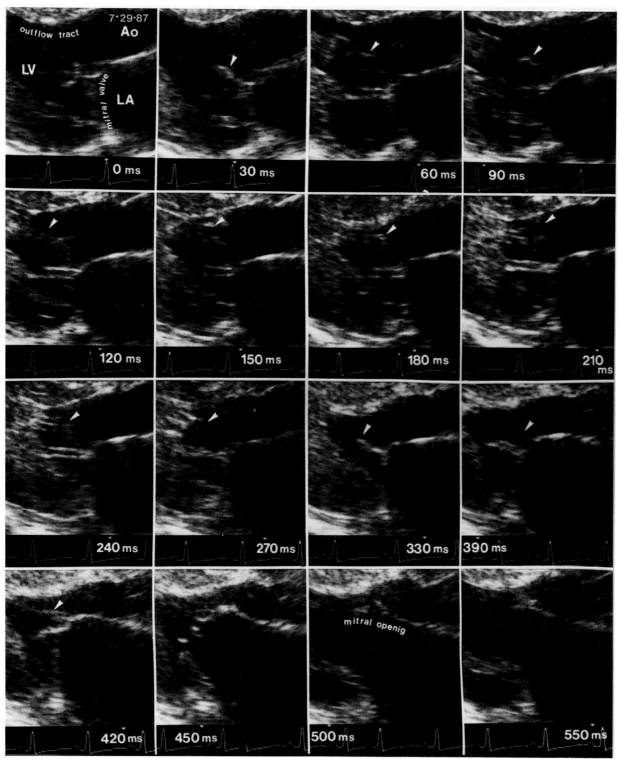

Fig. 8-2. *(Continued)* **B**, Systolic anterior movement (SAM) is a prominent echo feature of HOCM. Serial long-axis 2D-echoes focused on the mitral and the aortic orifices of the same patient disclose the nature of the SAM. The value in milliseconds (ms) indicates a delay from the peak of the R wave in the ECG which is the end-diastolic period. At 0 ms, the mitral valve is closed. From 30 ms to 270 ms, the mitral valve remains closed; however, a structure seems to be attached to the anterior mitral leaflet (AML), approaches the IVS, and crosses the LVOT (arrowhead). At 420 ms the mitral valve is ready to open, and at 500 ms maximal opening occurs. During systole, from 30 ms to 330 ms, a cord-like structure remains in position anterosuperiorly which causes SAM and can be seen in the M-mode echo. This is probably caused by thickened chordae.

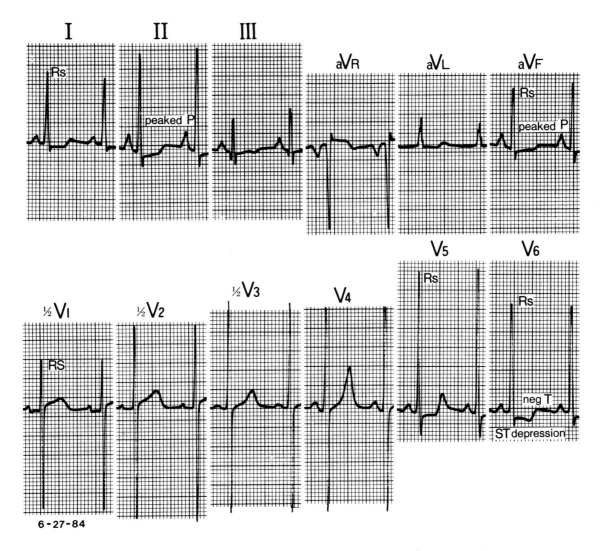

C

6-27-84

Fig. 8-2. *(Continued)* C, An ECG of the same patient shows a horizontal ST depression in leads I, II, aVF, and V$_5$ with tall and peaked P waves. There is no initial septal q wave in the LV leads but a tall R in V$_1$ due either to a hypertrophied septum or RVH. One may not be able to conclude that this is biventricular hypertrophy in spite of tall R waves in both right and left precordial leads.

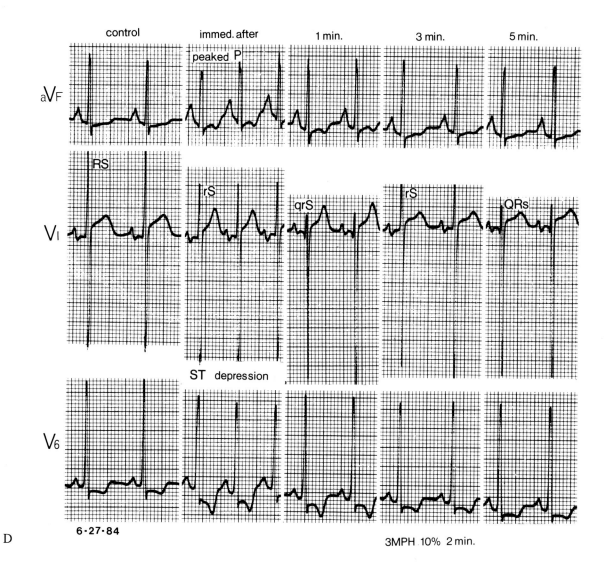

control   immed. after   1 min.   3 min.   5 min.

aVF

peaked P

V1

RS
rS
qrS
rS
QRs

ST depression

V6

D

6·27·84

3MPH 10% 2 min.

Fig. 8-2. *(Continued)* **D,** An exercise ECG shows further depression of the ST segments, and there is increased negativity of the T wave in aVF and V₆. The tall R wave in V₁ is decreased in amplitude and now shows a qRS pattern indicating a change in direction of the septal activation. Further ST depression and increased negativity of the T wave do not necessarily indicate myocardial ischemia in the presence of a conduction defect. The greater negativity of the terminal P wave in V₁ suggests LA overloading.

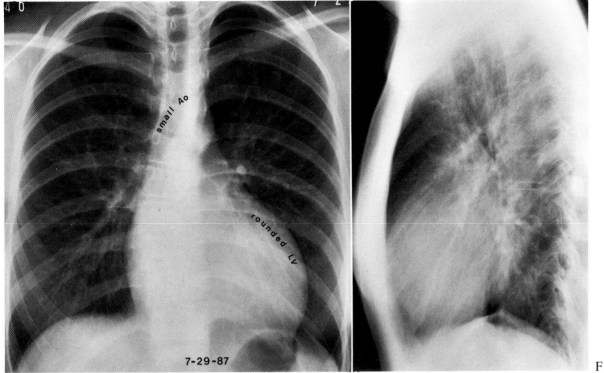

E

F

Fig. 8-2. *(Continued)* **E and F**, The recent chest x-rays of the same patient disclose a rounded LV segment suggestive of hypertrophy. The aortic arch is rather small, suggesting there is no increase in systemic flow.

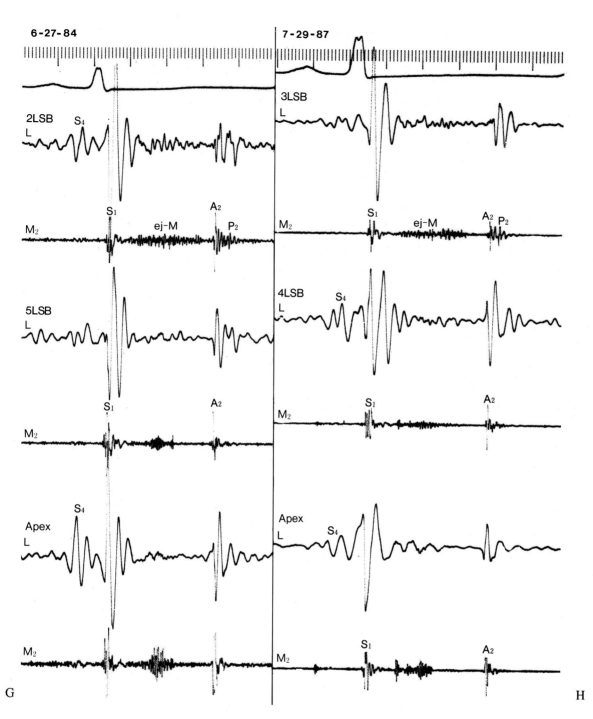

Fig. 8-2. *(Continued)* **G,** In the PCG, there is a prominent S$_4$ at the apex with a slight ejection murmur (ej-M) from the 2LSB to the apex. **H,** Three years later the findings are about the same, except for a reduced S$_4$ closer to the S$_1$.

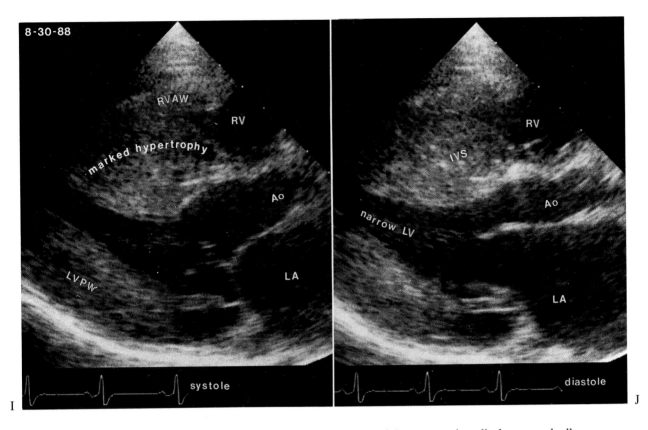

Fig. 8-2. *(Continued)* **I and J**, The most recent long-axis 2D-echoes of the same patient disclose a markedly hypertrophied IVS and LV posterior wall. The LV cavity is small. The delineation of the right ventricular anterior wall (RVAW) is not clear but it also appears to be hypertrophied.

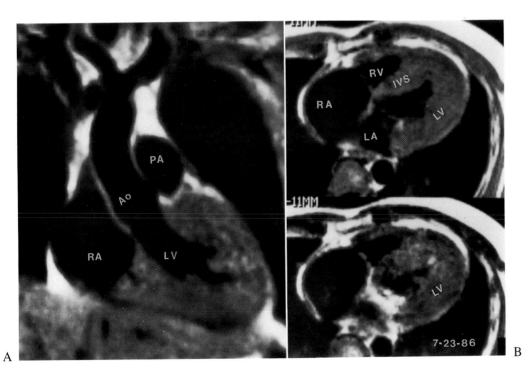

Fig. 8-3. A and B, This 38-year-old man had an abnormal ECG during an annual physical examination at his company. MRI shows hypertrophy of both IVS and LV. There is no obvious LVOT obstruction. There may be mild RV hypertrophy.

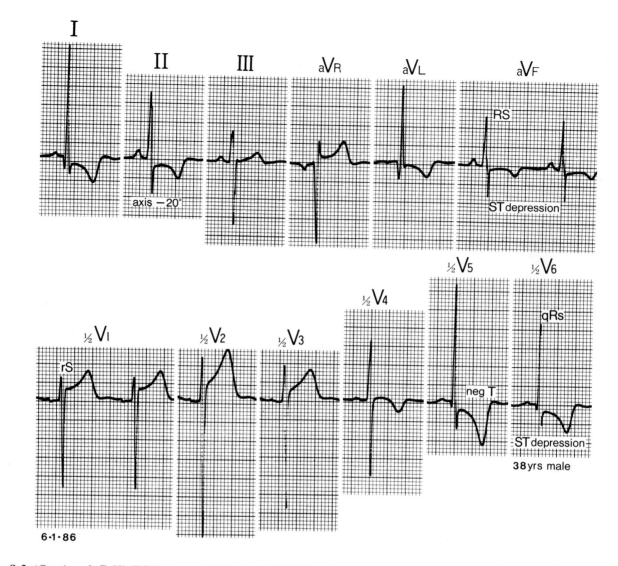

C 6·1·86

Fig. 8-3. *(Continued)* **C,** His ECG shows a QRS axis of –20°. There is a prominent Q wave in leads I and aV_L with ST depression and an inverted T wave (LVH strain pattern). Despite left ventricular hypertrophy, relatively tall R waves in the RV leads with a peaked P wave suggest coexisting RV overloading and/or a hypertrophied septum.

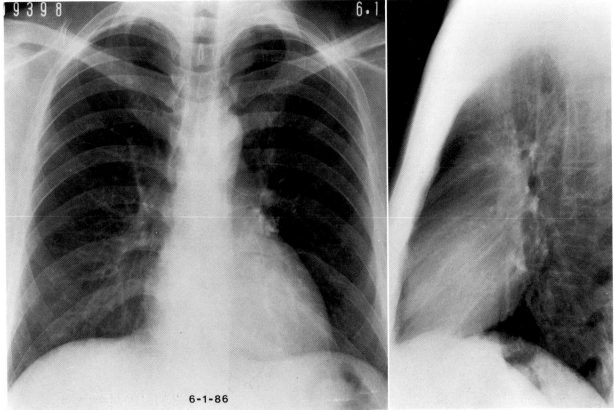

D

E

Fig. 8-3. *(Continued)* **D and E**, Chest x-rays of the same patient are unremarkable. An apparently abnormal ECG with an unremarkable chest x-ray is often seen in HCM.

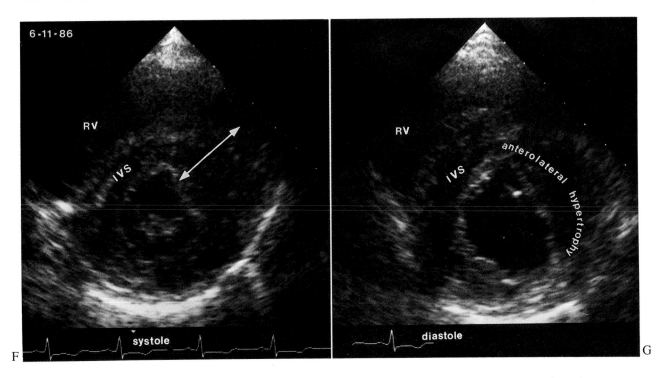

F

G

Fig. 8-3. *(Continued)* **F and G**, His short-axis 2D-echoes show hypertrophy of the IVS and the anterolateral wall of the LV as indicated by the distance between arrowheads.

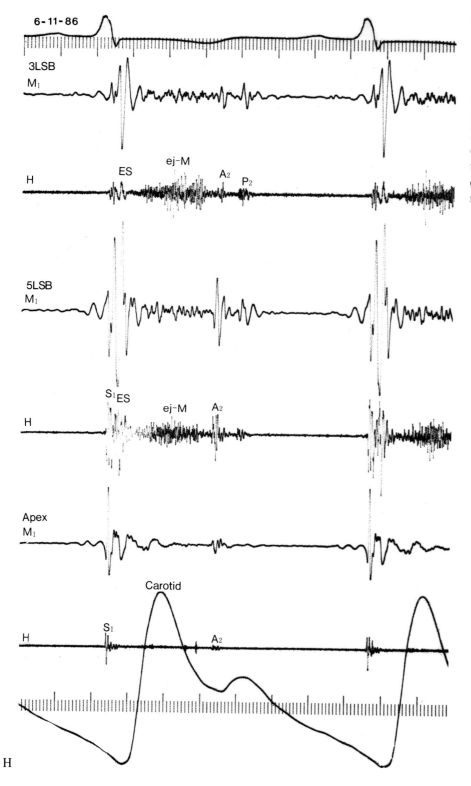

Fig. 8-3. *(Continued)* **H,** A PCG of the same patient discloses an ejection murmur (ej-M) which begins with an ejection sound (ES) and is loudest in the 3LSB to 5LSB. In the carotid pulse, there is no recognizable tidal wave. There is a widely split S_2 of about 0.05 sec. In HOCM, a prominent tidal wave often produces a palpably bifid pulse. In the present case, the cause of the ejection murmur can be attributed to rapid ejection.

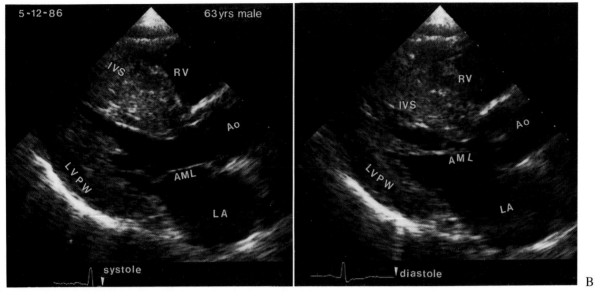

Fig. 8-4. A and B, These long axis 2D-echoes from a 63-year-old hypertensive man show marked hypertrophy of the septum as well as the LV posterior wall (LVPW). The thickness of the septum and the LV posterior wall did not vary between systole and diastole.

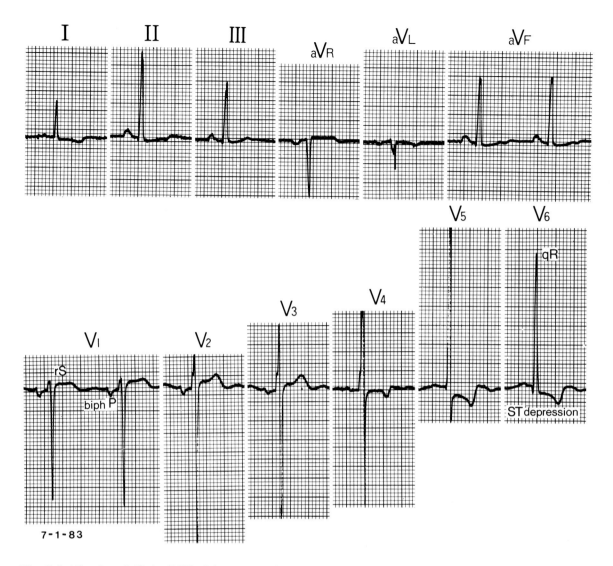

Fig. 8-4. *(Continued)* **C,** An ECG of the same patient shows severe systolic LV overloading as an LVH strain pattern and an index of Sokolow. A normal septal activation is indicated by an initial q wave in V₆.

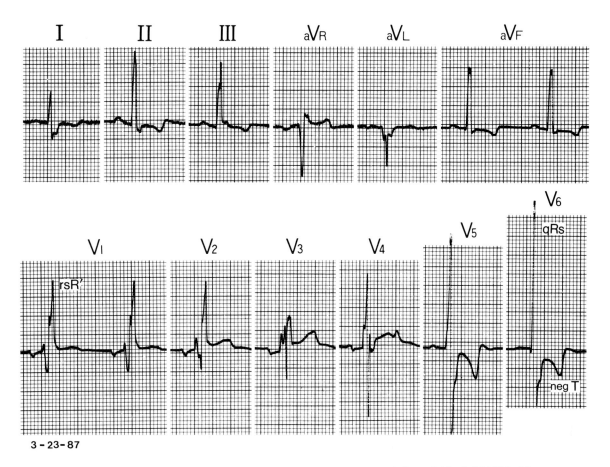

Fig. 8-4. *(Continued)* **D**, Two years later the patient's ECG shows right bundle branch block (RBBB). The appearance of RBBB, especially with a notch on the tall R′, is most likely caused by ischemic changes or fibrosis in the hypertrophied septum. One should always be aware of the possibility of a coexisting pulmonary embolism when there is a sudden appearance of RBBB. Despite the RBBB, he still has LVH voltage by index of Sokolow.

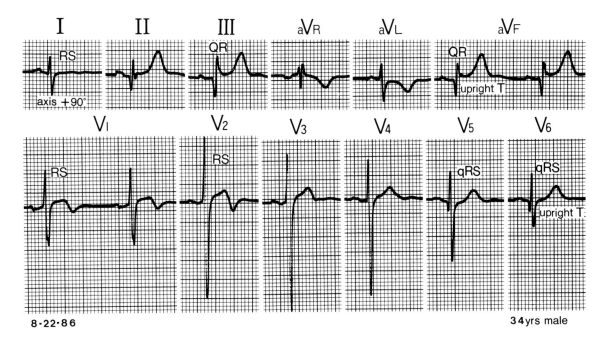

Fig. 8-5. A, ECG from a 34-year-old man who has many of the typical ECG findings of HOCM. There are deep Q waves in leads II, III, aV_F, and V_5 and V_6 associated with positive T waves and tall R waves in the right precordial leads; all are probably due to septal hypertrophy.

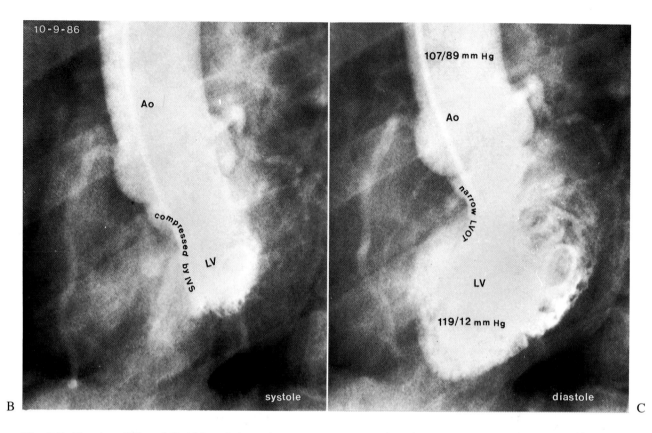

Fig. 8-5. *(Continued)* **B and C**, Although the patient was asymptomatic and there was no history to suggest a familial occurrence, LV angiography was performed because the results of an echo and cardiac CT were not helpful. The LV angiogram showed mild narrowing of the left ventricular outflow tract (LVOT) compressed by a hypertrophied IVS. There was neither a significant pressure gradient between the LV and the Ao nor hypertrophy of the LV free wall. Thus, asymmetric septal hypertrophy of a non-obstructive type is probable. Catheterization showed only a 10 mm Hg systolic gradient between the RV and main PA.

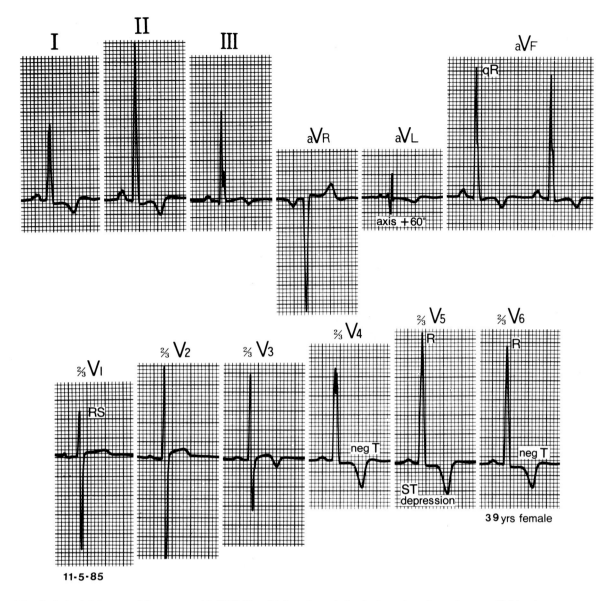

Fig. 8-6. A, A 39-year-old woman with HCM has high voltage in both the extremity and precordial leads. The absence of a septal q wave in V$_5$ or V$_6$ suggests a conduction abnormality similar to that seen in incomplete left bundle-branch block (LBBB). The inverted T wave and ST depressions are probably secondary to fibrosis. There are tall R waves in leads V$_1$ to V$_3$ suggesting concomitant RV overloading or septal hypertrophy.

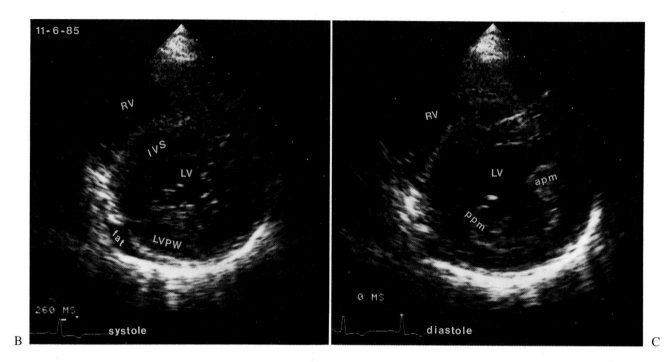

Fig. 8-6. *(Continued)* **B and C**, Short-axis 2D-echoes of the same patient disclose septal and lateral wall hypertrophy. Because the echo beam crosses different levels of the LV cavity during systole and diastole, the papillary muscles are scarely imaged in systole but clearly identified as anterior papillary muscle (apm) and posterior papillary muscle (ppm) in diastole. There is an extra echo space behind the LV posteromedially. In the past, this was thought to be caused by pericardial fluid, but recent studies have shown it is more likely due to subepicardial fat.

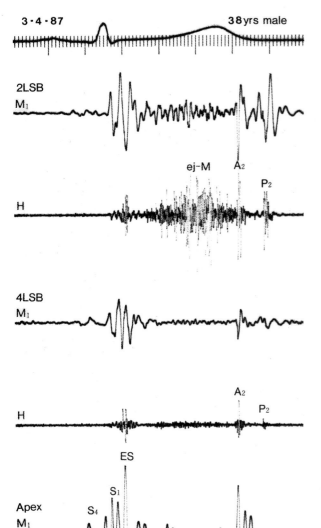

3·4·87   38yrs male

2LSB
M₁

ej-M   A₂

H   P₂

4LSB
M₁

A₂

H   P₂

ES

S₁

Apex
M₁   S₄

A H

Fig. 8-7. A, By auscultation, this 38-year-old male was suspected of having an atrial septal defect (ASD). A PCG shows wide splitting of the S_2 with an ejection murmur (ej-M) at the base of the heart with an enhancement toward the end of systole, which suggests that the murmur is of pulmonary origin. However, the P_2 is not accentuated since it is not transmitted to the apex. The splitting is wide but not fixed in a long continuous recording. There is a soft S_4 at the apex.

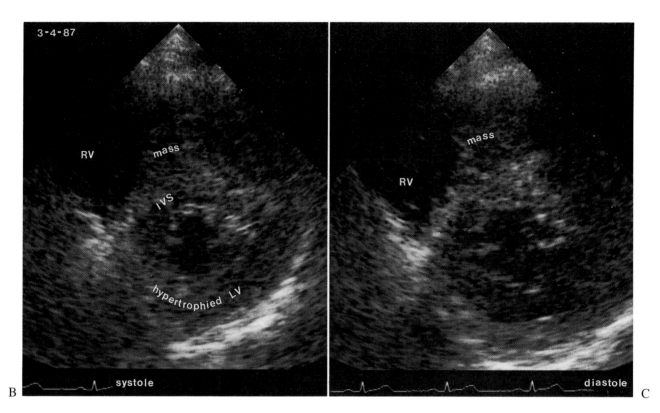

Fig. 8-7. *(Continued)* **B and C**, Short-axis 2D-echoes of the same patient disclose a mass in the RV cavity, seemingly attached to the IVS, both in systole and diastole. This is compatible with a cardiac tumor arising from the hypertrophied septum.

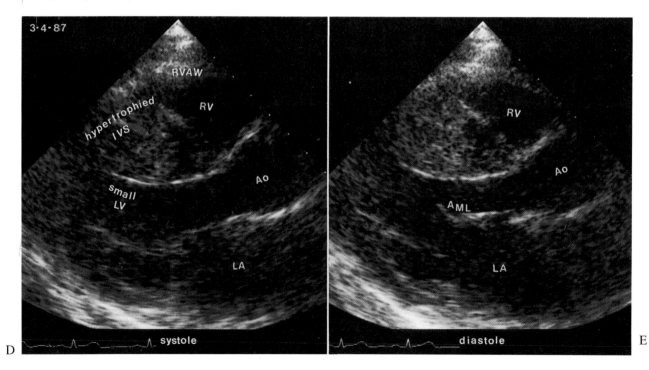

Fig. 8-7. *(Continued)* **D and E**, However, as the long axis echoes show, there are no apparent masses in the RV cavity connected with the septum. It looks rather like a hypertrophied IVS with some prominent trabeculae in the RV cavity. The thickness of the septum does not change between systole and diastole.

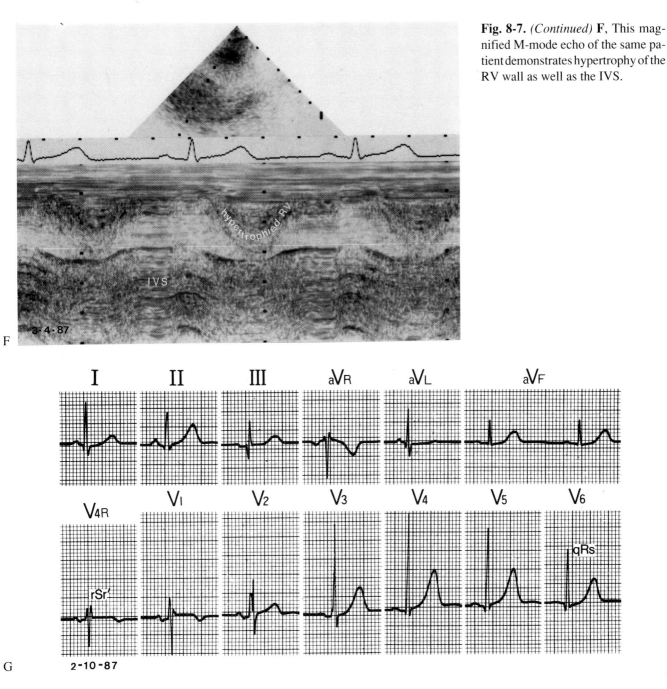

Fig. 8-7. *(Continued)* **F,** This magnified M-mode echo of the same patient demonstrates hypertrophy of the RV wall as well as the IVS.

Fig. 8-7. *(Continued)* **G,** The patient's ECG shows an rSr′ pattern in $V_1 \sim V_2$ which may be the result of RV overloading. However, there is no right-axis deviation and the overall findings are within normal limits. In this case, LV voltage may have been masked by the loss of terminal LV forces which were taken over by the outflow tract of the RV which caused the rSr′ pattern.

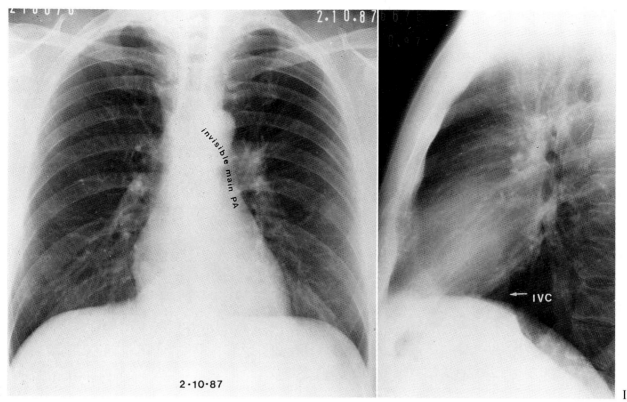

H   I

Fig. 8-7. *(Continued)* **H and I**, Chest x-rays are not remarkable except for an invisible main pulmonary artery suggesting counterclockwise rotation of the heart.

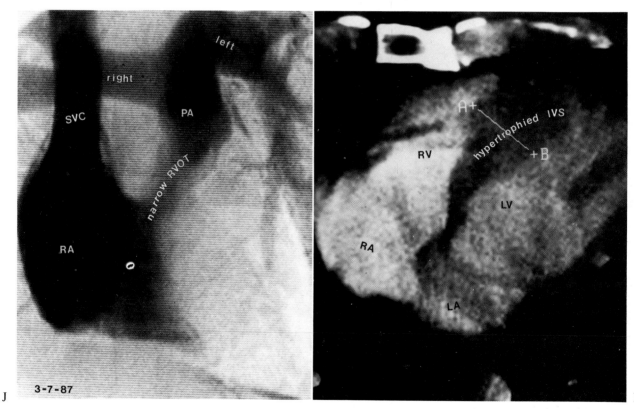

J   K

Fig. 8-7. *(Continued)* **J**, DSA shows narrowing of the RV outflow tract from compression by the hypertrophied septum. **K**, The cardiac CT shows marked hypertrophy of the IVS. The LV cavity appears to be small, but the LV free wall is not clear enough to determine its thickness.

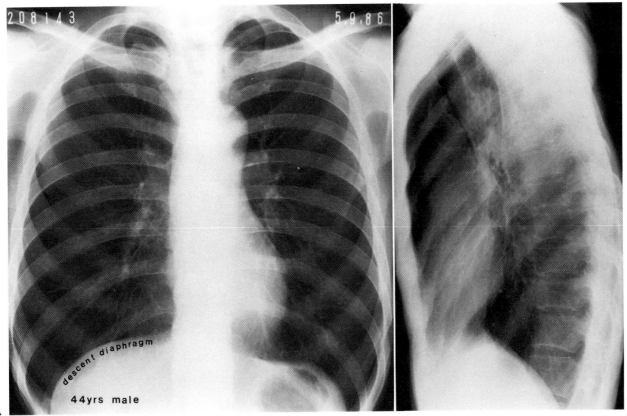

Fig. 8-8. A and B, Chest x-rays of a 44-year-old man with hypertension and emphysema, showing a low diaphragm with decreased pulmonary vascularity, indicating emphysema. The prominent aortic arch is probably caused by hypertension.

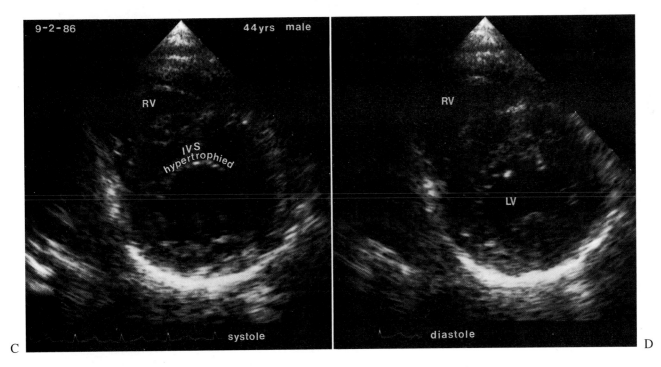

Fig. 8-8. *(Continued)* **C and D**, Short-axis echoes of the same patient unexpectedly show hypertrophy of the IVS.

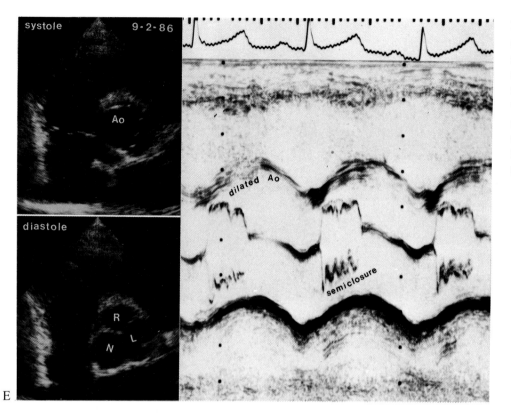

E

Fig. 8-8. *(Continued)* E, Short-axis echoes of the Ao show relatively limited opening clearly seen in the M-mode echo. The Ao is dilated and its valvular opening has semiclosures and does not reach the aortic wall, which suggests incomplete opening from possible HOCM.

Fig. 8-9. A, M-mode echo of the Ao from a 48-year-old man with HOCM. It shows semiclosure of the aortic valve during systole caused by LVOT obstruction. A normal M-mode echo of the aortic valve should show an abrupt opening; the valve should remain parallel to both the anterior and posterior aortic wall throughout systole. On the contrary, in this case the configuration resembles a bow tie. This tendency to close during mid-systole is seen in HOCM.

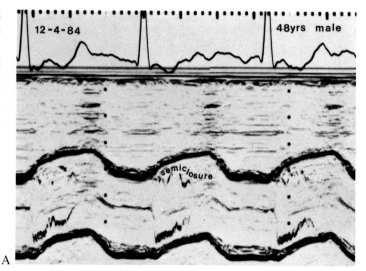

A

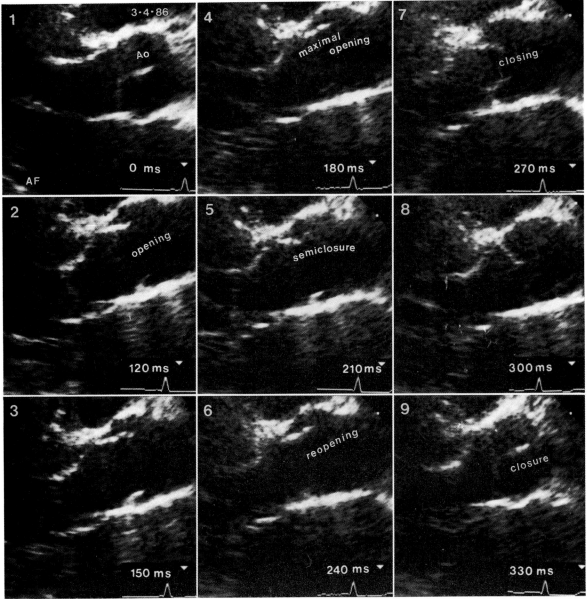

Fig. 8-9. *(Continued)* **B,** For clarification, serial tracings of long-axis 2D echoes focused on the aortic valve were recorded on the same patient. The patient has atrial fibrillation, and the values in milliseconds (ms) indicate a delay from the top of the R wave in the ECG. Illustration 1 is near end-diastole and shows a closed aortic valve while the mitral valve remains open. The maximal aortic valvular opening occurs at 180 ms in 4; the mid-systolic closing occurs at 210 ms in 5. The aortic valve reopens widely at 240 ms in 6. Thereafter, 7 to 9 show the final closing of the aortic valve. Normally, the semiclosure observed at 210 ms would never occur.

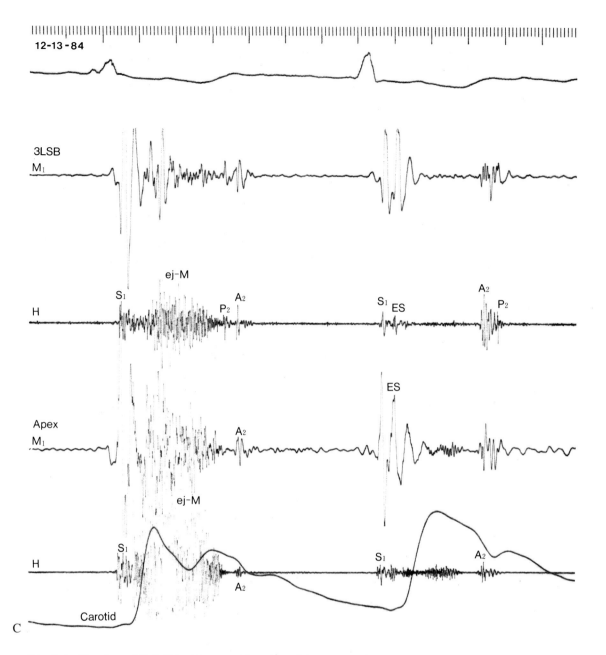

Fig. 8-9. *(Continued)* **C,** PCG with a carotid tracing of the same patient reveals a mid-systolic ejection murmur (ej-M) heard best at the apex. The S_2 is splitting paradoxically and the carotid tracing shows a prominent tidal wave (late systolic wave) in the first beat which produces a bifid configuration known as a bisferious pulse. The echo finding of semiclosure probably occurs simultaneously with the trough of the bifid pulse. The loudness of the ejection murmur is changing probably because of a longer diastolic pause preceding the first cardiac cycle. Usually a larger volume of the LV will decrease the LVOT obstruction; however, in this case, a forceful contraction of the postextrasystolic beat produces a stronger contraction resulting in a greater obstruction of the LVOT, which in turn causes a louder ejection murmur.

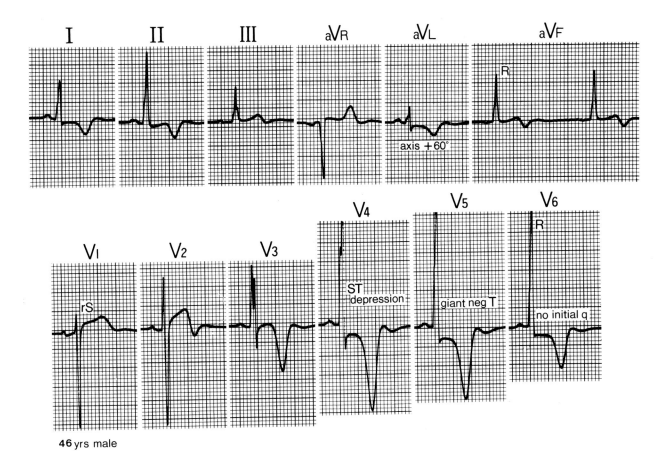

I II III aVR aVL aVF

axis +60°

V1 V2 V3 V4 V5 V6

rS

ST depression

giant neg T

R

no initial q

46 yrs male

Fig. 8-10. An ECG typical of HCM in a 46-year-old man. There are tall R waves with giant negative T waves in V_3 to V_6. The absent q wave in V_4 to V_6 together with a slightly short PR interval may be indicative of preexcitation, especially since the initial upstrokes of the R waves in leads II, aVF and $V_5 \sim V_6$ show some slurring, suggesting a delta wave. But slow conduction through a thick IVS may mimic a delta wave. These giant negative T waves and marked ST depressions varied from day to day, but the patient's condition remained unchanged. Therefore, it is unlikely that they are due to myocardial ischemia. This type of ECG is characteristic of hypertrophy localized to the apical area.

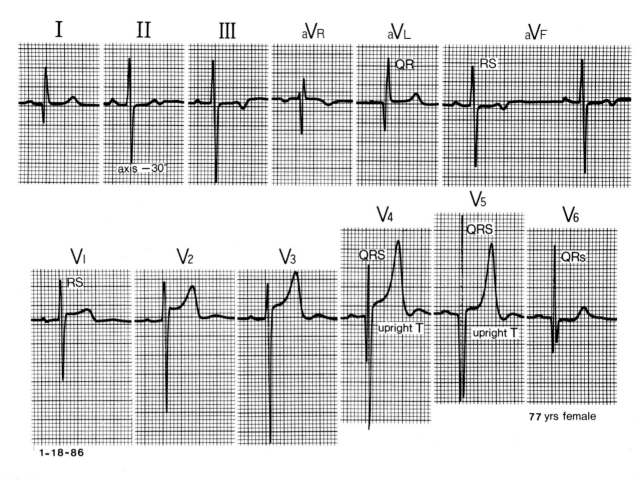

Fig. 8-11. ECG from a 77-year-old woman with HCM shows a narrow but deep Q wave in leads I, aVL and V₄ to V₆ with positive T waves. These Q waves represent abnormal activation of a thick IVS. The QRS axis is –30° due to an anterior divisional block. The cardiac CT demonstrated a hypertrophied IVS.

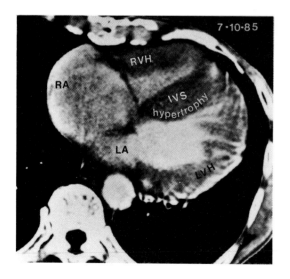

Fig. 8-12. A, The cardiac CT section near the mitral ring of this 73-year-old man with HCM shows hypertrophy of the RV in addition to the IVS and the LV. The patient occasionally developed congestive heart failure, but promptly recovered using digitalis and diuretics. His ECG showed RBBB.

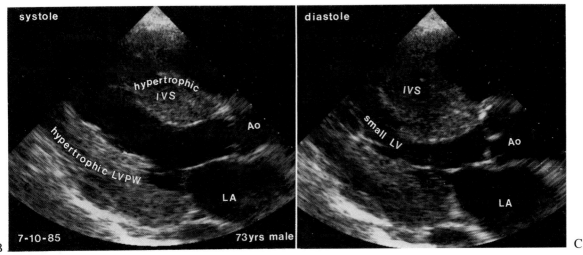

Fig. 8-12. *(Continued)* **B and C**, Long-axis 2D-echoes of the same patient show both IVS and LV free wall hypertrophy. The narrow extra echo space behind the LV posterior wall (LVPW) is probably caused by subepicardial fat rather than an effusion. Both the IVS and the LV posterior wall do not vary in thickness during different cardiac phases.

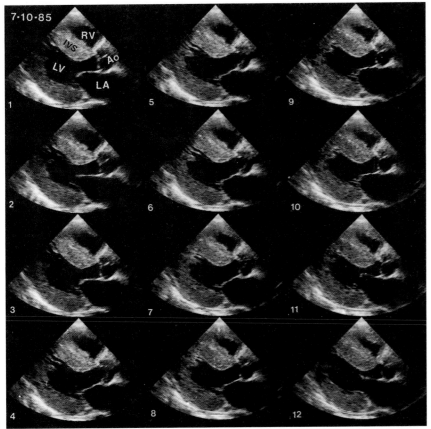

Fig. 8-12. *(Continued)* **D**, Serial long-axis echoes of the same patient, Figures 1 to 3 are during diastole, as indicated by a closed aortic valve and an open mitral valve. Figures 4 to 7 indicate systole since the aortic valve is open. The isovolumic relaxation period is shown in Figures 8 to 10 during which both the aortic and mitral valves are closed. In Figures 11 and 12, the mitral valve is open and indicates diastole. These serial recordings show only a slight measurable change in the thickness of the IVS or the LV. In Figures 5 to 7, the septums are slightly thicker than in Figures 1 to 3. However, any slight change in thickness on the M-mode recording may be the result of an anterior to posterior or superior to inferior rotation of the heart, and do not necessarily indicate a true change in the thickness of the IVS and/ or the LV.

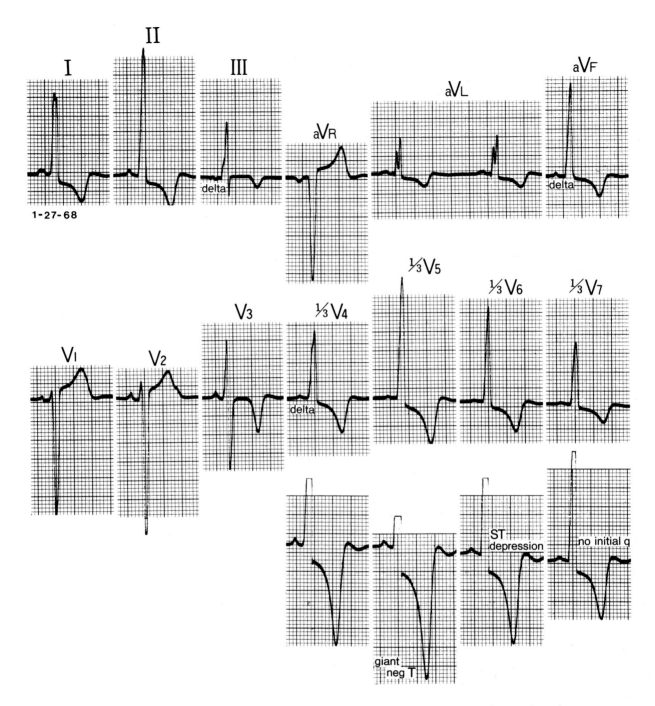

Fig. 8-13. **A,** ECG of a 41-year-old man with a history of alcoholism since age 15. The author has conducted his follow-up examinations for 15 years. On his initial visit for gastritis, his ECG showed a generalized increase in amplitude, so that the precordial leads had to be made using 1/3 the normal standardization. There was a transitional zone between V_3 and V_4, and there were no septal q waves in V_4 to V_7. The T waves were negative from V_3 and V_7. A tracing of V_5 made at normal standardization revealed a giant negative (35 mm) T wave with an ST depression of nearly 7 mm. Chest x-rays showed both marked LV hypertrophy and dilatation and either HCM or HOCM was suspected.

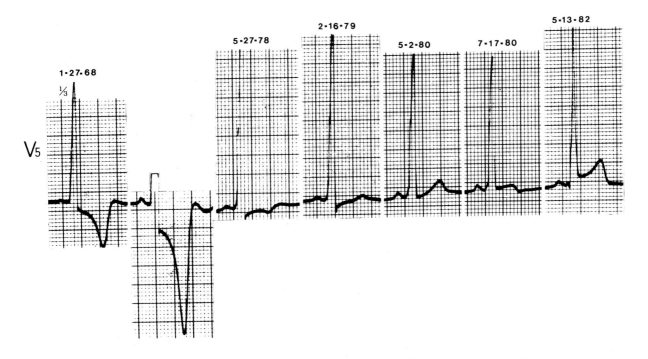

V_5

B

Fig. 8-13. *(Continued)* **B,** The patient reluctantly reported to us, mainly for his gastric complaints. He was found to have mild hypertension. For several years his ECG showed no changes, but chest x-rays showed further cardiac enlargement, partially from a weight gain of 15 kg. The patient did not visit us for 10 years, after which his ECGs showed a tall R wave associated with a delta wave in V_5. The R wave was tall but was decreased in amplitude compared to previous tracings. The T wave was low and, over the next 4 years, gradually became upright with slight ST elevation. The delta wave became more prominent. Although an ECG on 5–13–82 apparently had an initial q wave in V_5, it was actually an rsR′ pattern confirmed by its simultaneous recording in other leads. Unfortunately the patient died suddenly at home and no autopsy was performed.

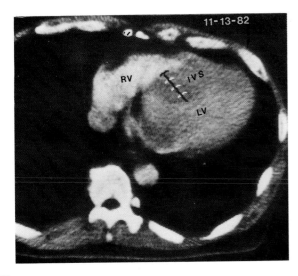

Fig. 8-13. *(Continued)* **C,** Cardiac CT 2 months prior to his death showed marked hypertrophy of the IVS and asymmetric hypertrophy of the LV. There was no evidence of LV outflow tract obstruction.

C

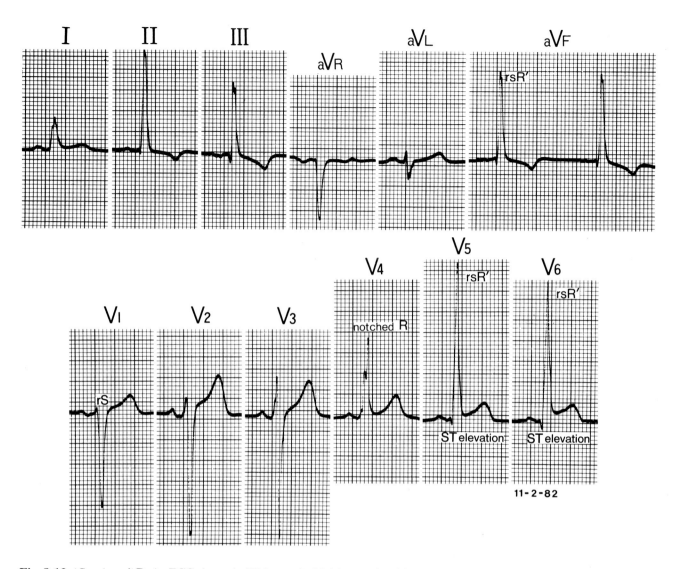

Fig. 8-13. *(Continued)* **D**, An ECG showed a PR interval of 0.16 seconds with a delta wave clearly visible in leads $V_3 \sim V_4$. However, a very small r wave mimicking a q wave in $V_5 \sim V_6$ could lead to an erroneous impression. The cause of the ST elevation and the positive T waves in the LV leads is uncertain. Since they varied from time to time, the degree of fusion between the normal and preexcitation path may have played a role.

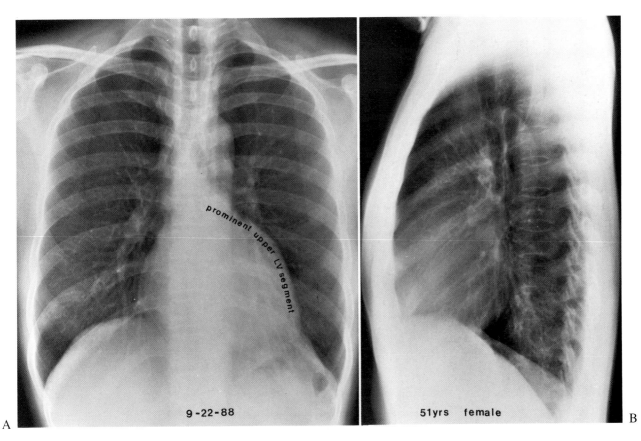

A   9-22-88   51yrs female   B

Fig. 8-14. A, A 51-year-old woman had recurrent attacks of congestive heart failure (CHF) over the past few years. Finally a lymph node biopsy from the right scalenous anticus muscle region disclosed sarcoidosis. Her chest x-rays show a prominent upper LV segment. In B, the anterior margin of the heart which abuts more than one-third of the sternum suggests right-sided heart enlargement.

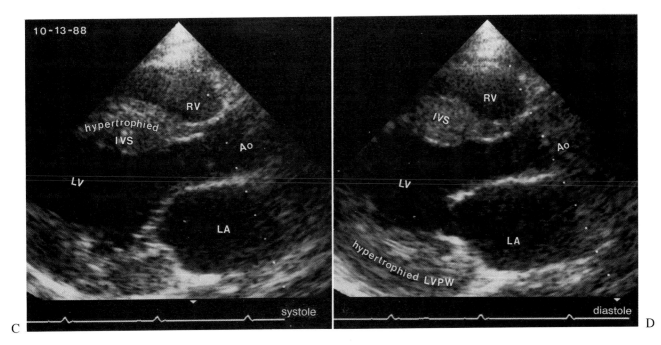

C   systole   diastole   D

Fig. 8-14. *(Continued)* **C and D**, Long-axis echoes show a hypertrophied IVS and a left ventricular posterior wall (LVPW) which contains granular echoes. This finding may suggest sarcoid involvement of the myocardium.

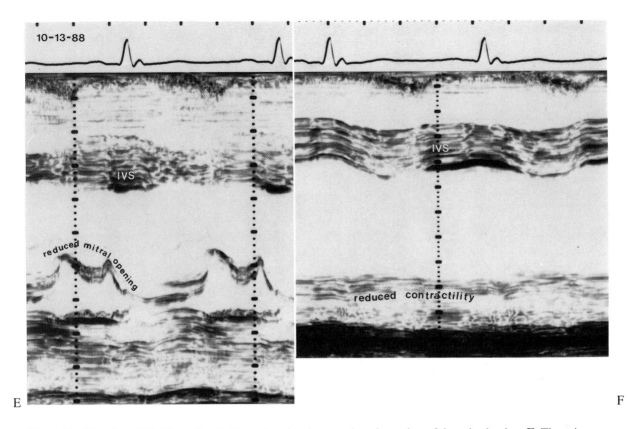

E

F

Fig. 8-14. *(Continued)* **E**, The patient's M-mode echo shows reduced opening of the mitral valve; **F**. There is markedly decreased LV posterior wall movement.

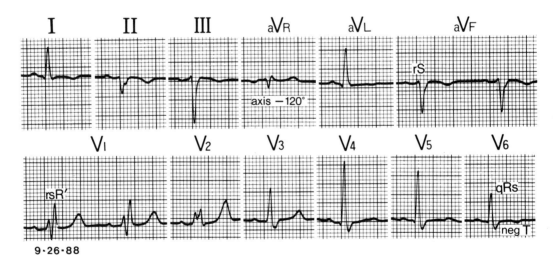

G

9·26·88

Fig. 8-14. *(Continued)* **G**, ECG of the same patient shows left-axis deviation of about −120°. There is an rsR′ pattern in V₁ with a positive T wave which is rather unusual. The T waves in the LV leads are either flat or negative, indicating myocardial damage.

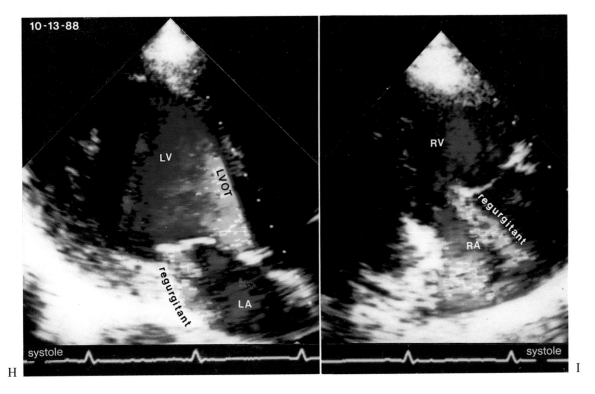

Fig. 8-14. *(Continued)* **H**, Her 2D-color Doppler echoes show mitral regurgitant flow indicated by a blue and orange mosaic pattern. In **I**, tricuspid regurgitant flow is also evident.

Chapter 9　Dilated Cardiomyopathy

Pathophysiology and Clinical Clues

In contrast to hypertrophic cardiomyopathy (HCM) or hypertrophic obstructive cardiomyopathy (HOCM), patients with dilated cardiomyopathy (DCM), or congestive cardiomyopathy, show enlargement of the left ventricular (LV) cavity with a normal or, occasionally, even thin interventricular septum (IVS) and LV free walls. Their LV movements are limited and show little change in their volumes between systole and diastole. The cause of the DCM is usually idiopathic; probably the end result of a viral mycarditis. In rare cases it may be the end stage of a hypertrophic cardiomyopathy.

The clinical findings of DCM are as follows:

★★★★　The echo shows dilatation of the LV cavity with reduced movements of the LV wall and IVS. Usually both the LV wall and IVS are normal in thickness and they may show some strong echoes due to myocardial degeneration.*

★★★★　On chest x-ray, there is cardiac enlargement with a small aortic arch.

★★★★　On the ECG, conduction disturbances such as bundle-branch block and anterior divisional block are common. A low-voltage QRS complex is often observed.

★★★★　On auscultation, an S_3 is common, and a mitral regurgitant murmur from LV dilatation may be present.

---

* A difficulty in the closure of the mitral valve can be observed in M-mode echo as a B-B′ step or shoulder on the anterior mitral leaflet.

Fig. 9-1. A, This 40-year-old man was admitted for congestive heart failure (CHF). The patient was known to have mild hypertension but no history of upper respiratory infection prior to the onset of CHF. His frontal chest x-ray shows marked cardiomegaly with pulmonary congestion. There is some pleural effusion on the right. Although the aorta (Ao) is elongated, there is no dilatation.

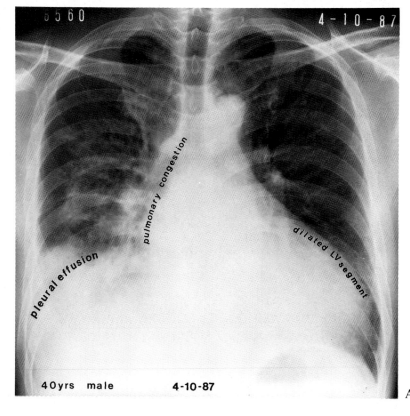

Fig. 9-1. *(Continued)* **B**, Frontal chest x-ray nearly 7 weeks later shows only an elongated Ao with very minimal right pleural effusion. His recovery was gradual.

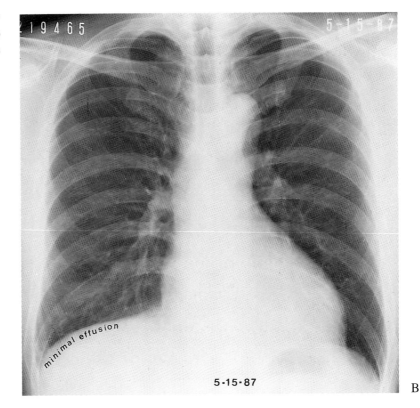

B

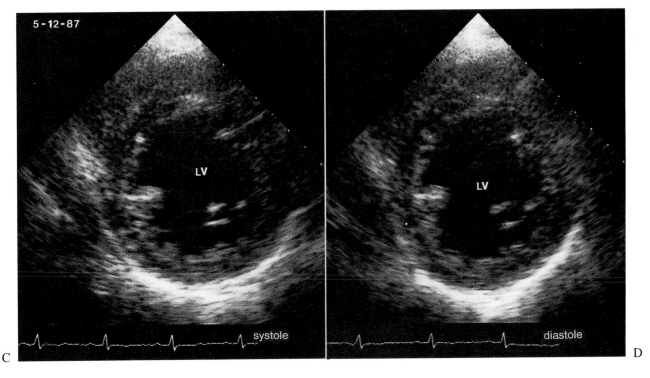

C

D

Fig. 9-1. *(Continued)* **C and D**, Since the papillary muscles vary in their positions depending on whether the picture is in systole or diastole, accurate comparisons of the LV cavity are difficult. However, the short-axis 2D-echoes made 3 days earlier than the last chest x-ray show some reduction in size of the LV cavity compared to that made earlier. Both the IVS and left ventricular posterior wall (LVPW) are relatively thin.

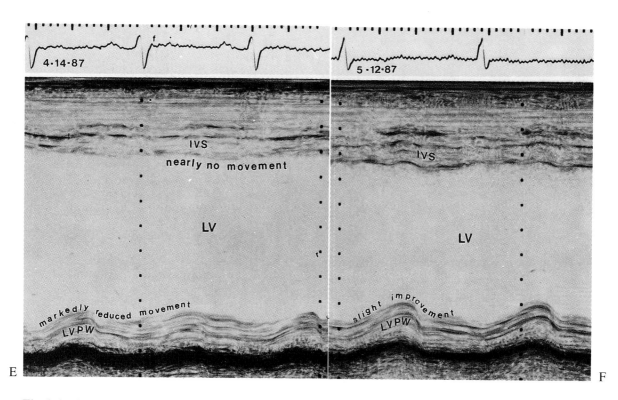

Fig. 9-1. *(Continued)* **E** and **F**, Comparison of M-mode tracings made 1 month apart shows a reduction in size of the LV cavity with some improvement in both IVS and LVPW movements.

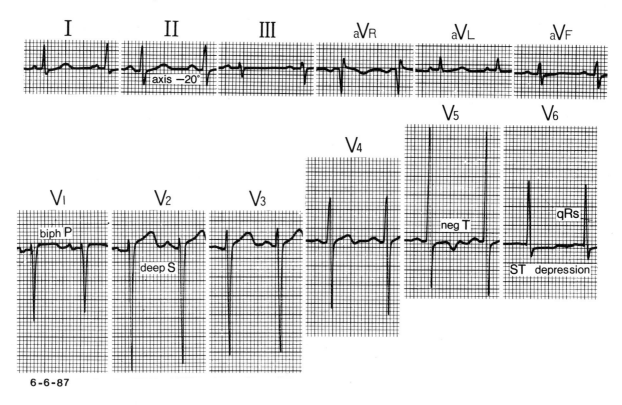

Fig. 9-1. *(Continued)* **G**, An ECG made 1 month later shows a sinus rhythm rate of 110. The QRS in aVF is negative and lead II shows positive indicating an axis of –20°. A large area of terminal P negativity in V₁ shows LA overloading from the CHF. The inverted T waves in the LV leads indicate LV myocardial damage, probably caused by fibrosis.

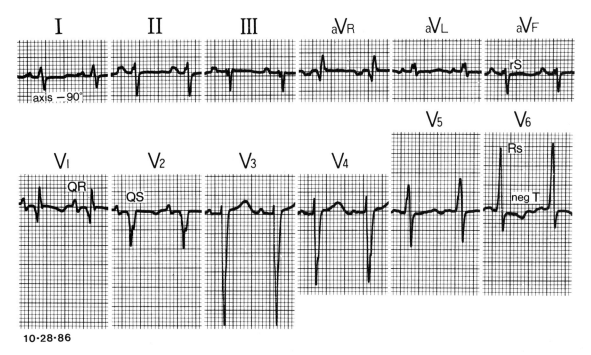

Fig. 9-1. *(Continued)* **H,** An ECG more than 4 months later shows more left axis deviation of about −90°. V₁ now shows QR and V₂ has a QS pattern. There is no previously noted septal q wave in V₆ due either to marked clockwise rotation of the heart caused by dilatation of the RV or loss of septal left-right forces from septal fibrosis. These findings indicate that there is severe myocardial damage.

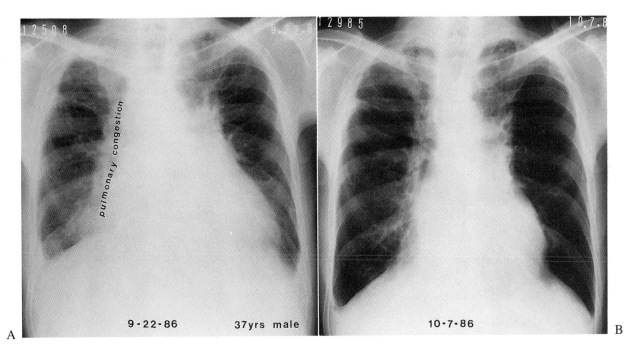

Fig. 9-2. A, A 37-year-old asthmatic man was admitted because of acute dyspnea. Prior to admission the patient suffered from an upper respiratory infection and noted that this dyspnea differed from his usual asthmatic attacks. His frontal chest x-ray shows marked cardiomegaly with bilateral pleural effusions. The pulmonary vascularity is congested. **B,** A chest x-ray 2 weeks later shows reduction in size of the cardiac silhouette and a minimal pleural effusion on the right. Both upper lobes of the lungs show some fibrotic changes and elevation of the minor fissure. The diaphragm is relatively low with considerable volume loss, indicating emphysema. The aortic arch is small.

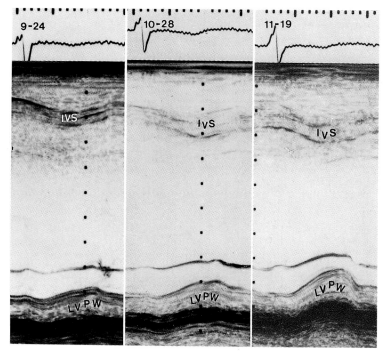

Fig. 9-2. *(Continued)* **C,** Comparison of the 3 M-mode echoes made 1 month apart shows that hypokinesis of the LV movements improved under the oral isoproterenol. The LV dilatation remained, but the nearly noncontractile left ventricular posterior wall (LVPW) now shows some movement. The IVS is thin.

Fig. 9-2. *(Continued)* **D,** M-mode echo shows limited mitral valvular movement. There is decrease in the height of the E wave and development of B-B′ step formation. This B-B′ step is evidence of elevated LA pressure with low ejection fraction and correlates with an S_4. **E,** About 5 months later, the mitral valvular movement became nearly normal and the previously noted B-B′ step had resolved.

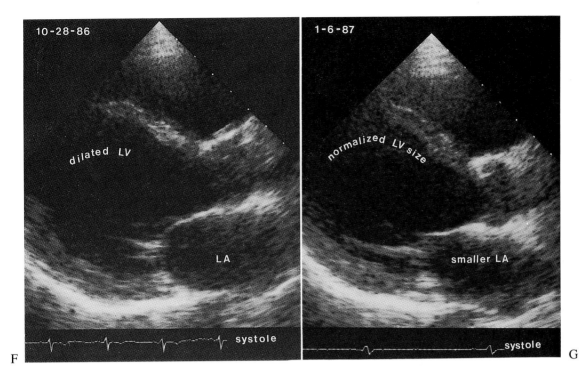

Fig. 9-2. *(Continued)* **F**, Long-axis echoes made 3 months apart. In an earlier stage, the LV cavity was very large and there was some dilatation of the RV. **G**, These changes became much less severe in the second study.

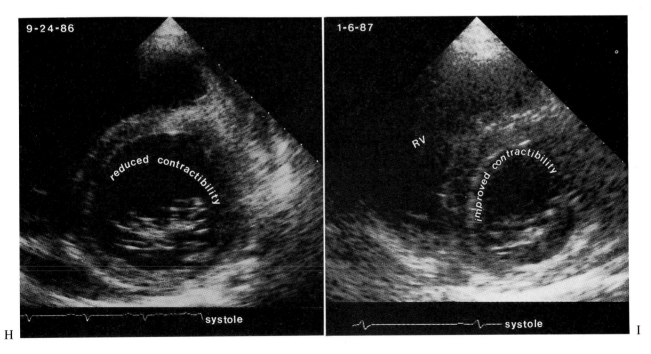

Fig. 9-2. *(Continued)* **H and I**, Short-axis echoes clearly show reduction of the LV cavity and improvement of LV movement.

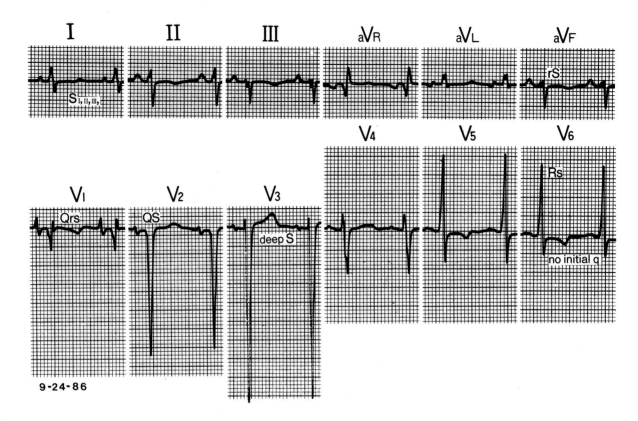

I   II   III   aVR   aVL   aVF

$S_{I, II, III,}$ rS

V4   V5   V6

Rs

V1   V2   V3

Qrs   QS   deep S   no initial q

9-24-86

J

Fig. 9-2. *(Continued)* **J,** An ECG taken on admission shows an $S_{I, II, III}$ pattern which is a sign of right ventricular overloading frequently observed in emphysema. There is also a tall peaked P wave in V_1. The QRS axis is indeterminate.* Inverted T waves in the LV leads are indicative of myocardial damage. V_1 shows a Qrs and V_2 a QS pattern. An initial septal q wave is absent in LV leads suggesting that the septal activation is simultaneous from both directions or dominant from right to left. Therefore, the presence of a Q wave in $V_1 \sim V_2$ does not necessarily indicate myocardial necrosis. Right precordial QS waves may be caused by emphysema because of the low position of the diaphragm. Abnormal QS waves in such cases are explained by the fact that the precordial leads may be located above the electrical center of the heart to an abnormal degree, similar to that of aVR.

* If 2 QRS complexes in the frontal plane are equiphasic (I and aVR, here) an axis cannot be determined accurately.

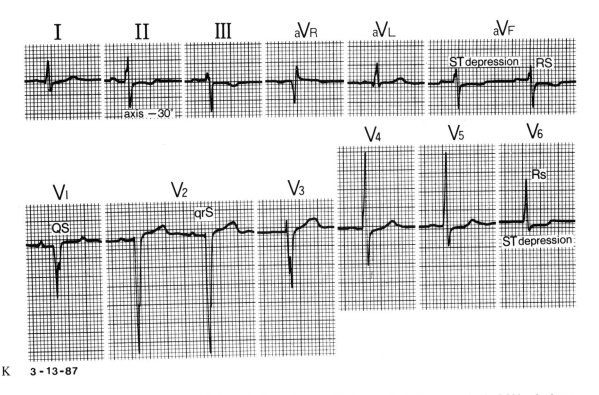

K   3-13-87

Fig. 9-2. *(Continued)* **K,** An ECG 6 months later shows a QRS axis of −30°, T waves in the LV leads show some improvement. The S in lead I and the notched QS in V₁ suggest an atypical incomplete right bundle-branch block (RBBB) pattern, and probably is caused by either concomitant RV overloading or fibrotic changes in the IVS.

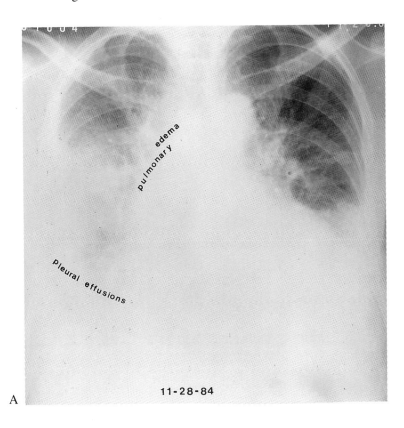

A

Fig. 9-3. A, This 54-year-old man had renal hypertension and developed acute dyspnea. On admission, his frontal portable chest x-ray showed marked cardiomegaly with blurring of the pulmonary vessels and bilateral pleural effusions indicating pulmonary edema.

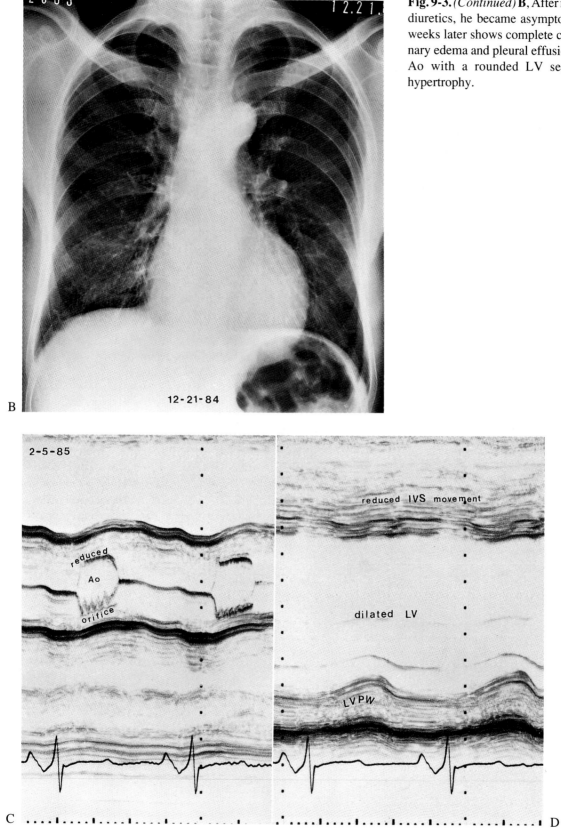

Fig. 9-3. *(Continued)* **B**, After receiving digitalis and diuretics, he became asymptomatic. Chest x-ray 4 weeks later shows complete clearing of the pulmonary edema and pleural effusions. But an elongated Ao with a rounded LV segment suggests LV hypertrophy.

Fig. 9-3. *(Continued)* **C and D**, M-mode echoes made 6 weeks later reveal an enlarged LV cavity. Movements of both the IVS and LV posterior wall are limited. The IVS is thick. A decreased opening of the aortic valve is noted.

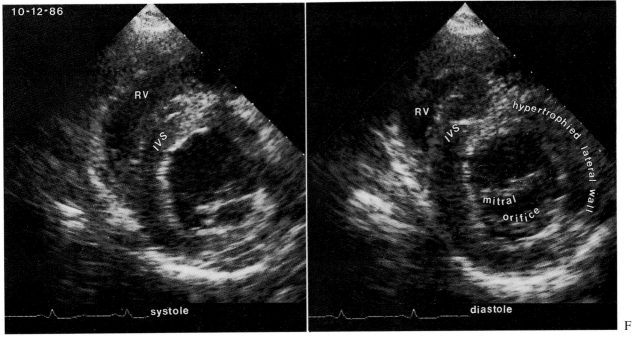

Fig. 9-3. *(Continued)* **E and F**, Short-axis echoes 20 months later show localized thickening of the lateral wall of the LV. Thus this seems to be a case of asymmetric hypertrophic cardiomyopathy (ASH) with acute CHF.

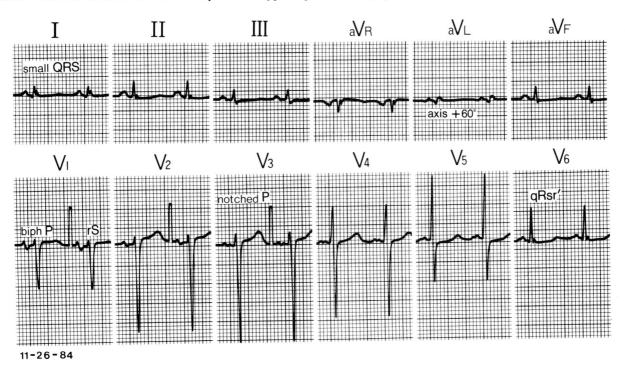

Fig. 9-3. *(Continued)* **G**, An ECG made on admission shows a QRS axis of +60°. The flat ST depression in V_6 is compatible with LV myocardial damage. The widely notched P wave in V_3 and a biphasic P wave with greater negativity in V_1 indicate LA overloading and damage.

9. Dilated Cardiomyopathy   *175*

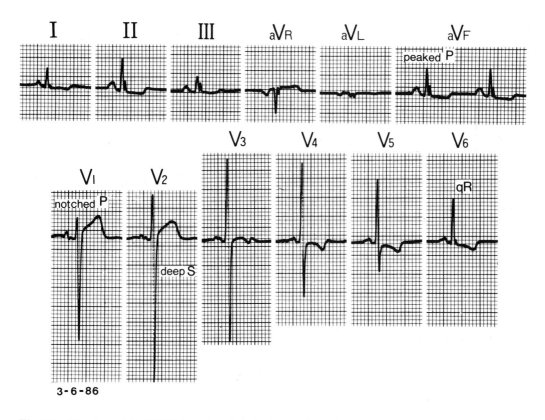

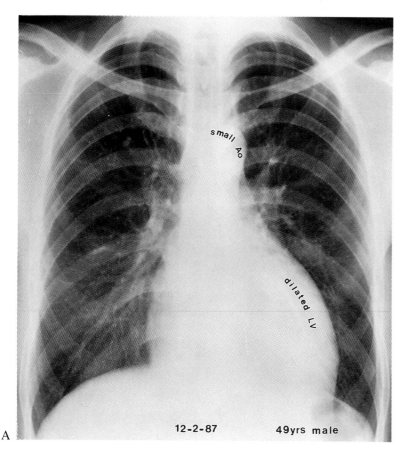

Fig. 9-3. *(Continued)* **H,** ECG 4 months after admission shows increased QRS amplitude in the extremity and the precordial leads indicating decreased pericardial effusion and less skin resistance with loss of edema. The inverted T waves in V_4 to V_6 represent LVH strain pattern which can be brought out by digitalis. The widely notched P in V_3 to V_6 reflect LA damage. Patient had recurrent attacks of CHF, and we assume that he has a transitional type of HCM that may be progressing to DCM.

Fig. 9-4. A, Frontal chest x-ray from a 49-year-old man with DCM showing moderate cardiac dilatation with a small aortic arch (Ao). The pulmonary vascularity is rather scant, indicating absence of CHF. Although this is a typical example of DCM, such chest x-ray findings may also be seen in Ebstein's anomaly or in pericardial effusion.

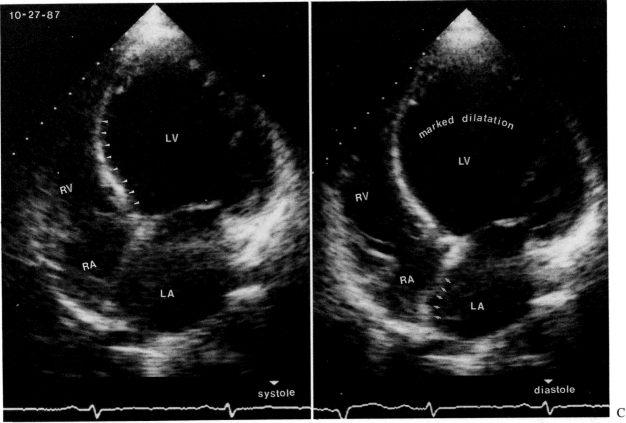

Fig. 9-4. *(Continued)* **B,** Apical four-chamber views show a markedly dilated LV cavity which is compressing the RV (arrowheads). **C,** Increased LA pressure is also evident by the fact that the interatrial septum is bulging toward the RA (small arrows).

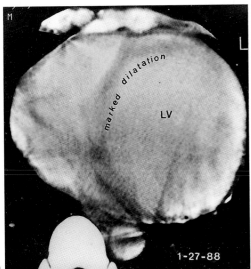

Fig. 9-4. *(Continued)* **D,** An enhanced cardiac CT of the same patient shows marked dilatation of the LV cavity with a relatively thin IVS.

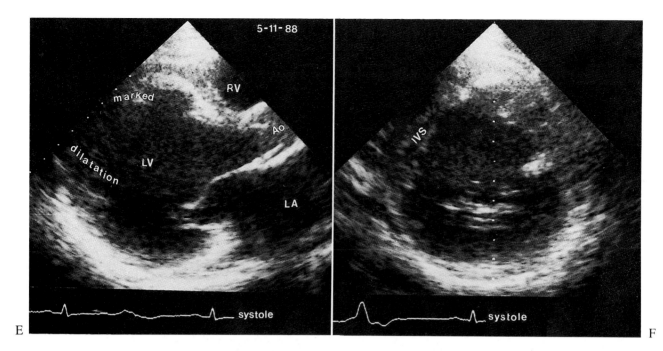

E   F

Fig. 9-4. *(Continued)* **E and F**, Long and short-axis echoes show marked dilatation of the LV and LA. The IVS is shifted upward against the RV resulting in a deformed LV cavity.

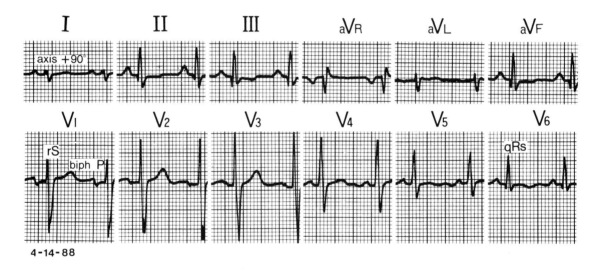

G

Fig. 9-4. *(Continued)* **G**, ECG shows generalized low voltage with a QRS axis of about +90°. A large P wave with terminal negativity in V₁ indicates LA overloading. Since there is no evidence of pericardial effusion by echo and CT, the generalized low voltage suggests myocardial damage.

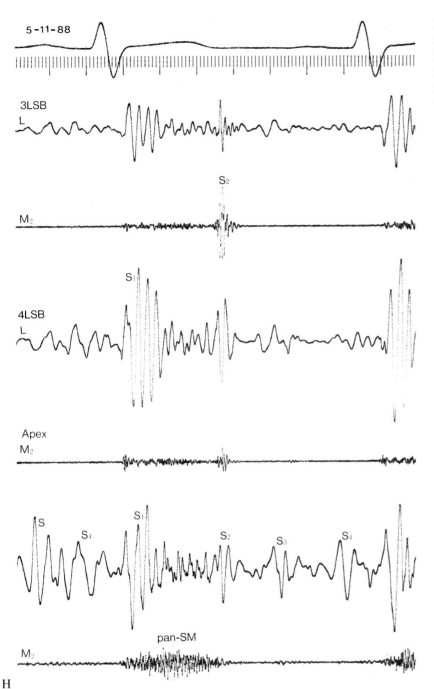

5-11-88

3LSB
L

S_2

M₂

S_1

4LSB
L

Apex
M₂

S S_4 S_1 S_2 S_3 S_4

pan-SM

M₂

H

Fig. 9-4. *(Continued)* **H**, The patient frequently developed CHF during which time his PCG often showed an S_3 and S_4 quadruple rhythm with a mitral regurgitation (MR) murmur. Unfortunately the patient died a few weeks after this PCG was made.

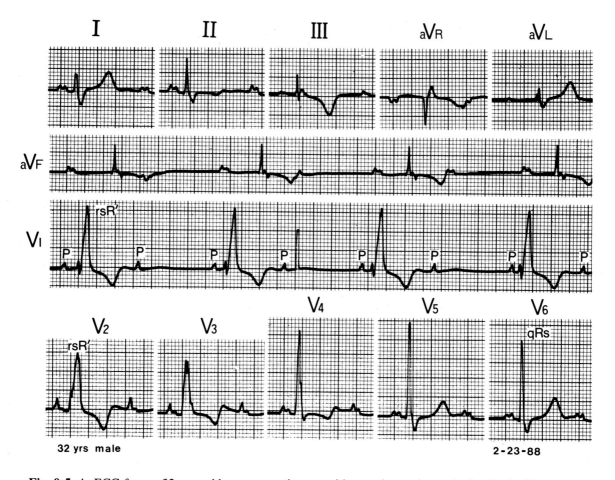

I   II   III   aVR   aVL

aVF

V₁

rsR'

P   P   P   P   P   P   P

V₂   V₃   V₄   V₅   V₆

rsR'   qRs

A   **32 yrs male**   **2-23-88**

Fig. 9-5. A, ECG from a 32-year-old asymptomatic man with complete atrioventricular block. He has never experienced any symptoms related to his cardiac condition. The P wave is notched and tall. The QRS axis is about +90°. There is rsR' pattern with a broad QRS indicating RBBB. This type of RBBB is seen in ischemic heart disease and/or DCM.

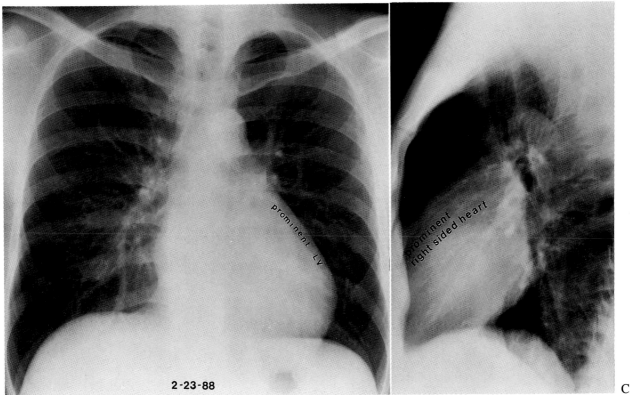

B   2-23-88   C

Fig. 9-5. *(Continued)* **B**, The frontal chest x-ray of the same patient shows an apparently prominent left-sided heart. However, the lateral view, **C**, reveals increased contact of the heart with the sternum, suggesting right-sided heart enlargement.

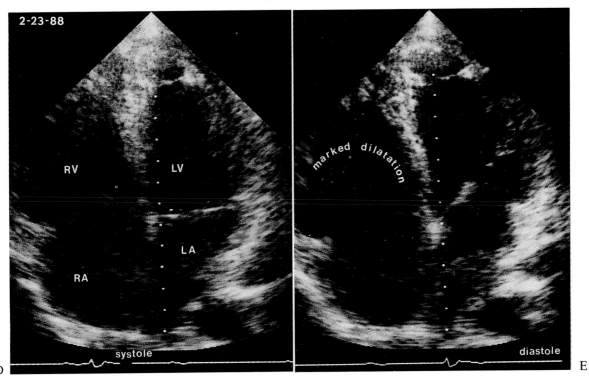

D   E

Fig. 9-5. *(Continued)* **D and E**, The echoes in the apical four-chamber view of the same patient show marked dilatation of both RA and RV.

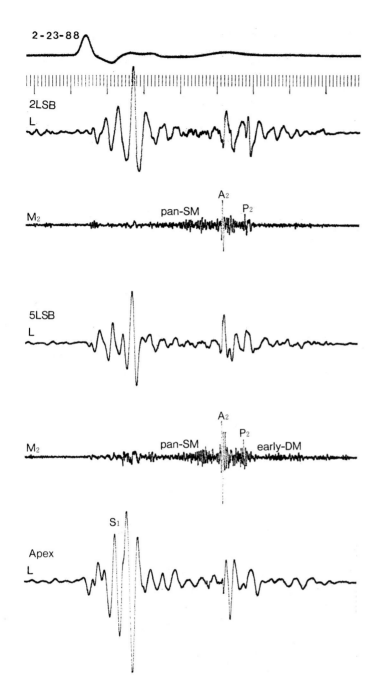

2-23-88

2LSB
L

M₂   pan-SM   A₂   P₂

5LSB
L

M₂   pan-SM   A₂   P₂   early-DM

S₁

Apex
L

M₂

F

Fig. 9-5. *(Continued)* **F,** PCG reveals a soft crescendo pansystolic murmur (pan-SM) of tricuspid regurgitation which is maximum at the 5LSB. There is also a soft, short early diastolic murmur (early DM) of probable pulmonary regurgitation (PR). Both murmurs were heard much better on auscultation than were recorded on the PCG. The murmurs were enhanced with inspiration indicating that they were right-sided in origin. Since the patient had no history to suggest myocarditis and refused to have coronary angiography, a definitive diagnosis was uncertain. However, the findings suggest right-sided heart involvement and may represent a right-sided DCM.

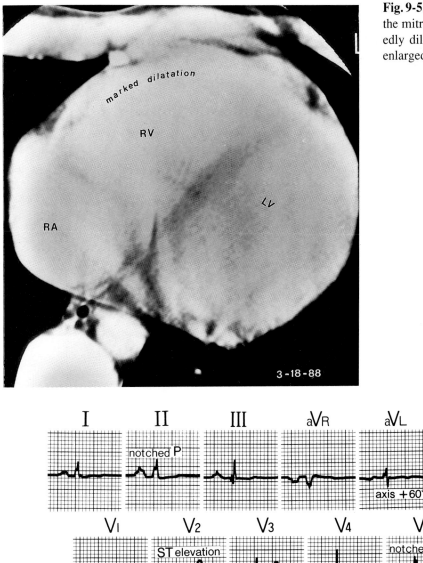

Fig. 9-5. *(Continued)* **G,** A cardiac CT section below the mitral valve of the same patient shows a markedly dilated RV and RA. The LV is also slightly enlarged in this section.

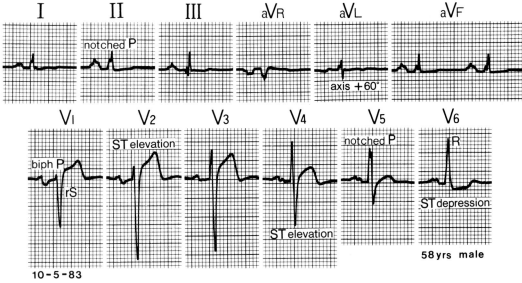

Fig. 9-6. A, ECG from a 58-year-old physician who gradually developed dyspnea. There was no history to suggest myocarditis. The P wave in V₁ shows a large area of terminal negativity indicating LA overload. There are slight ST elevations in V₁ to V₅ which is upwardly convex in V₄ to V₅ suggesting myocardial injury and/or aneurysm. Although the patient had no angina, coronary angiography was performed to rule out the possibility of an anterior aneurysm.

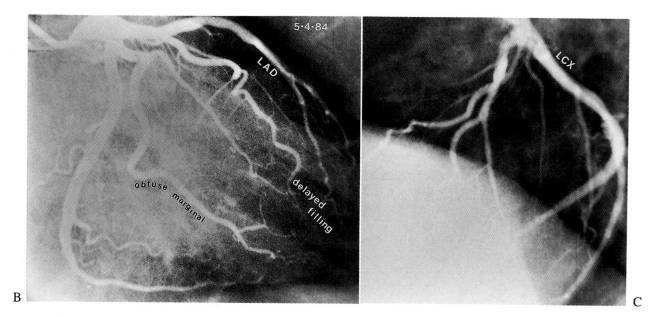

B

C

Fig. 9-6. *(Continued)* **B and C,** Coronary angiogram shows no stenosis or aneurysm. However, the flow in the distal portion of the left anterior descending artery (LAD) is delayed. This suggests an increase in resistance of the peripheral arterioles due to coronary arteriolar disease or recanalization of a previously occluded LAD.

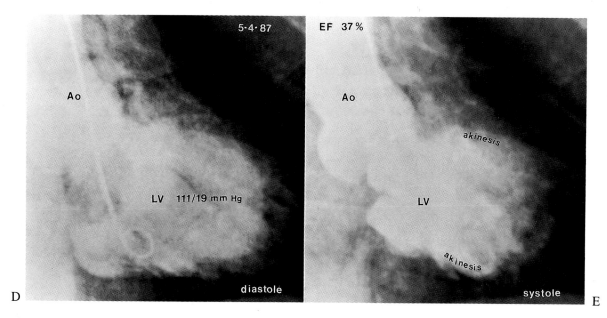

D

E

Fig. 9-6. *(Continued)* **D,** His left ventriculogram showed hypokinetic areas at the apex and high lateral wall and an ejection fraction (EF) of only 37% (normal 55 to 75%). **E,** Apical akinesis is assumed to be the cause of the ST elevation in V_1 to V_5. Since the coronary arteries were not stenotic, it may be postulated that this presents a postmyocarditis cardiomyopathy. Patients with DCM commonly have no apparent history of myocarditis.

Chapter 10 Pulmonary Thromboembolism

Pathophysiology and Clinical Clues

The diagnosis of pulmonary thromboembolism (PTE) is relatively difficult; it is mimicked by many conditions but especially by myocardial infarction (MI), and the dyspnea of chronic pulmonary disease and pleurisy. Pulmonary thromboembolism is caused by venous stasis, damaged vessel walls, and increased coagulability of the blood. Hypercoagulability often occurs postoperatively and postpartum. Congestive heart failure, prolonged bed rest especially after MI, chronic pulmonary disease, carcinoma, and removal of a cast from a lower extremity are common precipitating factors. PTE is often found in congenital pulmonary hypertension, aortitis syndrome, and/or Eisenmenger's syndrome. Because PTE produces a region of lung which can be ventilated but not perfused, it may result in cyanosis which persists even after oxygen administration. Dyspnea, cough, hemoptysis, pleuritic chest pain, palpitations, and tachycardia may occur.

The clinical approaches to diagnosing PTE are as follows:

★★★★ The chest x-ray may show unilateral elevation of the diaphragm, an abnormal vascular distribution, enlarged central arteries with a radiolucency in the peripheral portions of the lung fields, or a peripheral wedge-shaped opacity. Right-sided cardiac enlargement is also common.

★★★★ The ECG may show sinus tachycardia with peaked P waves, an rSr′ pattern in V_1 with slight ST elevation, and right-axis deviation with inverted T waves in the right precordial leads. Infrequently left-axis deviation, and occasionally an S_1, Q_{III} pattern when the involved region is large, may appear.

★★★★ On auscultation there may be an accentuated P_2 with wide splitting of S_2, an ejection murmur at the base of the heart, a friction rub, or a right-sided S_3 and/or S_4 due to RV overloading.

★★ An echo may show enlargement of the RV cavity.

Pulmonary blood-flow images and ventilation images by scintigraphy and/or angiography may be necessary for making the diagnosis.

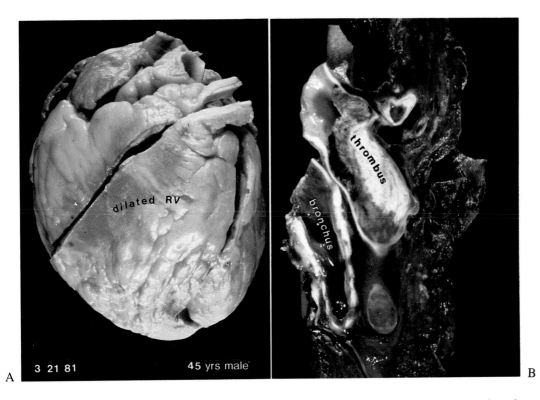

dilated RV

3 21 81   45 yrs male

A

thrombus

bronchus

B

Fig. 10-1. A and B, Autopsy specimen from a 45-year-old man with recurrent pulmonary thromboembolism (PTE) attacks. Multiple new and old PTE are observed.

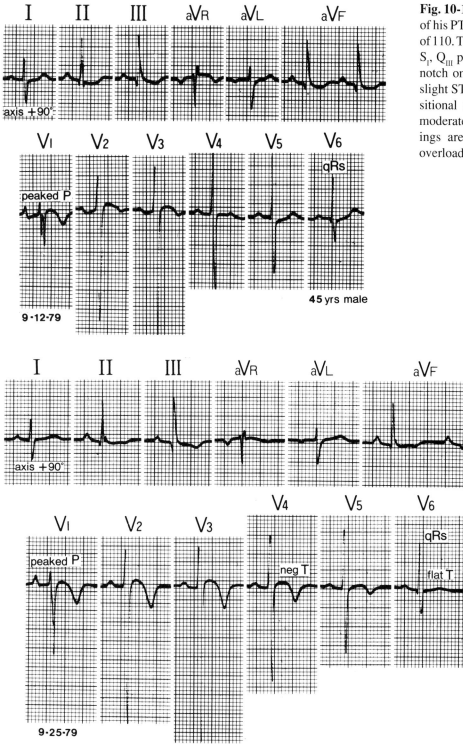

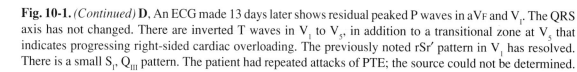

Fig. 10-1. (Continued) **C,** ECG made during one of his PTE episodes. It shows a sinus tachycardia of 110. The QRS axis is indeterminate. There is an S_I, Q_{III} pattern. There is an rS in V_1 with a deep notch on the ascending limb of the S wave. A slight ST elevation is seen in V_1 to V_3. The transitional zone is between V_4 and V_5 showing moderate clockwise rotation. The overall findings are compatible with right-sided cardiac overloading.

Fig. 10-1. (Continued) **D,** An ECG made 13 days later shows residual peaked P waves in aVF and V_1. The QRS axis has not changed. There are inverted T waves in V_1 to V_5, in addition to a transitional zone at V_5 that indicates progressing right-sided cardiac overloading. The previously noted rSr' pattern in V_1 has resolved. There is a small S_I, Q_{III} pattern. The patient had repeated attacks of PTE; the source could not be determined.

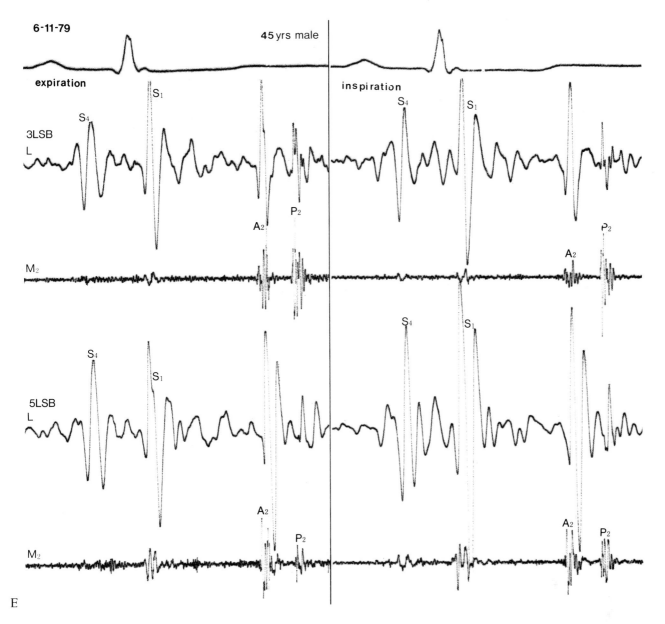

Fig. 10-1. *(Continued)* **E**, His PCG during a PTE attack shows wide splitting of S_2 with an accentuated P_2 as shown by its appearance at the apex and by being louder than the A_2 at high frequency. An S_4 is present and is enhanced by inspiration, suggesting right-sided heart origin.

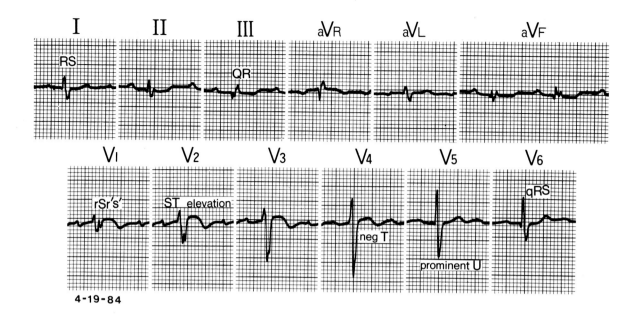

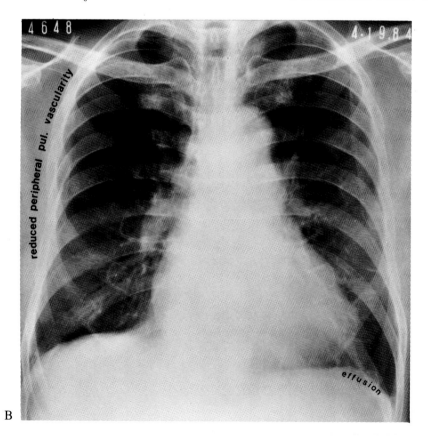

Fig. 10-2. A, This 72-year-old man experienced acute dyspnea. An S$_I$, Q$_{III}$ pattern and an rsr's' pattern in V$_1$ with slight ST elevation in V$_1$ to V$_3$ are compatible with PTE. The negative T waves and transitional zone shift to the left at V$_6$ correlate well with clockwise rotation of the heart seen with RV overloading.

Fig. 10-2. *(Continued)* **B,** Frontal chest x-ray of the same patient shows an enlarged aortic arch, probably from hypertension. Prominent central arteries with reduced peripheral vascular markings, especially in both upper lung fields, suggest PTE. There apparently is a small pleural effusion on the left which is different from the usual pleural effusion of congestive heart failure which occurs most often on the right.

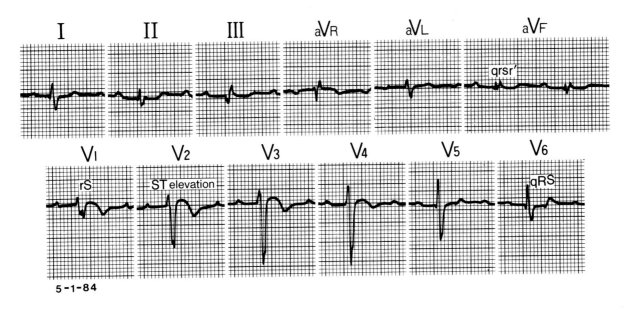

I   II   III   aVR   aVL   aVF

qrsr'

V1   V2   V3   V4   V5   V6

rS   ST elevation   qRS

C   5-1-84

Fig. 10-2. *(Continued)* **C,** ECG made 3 weeks after onset shows nearly the same findings with the ST segment elevations in leads V₁ to V₃, possibly due to adjacent pericarditis. V₁ now shows an rS pattern.

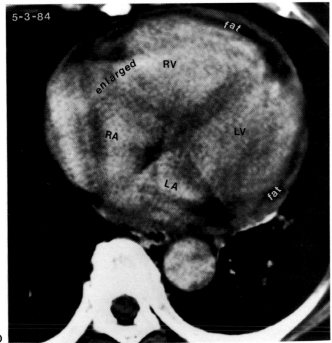

5-3-84

fat

enlarged   RV

RA   LV

LA   fat

D

Fig. 10-2. *(Continued)* **D,** A cardiac CT scan of the same patient shows an enlarged RA and RV. A prominent subepicardial fat layer is observed in both the anterior and posterior portions of the heart. There may be a small associated pericardial effusion as well.

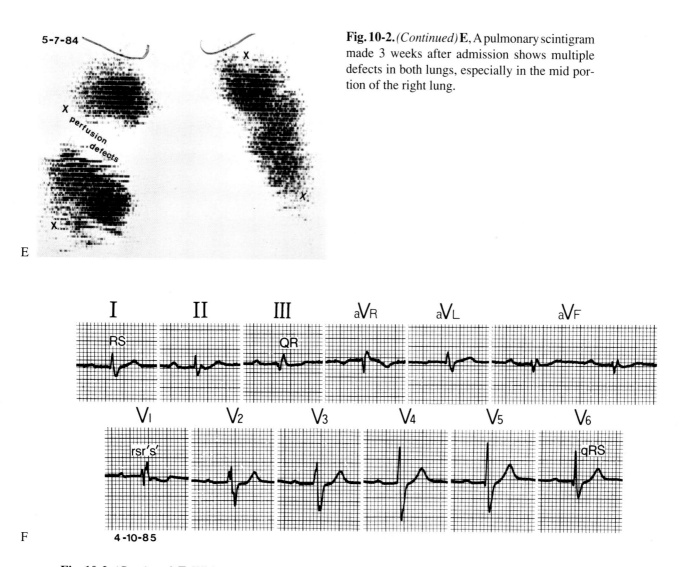

5-7-84

X
X perfusion defects
X

X

Fig. 10-2. *(Continued)* **E,** A pulmonary scintigram made 3 weeks after admission shows multiple defects in both lungs, especially in the mid portion of the right lung.

E

I II III aVR aVL aVF
RS   QR

V₁ V₂ V₃ V₄ V₅ V₆
rsr's'   qRS

4-10-85

F

Fig. 10-2. *(Continued)* **F,** With conservative treatment, the patient recovered from the PTE uneventfully. His ECG about 1 year after the original attack shows an rsr's' pattern in V₁ with normalization of the previously elevated ST segments and negative T waves in V₂ to V₄ becoming upright, indicating some resolution of the RV overloading.

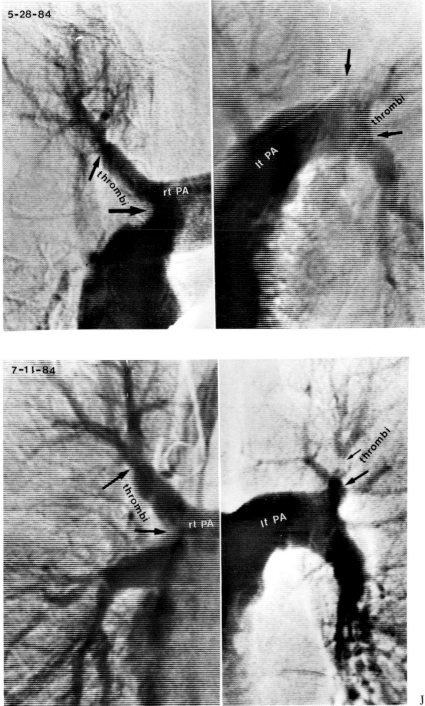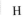

Fig. 10-2. *(Continued)* **G and H**, A DSA 40 days after admission, shows either occlusion or narrowing of the pulmonary arteries. Indentations outlined by arrows indicate thrombi.

Fig. 10-2. *(Continued)* **I and J**, A follow-up DSA about 3 months after the onset of PTE shows some resolution of the thrombi especially in the right lower pulmonary artery and in both the upper and lower left PA where branching is now visible.

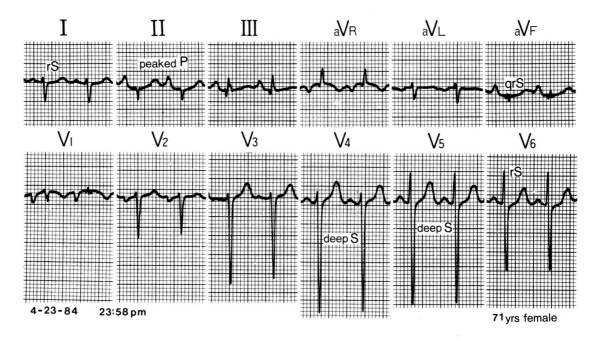

Fig. 10-3. A, This ECG of a 71-year-old woman with acute dyspnea and fever shows an $S_I\,Q_{III}$ pattern. Peaked P waves are seen in aVF, and a negative P wave in V_1. The QRS axis is +180° (equiphasic in aVF). The transitional zone is shifted far to the left with a deep S wave in V_6 indicating that the axis is posterior and to the right, as is occasionally seen in chronic obstructive pulmonary disease (COPD) with clockwise rotation of the heart. Sinus tachycardia of 125 with peaked P waves and marked clockwise rotation suggest that PTE may be superimposed on chronic obstructive pulmonary disease.

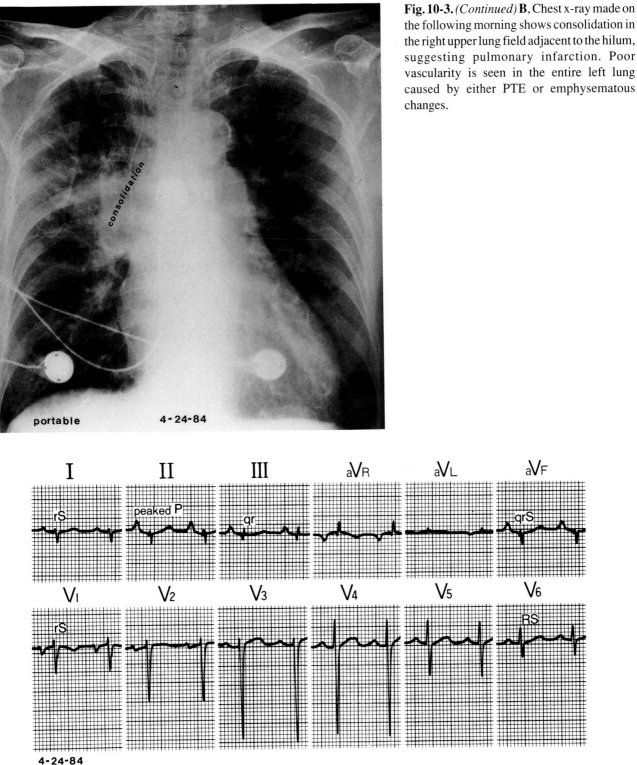

Fig. 10-3. *(Continued)* **B,** Chest x-ray made on the following morning shows consolidation in the right upper lung field adjacent to the hilum, suggesting pulmonary infarction. Poor vascularity is seen in the entire left lung caused by either PTE or emphysematous changes.

Fig. 10-3. *(Continued)* **C,** Sixteen hours after admission she shows an S in III and aVF suggesting a superior and rightward terminal force travelling up the right ventricular outflow tract at –140°. There is no negative T wave in the right precordial leads to suggest RV pressure overloading.

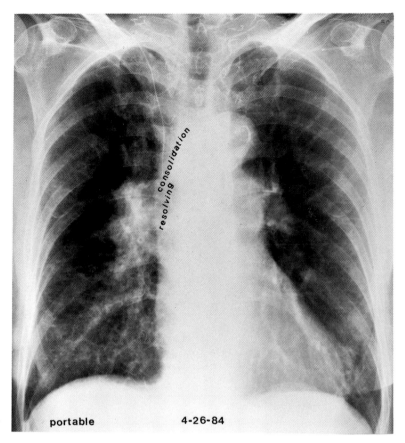

Fig. 10-3. *(Continued)* **D**, Chest x-ray 4 days after admission shows that the previously noted consolidation in the right upper lobe has resolved, leaving enlarged central arteries with poor peripheral vascular markings. By this time, the fever resolved and the patient was asymptomatic. Her ECG showed no changes.

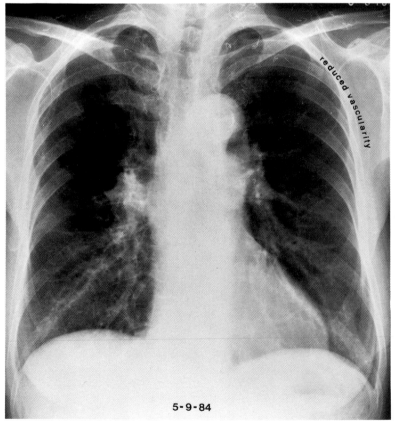

Fig. 10-3. *(Continued)* **E**, Chest x-ray 2 weeks later showed reduced size of the central arteries and increased radiolucency in both upper lung fields.

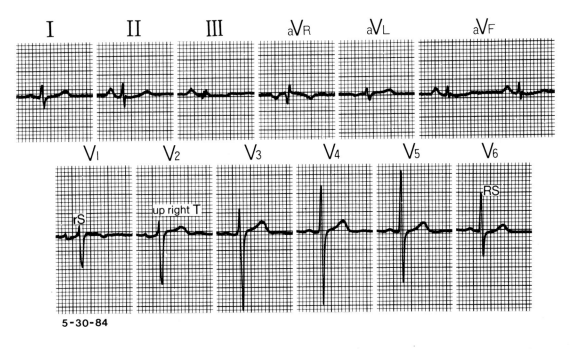

F

Fig. 10-3. *(Continued)* **F,** An ECG 4 weeks later shows a lesser degree of right axis and the P waves have become less prominent. The late R wave in aVr has become smaller and the transition has shifted to V₅, suggesting some improvement in the RV overloading.

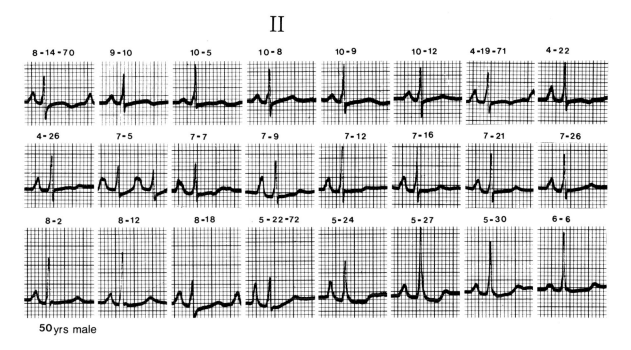

A

Fig. 10-4. A, These serial tracings of lead II from a 50-year-old man with renal hypertension show extremely tall peaked P waves during PTE attacks. During recurrent PTE attacks, his ECGs consistently showed peaked P waves which usually returned to the control level within 7 to 10 days after onset of PTE. The cause of the PTE was unknown.

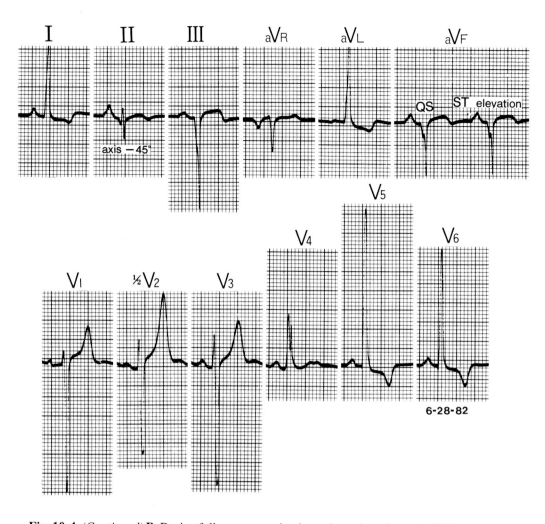

Fig. 10-4. *(Continued)* **B,** During follow-up examinations, the patient showed a QRS axis of −45° with a QS pattern and ST elevation in aVF together with tall T waves in V₁ to V₃. These indicate posteroinferior involvement.

Chapter 11 Pulmonary Hypertension

Pathophysiology and Clinical Clues

Pulmonary hypertension (PH) can be either acute or chronic. Primary PH, Eisenmenger's syndrome, the aortitis syndrome, mitral stenosis, chronic pulmonary disease, and recurrent pulmonary thromboembolic disease are the causes of chronic PH. Chronic PH is discussed in this chapter.

Clinical approaches to diagnosing PH are as follows:

★★★★ Chest x-ray may show marked enlargement of the right side of the heart, dilatation of the main and central pulmonary arteries, and reduced peripheral pulmonary vasculature.

★★★★ Echo may show dilatation and/or hypertrophy of the RV, a deformed LV cavity due to volume overloading of the RV, and semiclosure of the pulmonary valve.

★★★★ ECG often shows right axis deviation (RAD), tall and/or peaked P waves, and an rsR′ or Rs pattern in V_1 to indicate RV overloading.

★★★ Auscultation reveals an accentuated P_2, a right atrial S_4 and a pulmonary ejection murmur with or without an ejection sound.

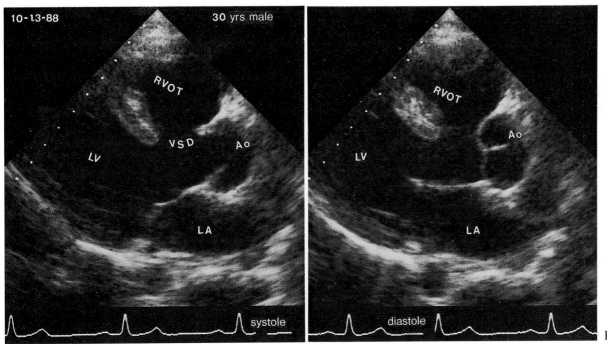

Fig. 11-1. A and B, This 30-year-old man with Eisenmenger's syndrome has the large VSD that was shown in Figure 1-4. At age 12, right heart catheterization was performed in a local hospital but no information was available. Presently he has cyanosis and clubbing of fingers and toes. He has been able to continue his work as a dental assistant. The long-axis echoes show a large VSD that separates the anterior aortic wall from the interventricular septum (IVS). There is no overriding of the Ao and the RV outflow tract (RVOT) is markedly dilated.

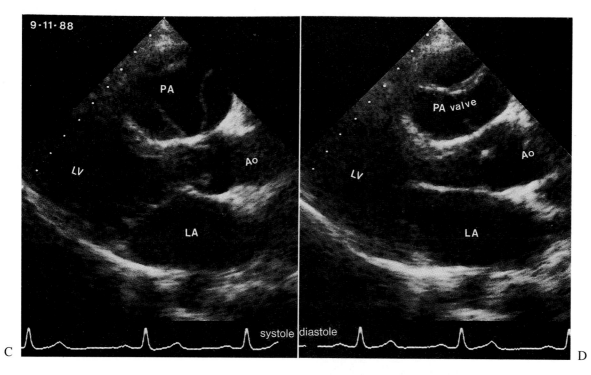

Fig. 11-1. *(Continued)* **C and D,** Slightly upward projection of long-axis echoes show a markedly dilated pulmonary ring with a visible pulmonary valve during both systole and diastole.

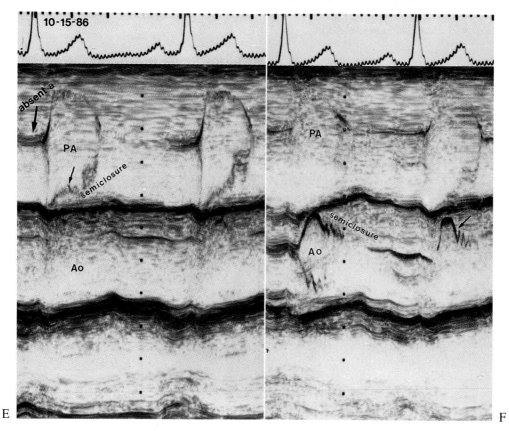

Fig. 11-1. *(Continued)* **E,** Because of the marked dilatation of the main PA, a simultaneous recording of both the Ao and the PA was possible, showing semiclosure of the valves (arrows). The semiclosure of the pulmonary valve occurring during systole together with an absent a wave are indicative of PH, also indicated by the flat diastolic period. **F,** The cause of semiclosure of the aortic valve is not clear. The angiographic study did not reveal the cause of the aneurysmal dilatation of the main PA, and it is assumed to be a congenital deformity. The severity of the PH made surgical correction impossible.

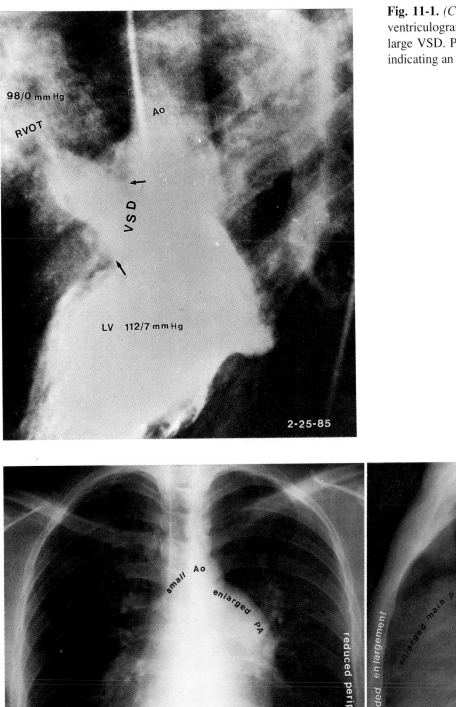

Fig. 11-1. *(Continued)* **G**, The same patient's left ventriculogram shows a LV to RV shunt through a large VSD. Pressure in the RV was 98/0 mm Hg, indicating an Eisenmenger syndrome.

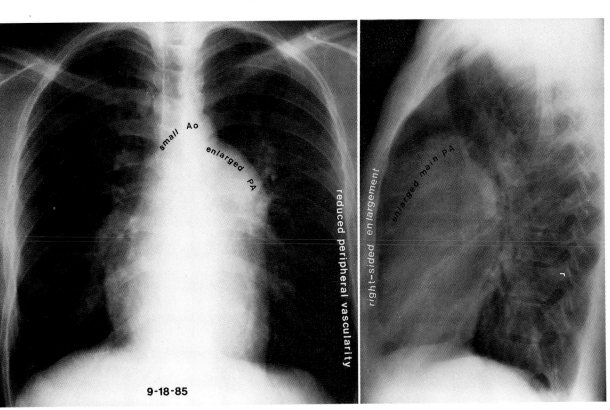

Fig. 11-1. *(Continued)* **H**, Chest x-rays show a prominent main PA due to aneurysmal dilatation. The central arteries are not enlarged as would be expected in PH, despite the poor peripheral vasculature. **I**, The lateral view shows an enlarged main PA occupying the retrosternal space.

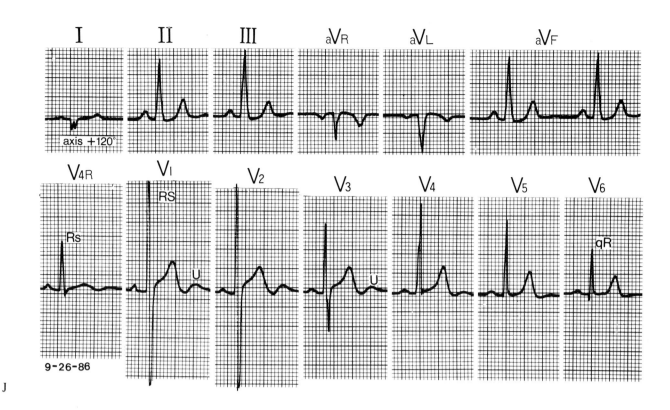

I   II   III   aVR   aVL   aVF

axis +120°

V4R   V1   V2   V3   V4   V5   V6

Rs   RS   U   U   qR

9-26-86

Fig. 11-1. *(Continued)* **J,** The patient's ECG shows right-axis deviation of nearly +120°. V_6 begins with an initial septal q wave indicating normal septal activation.* Despite a tall R wave in V_1, the T wave is upright.

*The Rs pattern in V_{4R} and the wide transitional zone located anywhere from V_1 to V_3 are compatible with RV overloading. The positive T waves in the RV leads and the absence of S waves in the LV leads are difficult to explain by the RV overloading alone and may represent biventricular overloading which is further suggested by the large biphasic complexes in V_1 and V_2.

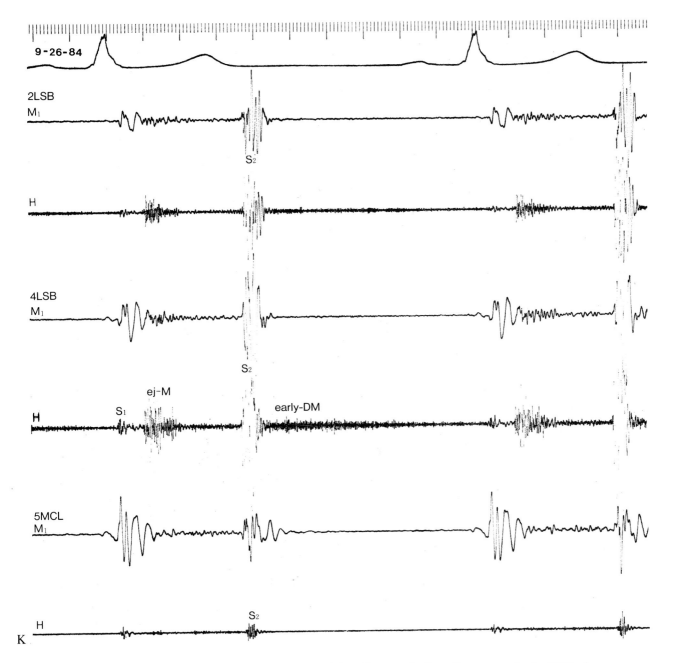

Fig. 11-1. *(Continued)* **K,** His PCG shows an accentuated S₂ with an early diastolic murmur (early DM) of probable pulmonary regurgitation (PR). This is the Graham-Steell murmur. There is also a soft, short ejection murmur (ej-M).

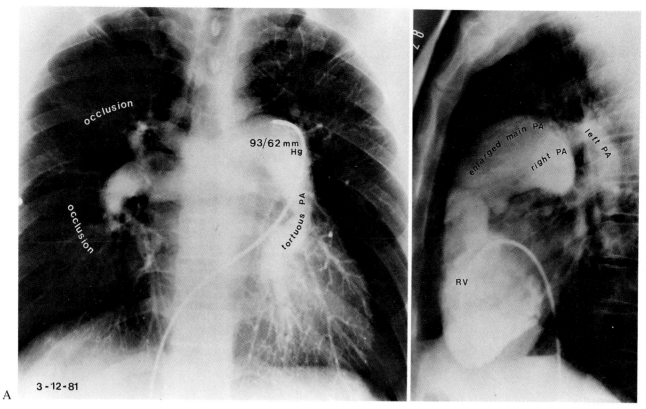

Fig. 11-2. This 38-year-old police detective shows marked dilatation of the main PA on his angiogram. **A**, His left PA is also dilated, with tortuous branches suggesting primary PH. Recurrent pulmonary embolism cannot be excluded. **B**, The lateral projection shows marked dilatation of the main PA which had a pressure of 93/62 mm Hg. The pulmonary capillary (PC) pressure was 17 mm Hg, indicating LV failure.

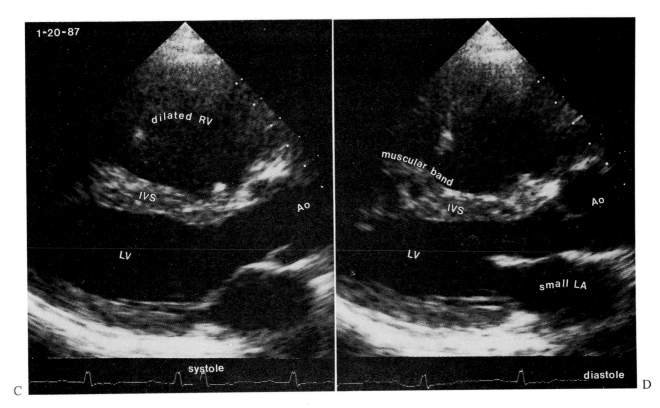

Fig. 11-2. *(Continued)* **C and D**, Long-axis echoes made 6 years after the first examination show an enlarged RV cavity with a hypertrophied muscular band separating it from the IVS appearing as a horizontal figure Y. Both the LV and the LA cavity are small due to their compression by the enlarged RV. His M-mode echo shows semiclosure of the pulmonary valve during systole, indicating PH. A concomitant flat diastolic phase also suggests PH.

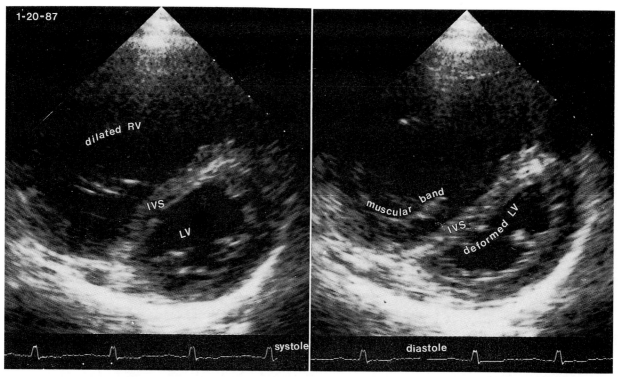

Fig. 11-2. *(Continued)* **E,** Short-axis echoes clearly demonstrate a deformed LV compressed by the enlarged RV. This case represents both pressure and volume overloading of the RV. **F,** The deformed LV is better seen during diastole, when the LV resembles a half moon. The cause of this deformed LV is due to volume overloading of the RV because an elevated pressure in the RV alone will not produce such a deformity.

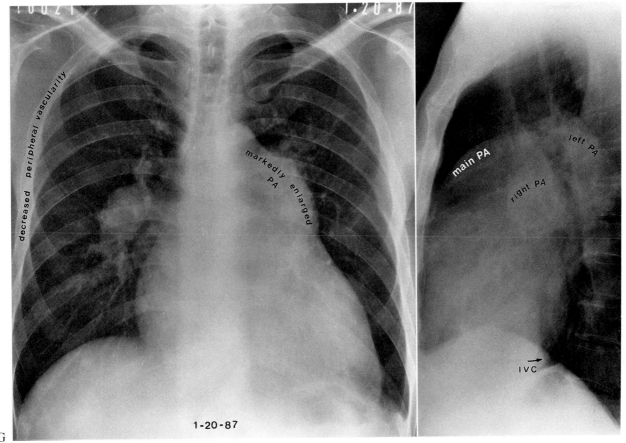

G

H

Fig. 11-2. *(Continued)* **G,** Chest x-rays on the same day as the echoes show generalized cardiomegaly with marked dilatation of the main PA. The right PA at the hilum is also enlarged with reduced peripheral vasculature. **H** shows the junction of the inferior vena cava (IVC) and the posterior cardiac border below the level of the diaphragm. This usually suggests LV enlargement, but in this case, the marked right-sided cardiac dilatation displaced the LV posteriorly, resembling LV enlargement.

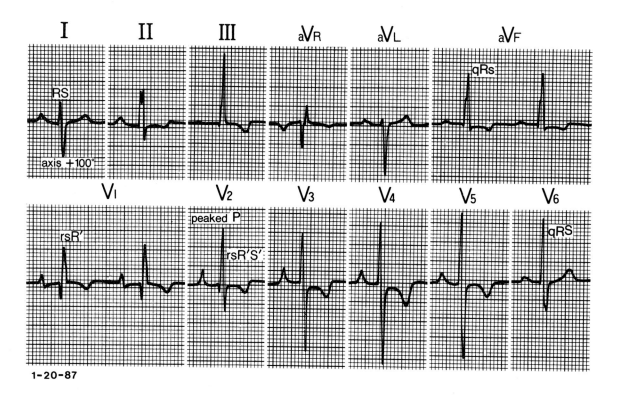

I

1-20-87

Fig. 11-2. *(Continued)* **I,** There is no change in the ECG since the initial examination of this patient 6 years before. There are peaked P waves in the precordial leads with a QRS axis of about +100°. An rsR′ pattern in V₁ with inverted T waves in V₁ to V₅ indicate systolic RV overloading.

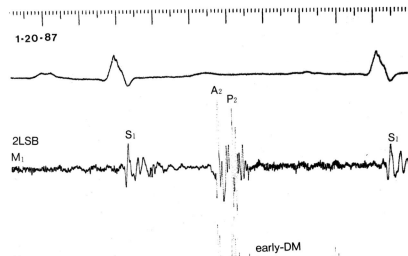

1·20·87

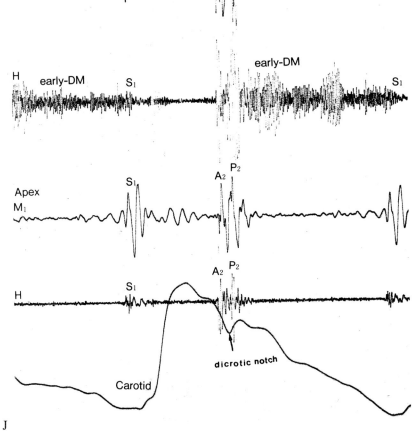

A₂ P₂

2LSB
M₁   S₁   S₁

H   early-DM   S₁   early-DM   S₁

Apex
M₁   S₁   A₂ P₂   S₁

H   S₁   A₂ P₂

dicrotic notch

Carotid

J

Fig. 11-2. *(Continued)* **J,** The S₂ is split from the 2LSB to the apex. The P₂ is accentuated in all areas. There is a pandiastolic murmur indicating pulmonary regurgitation (PR). This murmur has two crescendo-decrescendo components. It is a Graham-Steell murmur.*

*The murmur in the present case is not pure, and may contain friction rubs.

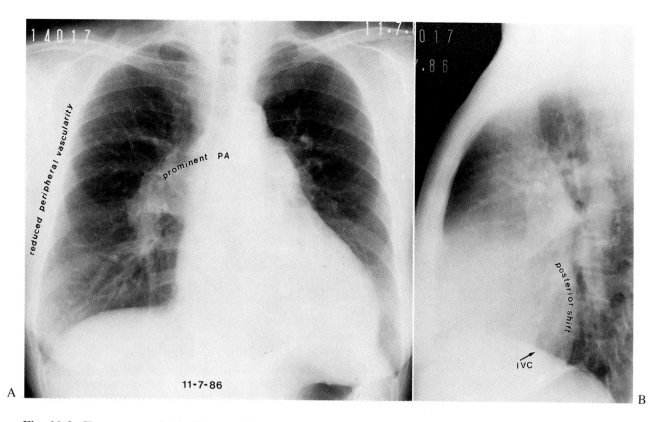

A

B

Fig. 11-3. Chest x-rays of this 52-year-old acyanotic woman with an atrial septal defect (ASD) show a prominent main PA, **A**, and marked dilatation of the central artery. The peripheral vasculature is still seen, but an abrupt narrowing of the right PA suggests the presence of PH. On the lateral view, **B**, anterior enlargement of the right cardiac silhouette displaces the LV posteriorly, and simulates a large LV.

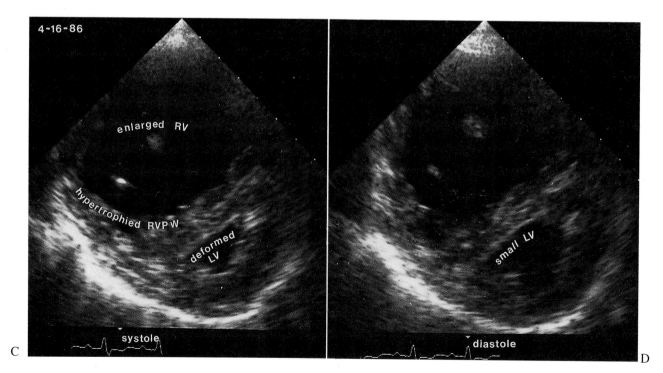

C

D

Fig. 11-3. *(Continued)* **C and D**, Short-axis echoes show enlargement and hypertrophy of the RV. The large amount of the blood in the dilated RV is compressing the LV causing a narrow cavity. This is typical of a volume-overloaded ASD with PH.

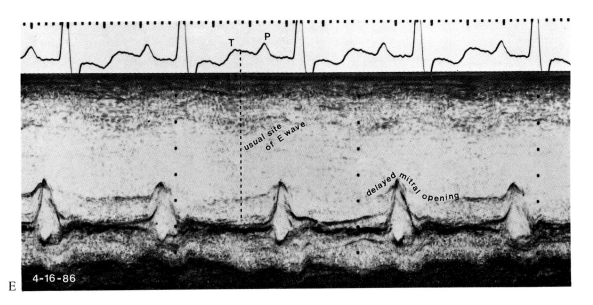

E

Fig. 11-3. *(Continued)* **E,** An M-mode echo recorded at the level of the mitral valve of the same patient shows a delta-like wave instead of the normally seen twin-peaked E and A waves. The delta wave is a mixture of E and A waves and is frequently observed in tachycardias. However, the estimated heart rate of this case is 93 per minute. It is unlikely that this slight tachycardia alone will produce a delta wave. The long PR interval is partly responsible for the early atrial contraction.

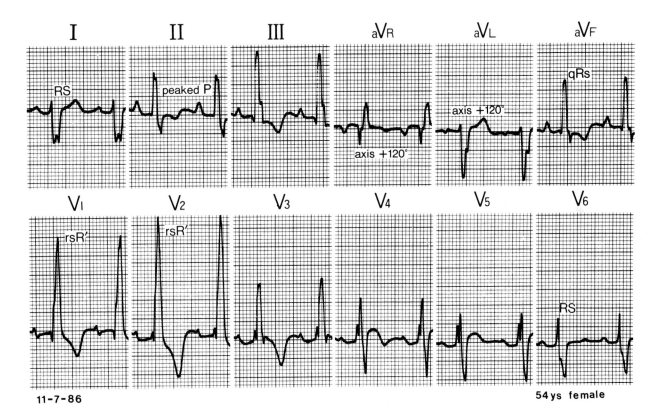

F

Fig. 11-3. *(Continued)* **F,** An ECG of the same patient shows peaked P waves in leads II, III and aVF indicating RA overloading. The QRS axis is nearly +120°. In the precordial leads, an rsR′ pattern with a tall R′ in V_2 indicates systolic RV overloading. The inverted T waves in V_1 to V_4 are compatible with PH. Normally the systolic RV overloading shows a narrower QRS complex than in this case. A wide QRS complex resembling RBBB with marked right axis deviation suggests that the RBBB is complicated by a posterior divisional block. However, the overall findings favor systolic RV overloading.

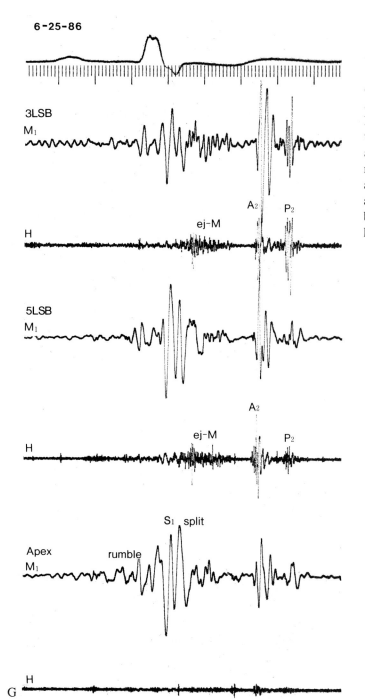

6-25-86

3LSB
M₁

H ej-M A₂ P₂

5LSB
M₁

H ej-M A₂ P₂

Apex
M₁ rumble S₁ split

G H

Fig. 11-3. *(Continued)* **G,** Her PCG shows a small ejection murmur (ej-M) in 3LSB to 5LSB. There may be a soft ejection sound (ES) or splitting of S_1. The S_2 is widely split which is at least partly due to the RBBB. Only one cardiac cycle is shown in the figure, but the splitting was confirmed as fixed. The height of P_2 is unexpectedly normal instead of high, suggesting some RV failure, but its transmission to the 5LSB and apex indicates dilatation of the RV. There is a presystolic rumble at the apex representing a flow murmur through the tricuspid orifice caused by the forceful atrial contraction. Since the patient refused invasive diagnostic procedures, no conclusive diagnosis is available but the presence of an ASD with PH seems to be the most likely.

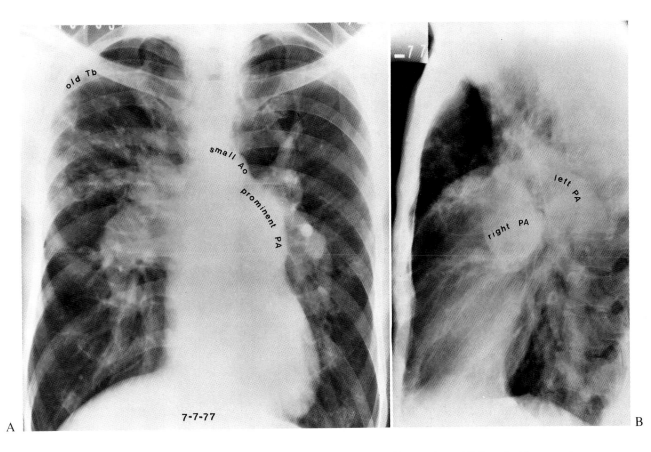

A   7-7-77   B

Fig. 11-4. This 41-year-old construction worker was known to have heart disease since childhood with cyanosis and clubbing of the fingers. In his youth, he suffered from pulmonary tuberculosis. The patient had a short ejection murmur and an accentuated single S_2 followed by an early diastolic murmur. His chest x-rays show marked dilatation of both the main PA, **A**, and central arteries. The peripheral pulmonary vasculature is decreased. **B**, Dilatation of the right and left PA is seen in the lateral view. The right side of his heart is enlarged anterosuperiorly. There is an old pulmonary tuberculous lesion in the right upper lung field.

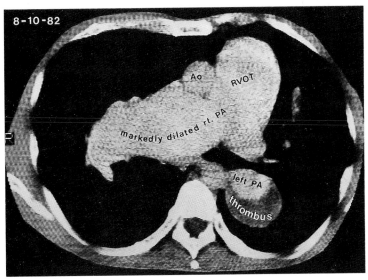

C

Fig. 11-4. *(Continued)* **C**, The patient was very anxious and uncooperative concerning any diagnostic procedures. He finally agreed to have an enhanced cardiac CT examination. Cardiac CT section at the level of the PA shows a marked dilatation of the RV outflow tract (RVOT) and of the PA bilaterally. The dilatation of the main PA extends through about three aortic diameters. A branch of the left PA shows formation of a large thrombus.

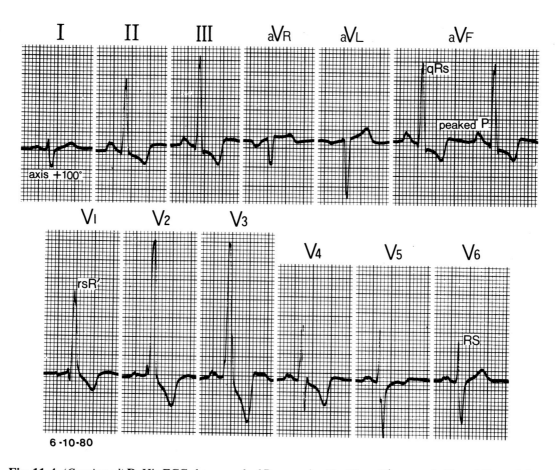

Fig. 11-4. *(Continued)* **D**, His ECG shows peaked P waves in aV$_F$. The rsR′ pattern in V$_1$ and V$_2$, and the QRS axis of more than +100° indicate systolic RV overloading. An S wave in V$_5$ and V$_6$ and inverted T waves in V$_1$ to V$_4$ are also signs compatible with systolic RV overloading.

Chapter 12 Pulmonary Stenosis

Pathophysiology and Clinical Clues

In pulmonary stenosis, (PS) there is an obstruction between the RV outflow tract (RVOT) and the pulmonary valve and/or obstruction at the pulmonary orifice.* With a narrowed RVOT and/or valvular PS, a coarse ejection murmur (usually with a late peak accentuation) is audible. The RV compensates by hypertrophy so that pulmonary flow is not diminished unless there is a right-to-left shunt or RV failure. Unless the PS is very severe, there are no symptoms.

Clinical approaches to the diagnosis of PS are as follows:

★★★★ Chest x-ray findings in PS consist of poststenotic dilatation of the main PA.† There is no PA enlargement at the hilum as is seen in ASD. The peripheral pulmonary vascularity is often normal. RA enlargement may be seen.

★★★★ The auscultatory finding consists of a coarse or crunchy ejection murmur at the 2LSB and 3LSB lasting until just before the soft P_2. A wide splitting of the S_2 is usually recorded on PCG, but it may not be audible.

★★★★ The ECG shows RV systolic overloading manifested by right-axis deviation and tall R waves in leads V_1 to V_3. Peaked P waves and negative T waves in the RV leads, and narrow S waves in the LV leads are common.

★★ The echo may reveal a hypertrophied RV wall, but no RV dilatation. The pulmonary valve is barely recordable.

* In the aortitis syndrome, a pulmonary artery branch may be obstructed.

† The characteristic enlargement of the main PA in PS merges into the left cardiac margin vertically in contrast to that of ASD, where the main PA tends to merge into the left cardiac margin diagonally.

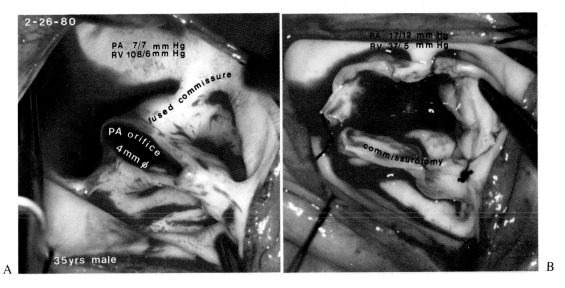

Fig. 12-1. This 35-year-old asymptomatic man had a coarse systolic murmur at the base of his heart since childhood. **A,** Right heart catheterization showed his PA pressure to be 7/7 and his RV pressure to be 108/6 mm Hg. At surgery, all pulmonary valvular cusps were hypertrophied and the commissures were fused. **B,** After a commissurotomy, the PA pressure was 17/12 and the RV pressure was 37/5 mm Hg.

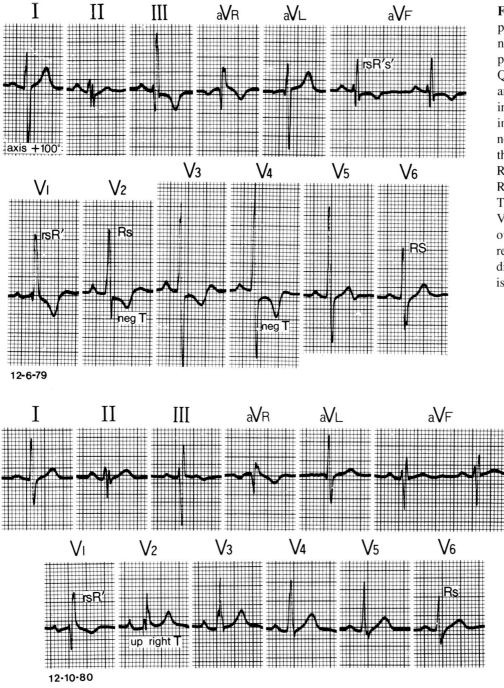

Fig. 12-1. *(Continued)* **C,** His preoperative ECG shows a slightly negative QRS in lead I with the positive QRS in aVF indicating a QRS axis of about +100°. There is an rsR′ pattern in V₁ with a tall R′ indicating systolic RV overloading. The entire QRS complex is not wide and there is no notch on the R′ which is typical of systolic RV overloading and differs from RBBB of ischemic heart disease. The T waves are negative in V₁ and V₄, also compatible with RV overloading. The QRS in aVF resembles V₁ suggesting that the diaphragmatic portion of his heart is compromised by the RV.

C   12-6-79

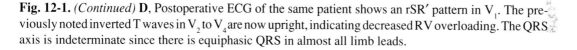

D   12·10·80

Fig. 12-1. *(Continued)* **D,** Postoperative ECG of the same patient shows an rSR′ pattern in V₁. The previously noted inverted T waves in V₂ to V₄ are now upright, indicating decreased RV overloading. The QRS axis is indeterminate since there is equiphasic QRS in almost all limb leads.

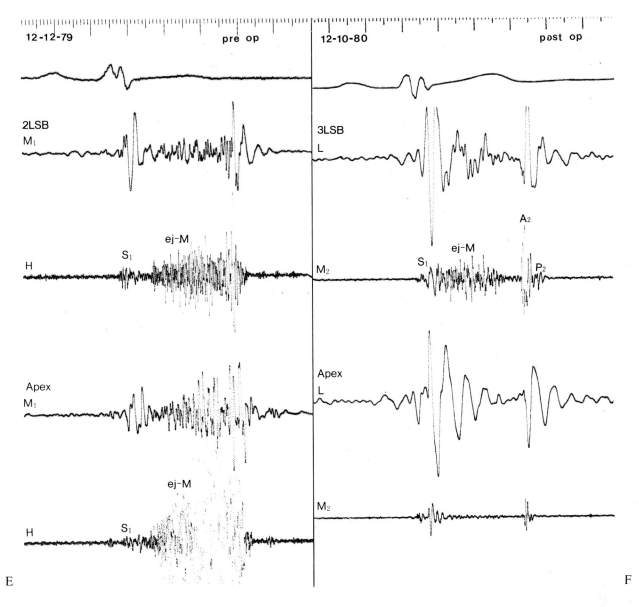

E   F

Fig. 12-1. *(Continued)* **E,** Preoperative PCG shows a coarse ejection murmur (ej-M) from the second left intercostal space (2LSB) to the apex. The splitting of the S_2 is not sharp and small vibrations after S_2 at the apex may represent an early diastolic murmur (early-DM) of pulmonary regurgitation. Postoperatively, **F,** PCG shows only a markedly diminished ejection murmur. A small vibration following the S_2 may be P_2.

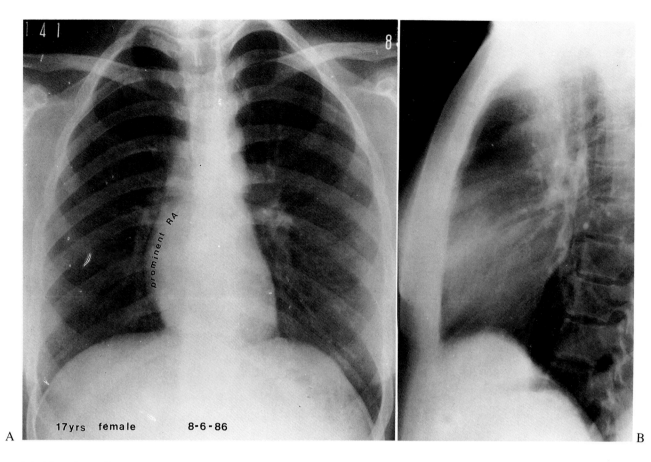

Fig 12-2. A and B, Chest x-rays of a 17-year-old asymptomatic retarded female show a centrally located cardiac silhouette with a prominent RA and an invisible main PA segment. There may be reduced peripheral vascularity, especially on the right, suggesting possible PS despite the absence of poststenotic dilatation of the main PA. She had a coarse systolic murmur at the base of her heart.

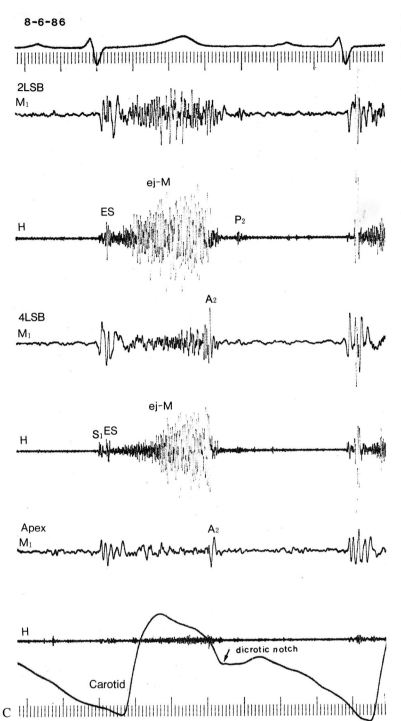

8-6-86

2LSB
M₁

ej-M

ES

H

P₂

4LSB
M₁

A₂

ej-M

H

S₁ ES

Apex
M₁

A₂

H

Carotid

dicrotic notch

C

Fig. 12-2. *(Continued)* C, Her PCG shows an ejection sound (ES) followed by a loud, coarse ejection murmur (ej-M) with late systolic accentuation terminating before soft P₂ in the 2LSB to 4LSB, all indicating that this murmur is caused by PS. But telling the difference between VSD and PS by auscultation is often difficult. On the carotid tracing an arrow indicates the dicrotic notch. Therefore, the S_2 component just before the dicrotic notch is A_2, and there is a 0.05 second splitting of the S_2.

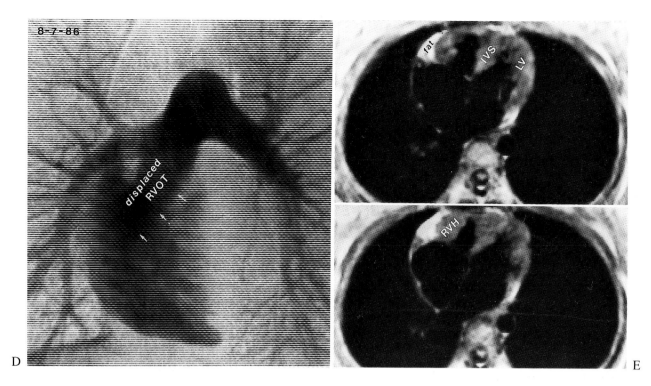

D

E

Fig. 12-2. *(Continued)* **D,** A DSA of the same patient (on the left) reveals a narrowed right ventricular outflow tract (RVOT) (white arrows). There is no evidence of valvular stenosis. **E,** An MRI demonstrates a hypertrophied RV and IVS. The zone anterolateral to the RV is subepicardial fat.*

* In an MRI with spin echo pulse sequence, fat appears white contrary to its radiolucent CT image.

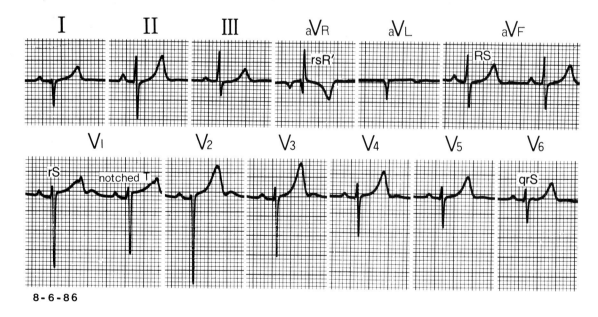

F

8-6-86

Fig. 12-2. *(Continued)* **F,** Her ECG shows marked right-axis deviation of about +180° (equiphasic aVF). The T waves are upright in all precordial leads. There is a marked shift of the transitional zone to the left and S waves are seen in V$_5$ and V$_6$ denoting a markedly posterior QRS. There is nothing to indicate RV overloading other than the marked right-axis deviation.

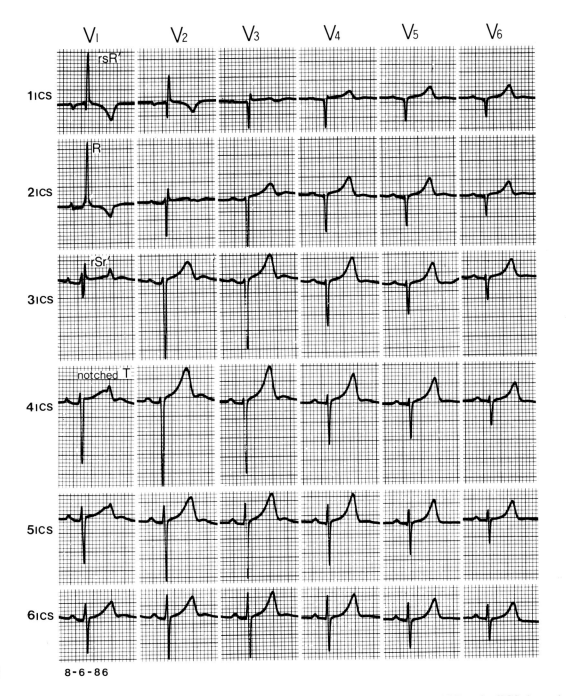

G   8-6-86

Fig. 12-2. *(Continued)* **G**, ECG tracings obtained from the first intercostal space (1ICS) to the 6ICS showed tall R waves along the parasternal regions in the right 1ICS and 3ICS, which suggests right ventricular outflow tract (RVOT) hypertrophy. This is a rather unusual case of infundibular PS in which a conventional ECG alone was not diagnostic.

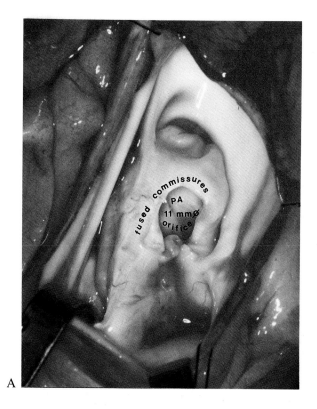

A

Fig. 12-3. A, This 23-year-old asymptomatic man had a cardiac murmur since childhood. A thorough study revealed moderately severe PS. At surgery, his pulmonary orifice was fish-mouth in appearance and 11 mm in diameter caused by hypertrophied cusps and fusion of the commissures. There was hypertrophy of the RV free wall and of anomalous muscle bands in the RV cavity.

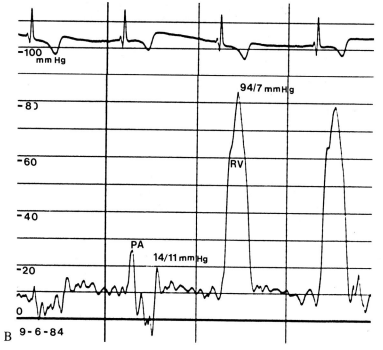

B

Fig. 12-3. *(Continued)* **B,** Catheterization revealed a RV pressure of 94/7 and a PA pressure of 14/11 mm Hg.

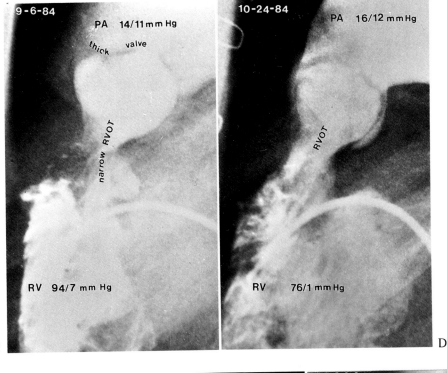

9-6-84

PA 14/11 mm Hg

thick valve

narrow RVOT

RV 94/7 mm Hg

C

10-24-84

PA 16/12 mm Hg

RVOT

RV 76/1 mm Hg

D

Fig. 12-3. *(Continued)* **C,** A preoperative angiogram showed narrowing of the RVOT and thickening and doming of the pulmonary valve. **D,** Four weeks postoperatively the angiogram shows some reduction of the RVOT obstruction. The pressures were 76/1 in the RV and 16/12 mm Hg in the PA.

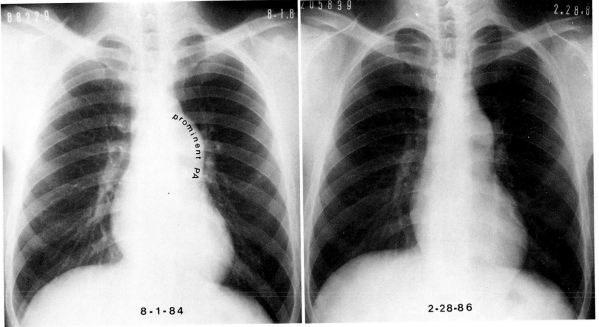

8.1.8

prominent PA

8-1-84

E

2.28.8

2-28-86

F

Fig. 12-3. *(Continued)* **E,** A preoperative frontal chest x-ray of the same patient shows poststenotic dilatation of the main PA which merges with the cardiac border almost vertically. The RA is prominent. **F,** The postoperative frontal chest x-ray 16 months later shows a decrease in the extent of the poststenotic dilatation of the main PA and a reduction in the size of the RA.

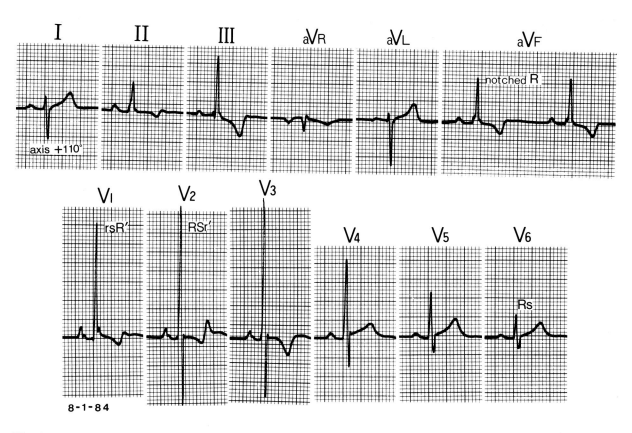

G

Fig. 12-3. *(Continued)* G, Preoperative ECG shows a negative QRS complex in lead I with positive QRS in aVF indicating about +110° right axis deviation. Peaked P waves in V_1 to V_4 with inverted T waves and an rsR′ pattern with a high amplitude of the R′ in V_1 indicates RV systolic overloading.

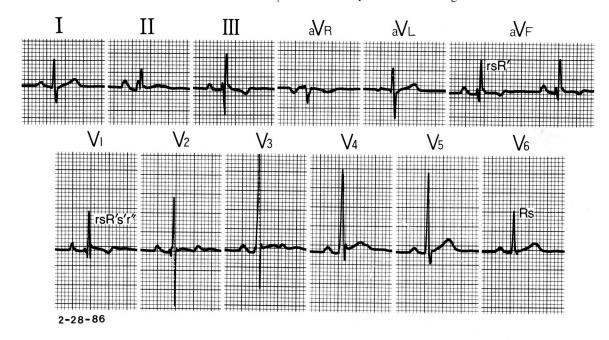

H

Fig. 12-3. *(Continued)* H, A postoperative ECG 16 months later shows resolution of the marked right-axis deviation; the axis is now about +80°. The QRS in V_1 now shows an rsR′s′r″ pattern with reduction of the R′ amplitude indicating a decrease in RV overloading. The previously noted negative T waves in V_2 to V_4 are now only negative in V_1. The peaked P wave is still observed in lead V_1.

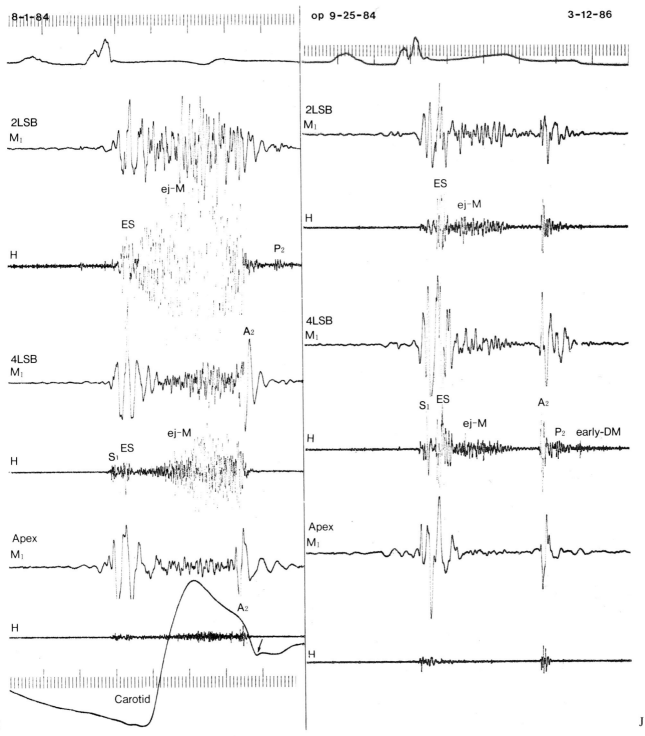

Fig. 12-3. *(Continued)* **I,** His preoperative PCG shows a loud ejection sound (ES) followed by a coarse ejection murmur (ej-M) maximum at the 2LSB which is transmitted to the 4LSB. This murmur has late systolic accentuation which suggests PS. A wide splitting of the S_2 was recorded only at the 2LSB. On the carotid tracing, an arrow indicates the dicrotic notch. Therefore, the S_2 component slightly before the dicrotic notch is A_2. Eighteen months postoperatively, **J,** the ES remained the same but the ejection murmur (ej-M) became very soft. The splitting of the S_2 is now narrow and there may be a soft early diastolic murmur (early DM) of pulmonary regurgitation at the 4LSB.

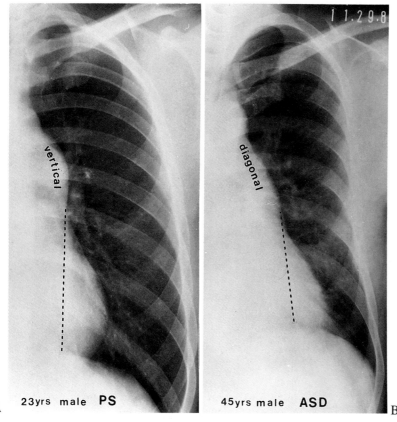

vertical

diagonal

A   23yrs male **PS**

45yrs male **ASD**   B

Fig. 12-4. These chest x-rays demonstrate the manifestations of various causes of a prominent main pulmonary artery (PA). On the left, **A**, is poststenotic dilatation of the main PA due to pulmonary stenosis. (Fig. 12-3E). The dilated main PA merges into the left cardiac border almost vertically, showing systolic overloading of the RV. This suggests that the cardiac apex is medially located. On the right, **B**, is a prominent main PA due to an ASD. In this case, the main PA merges into the cardiac border rather diagonally beause of diastolic RV overloading. This indicates that the cardiac apex is laterally displaced.

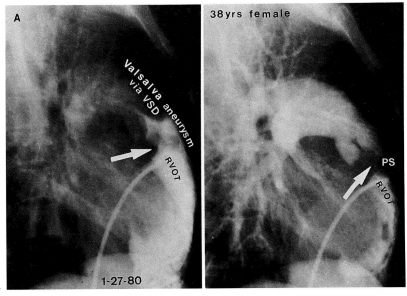

Fig. 12-5. Angiograms from a 38-year-old woman with a loud systolic murmur along the 3LSB to 5LSB. **A,** An early systolic phase shows a negative defect below the pulmonary valve. **B,** during late systole both RV and PA are imaged. A white arrow indicates a negative filling defect below the pulmonary valve causing PS. Defect was caused by aneurysmal dilation of one of the aortic sinuses of Valsalva. This is a case of supracristal VSD with aneurysmal dilatation of the right sinus of Valsalva protruding into the RVOT, causing the PS. The prolapsed right cusp occludes the VSD but produces the AR.

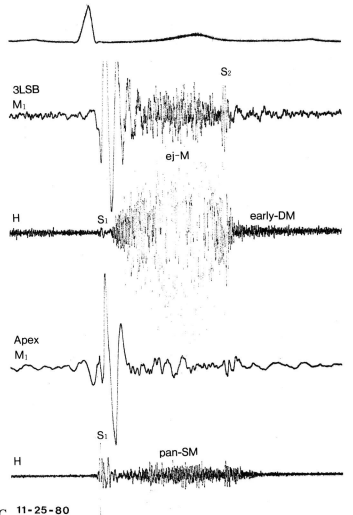

Fig. 12-5. *(Continued)* C, Her PCG shows a coarse ejection murmur (ej-M) which begins with a slight delay after the S_1 at the 3LSB and continues until S_2. Splitting of the S_2 is not seen. There is an early high frequency diastolic murmur (early DM) of AR beginning from S_2. This is a to-and-fro murmur due to PS and AR, but it may be misinterpreted as a continuous murmur on auscultation. The difference is that during systole, the continuous murmur has the maximum intensity around the S_2. There is an additional spindle-shaped pansystolic murmur at the apex denoting either the presence of MR possibly from mitral valve prolapse.

Chapter 13 Tetralogy of Fallot

Pathophysiology and Clinical Clues

Tetralogy of Fallot (T/F) is one of the most common congenital heart diseases in children; it is rarely seen in adults. It is characterized by PS and an Ao which overrides or straddles a large VSD. The pulmonary valve may be malformed and stenotic but right ventricular outflow tract (RVOT, or infundibular) obstruction is the usual cause of the PS and produces systolic overloading of the RV causing right ventricular hypertrophy. Cyanosis is common and depends on the degree of PS.

Clinical approaches to diagnosing T/F are as follows:

★★★★ ECG shows marked right-axis deviation, peaked P waves, and RVH as manifested by tall R waves in RV leads. However, the T waves may not be inverted in V₁ if LV volume is still normal as when the PS is only mild to moderate.

★★★★ Chest x-ray shows a prominent aortic arch with absence of the main PA segment. Peripheral pulmonary vascularity is diminished due to the reduced pulmonary flow caused by the R to L shunt. The cardiac apex is often elevated. There may be a right-sided aortic arch.

★★★★ The echo shows overriding of the Ao with a large VSD. A magnified echo may reveal RVH.

★★★★ A PCG shows a loud ejection murmur at the base of the heart due to the PS. A loud single S₂ is usual but a widely split S₂ may occasionally be seen even though the P₂ is barely audible. In some cases the ejection murmur of PS is overlapped by a regurgitant murmur of VSD.

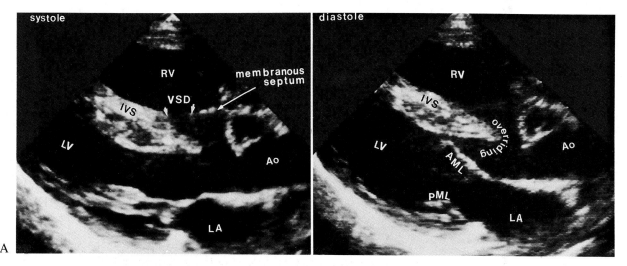

Fig. 13-1. This is an example of long-axis echoes in T/F. The patient is a 6-year-old cyanotic girl who had a loud cardiac murmur since birth. **A**, A discontinuity between the anterior aortic wall and the interventricular septum (IVS) is clearly seen. A thin cord-like structure valve continuous from the anterior aortic wall may represent a portion of membranous septum and/or muscular aspect of the basal region of the sinus of Valsalva or a portion of the tricuspid valve. **B**, A dilated Ao overrides a large VSD. The hypertrophy of the anterior RV wall is not clear. The LV free wall is relatively thin and its cavity is small indicating hypoplasia of the LV. (Courtesy of the Pediatric Department of Tokai University.)

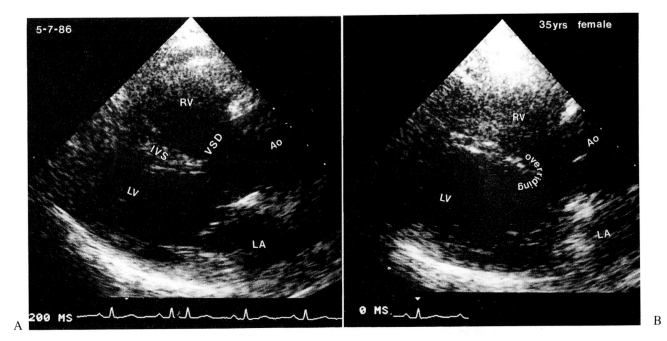

Fig. 13-2. These echoes are from a 35-year-old housewife and mother of 2 children. The patient is cyanotic and has clubbing of her fingers and toes. **A,** Her obesity and RVH resulted in long-axis echoes of poor quality. **B,** But they do show a large VSD, and her Ao overrides the IVS.

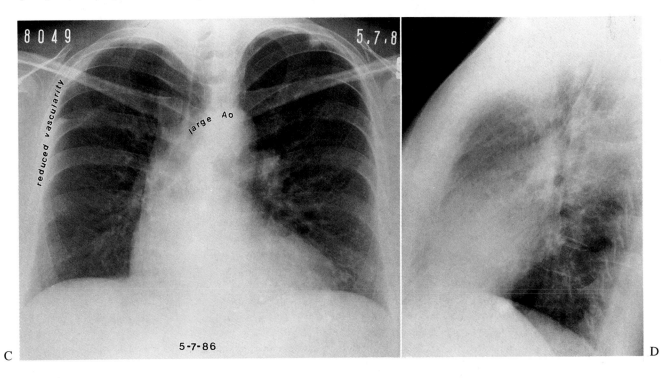

Fig. 13-2. *(Continued)* **C and D,** Chest x-rays of the same patient show an elevated diaphragm due to her obesity. Her cardiac silhouette is relatively horizontal in its orientation. There is a large aortic arch and a concave main PA segment. The central arteries are also small with reduced peripheral pulmonary vascularity. Because of the elevation of the diaphragm, a typical cardiac silhouette of a wooden shoe and/or number one wood golf club is not seen.

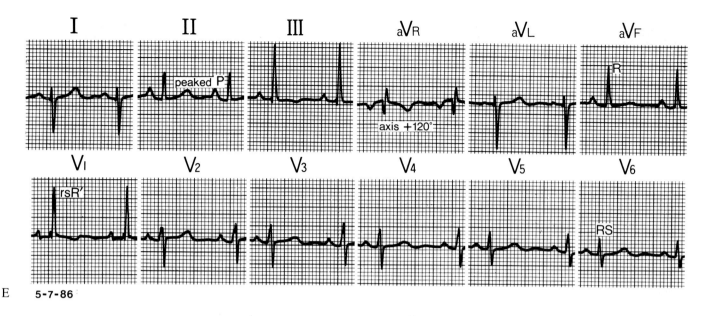

E   5-7-86

Fig. 13-2. *(Continued)* **E,** Her ECG shows an equiphasic QRS in aVʀ with a positive QRS in aVꜰ indicating +120° right-axis deviation. Peaked P waves are seen in leads V$_1$ and V$_2$. There is a narrow rsR′ pattern in V$_1$ with a negative T wave compatible with systolic RV overloading. The small r waves in V$_2$ to V$_6$ suggest hypoplasia of the LV. Except for a shallow negative T wave in V$_1$, there are positive T waves in the other RV leads which differ from those seen in pure PS probably because in T/F, RV pressures do not rise above systemic levels.

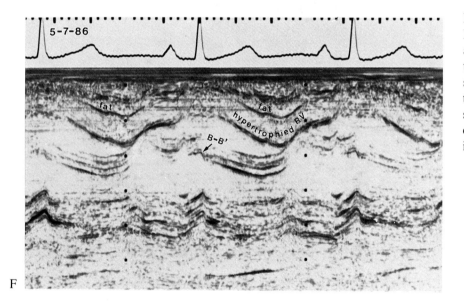

Fig. 13-2. *(Continued)* **F,** A magnified M-mode echo of the same patient shows a hypertrophic RV free wall with tricuspid valvular movement which shows B-B′ step formation. Although this usually suggests elevated RA pressure, catheterization showed pressures of 4 in the RA and 80/5 in the RV, 12/9 in the PA and 94/4 mm Hg in the LV.

F

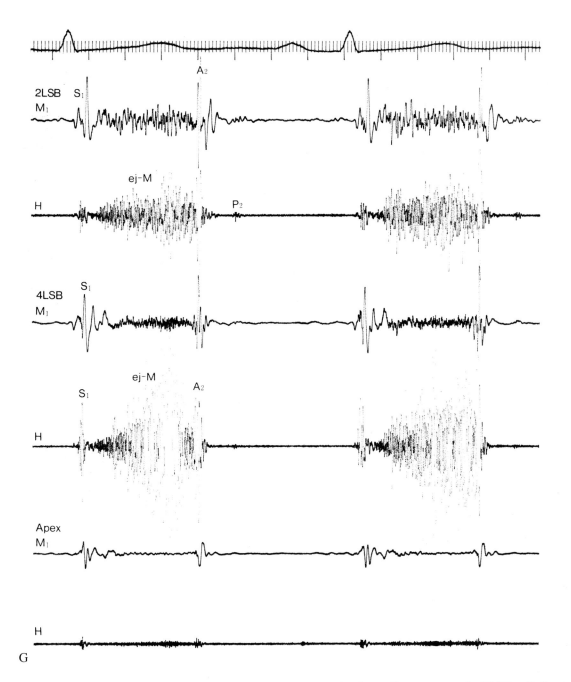

Fig. 13-2. *(Continued)* **G**, PCG of the same patient shows a loud systolic murmur at the 2LSB radiating to the 4LSB. The murmur begins slightly after the S_1 and extends beyond the A_2, but terminates before the P_2 indicating it is an ejection murmur (ej-M) of PS. This is typical of the T/F murmur which is due to the PS rather than the VSD.

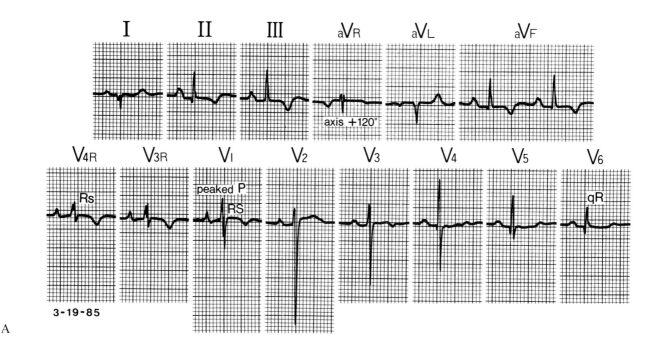

V4R V3R V1 V2 V3 V4 V5 V6

axis +120°

Rs

peaked P

RS

qR

3-19-85

A

Fig. 13-3. A, This 64-year-old housewife had clubbing of her fingers, minimal cyanosis, and hypertension (170/90). The patient was told that she had heart disease and was cyanotic in her childhood. At 18, she married and had 2 children. She has been asymptomatic. Her ECG shows an equiphasic QRS in aVR with a positive QRS in aVF, indicating a right-axis deviation of +120°. Peaked P waves are seen in leads II, III, aVF and V_{4R} to V_2. There is an RS pattern in V_1. These findings are compatible with systolic RV overloading.

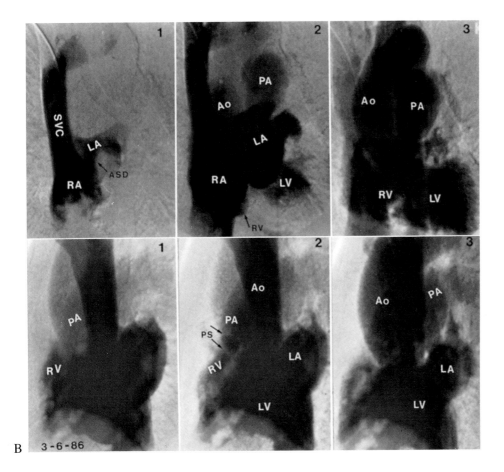

Fig. 13-3. *(Continued)* **B**, Her DSA on the upper row shows a RA to LA shunt through an ASD (1 to 2). In 3, the LV, Ao, and PA are clearly seen, but the RV is not. The lateral views in the lower row show a very small RV with right ventricular outflow (RVOT) obstruction in 1. There may be some valvular stenosis as indicated by arrows in 2 but there is no evidence of a LV to RV shunt.

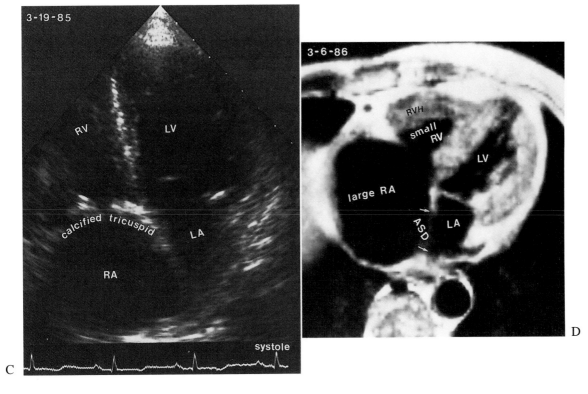

Fig. 13-3. *(Continued)* **C**, The echo in the apical four-chamber view of the same patient shows a large RA and LV. Both the LA and RV are relatively small. The strong echoes are seen at the sites of the tricuspid valve and its calcified annulus. **D**, Her MRI reveals a large RA. The RV is small and hypertrophied. Both IVS and LV are hypertrophied.

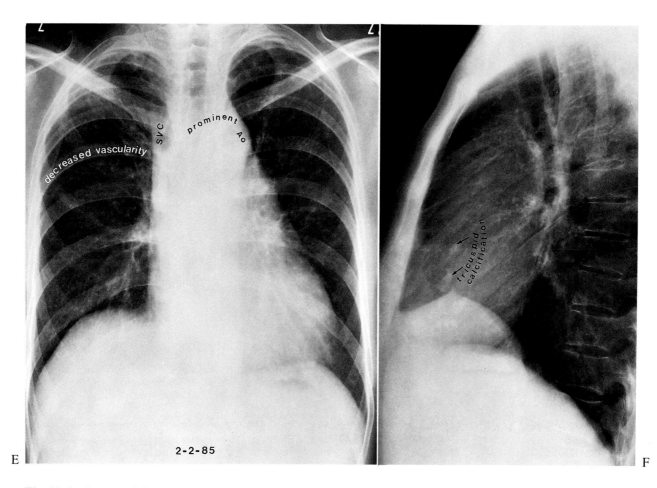

Fig. 13-3. *(Continued)* **E,** Her chest x-rays show a dilated superior vena cava (SVC) with decreased peripheral vascularity in her lung fields suggesting a reduced pulmonary flow. The aortic arch is relatively large, but the main PA is not clearly imaged. In **F,** calcifications in the tricuspid valve and its ring are present and indicated by arrows.

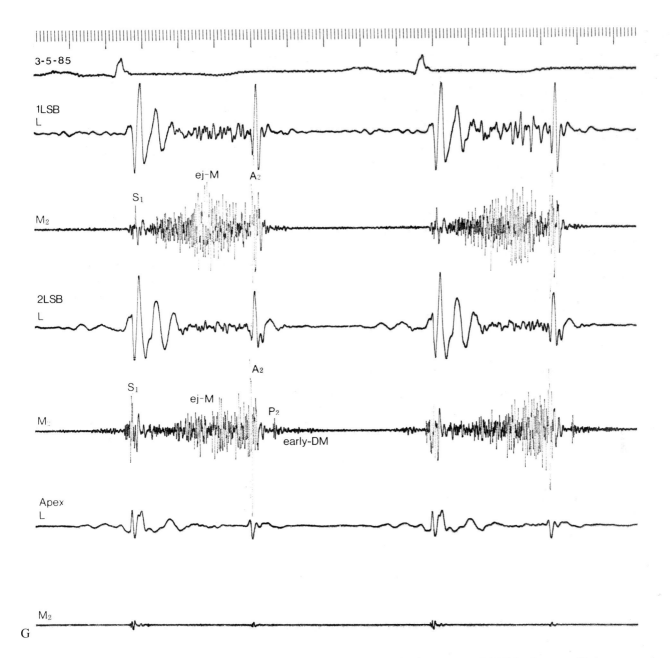

Fig. 13-3. *(Continued)* **G,** Her PCG shows wide splitting of S_2. A coarse ejection murmur (ej-M) has late systolic accentuation and finishes before the P_2. The murmur and wide splitting of S_2 suggest the presence of PS. At the 2LSB there is also a soft diastolic murmur (early DM) with a presystolic component. This murmur appears to begin with P_2, suggesting PR.

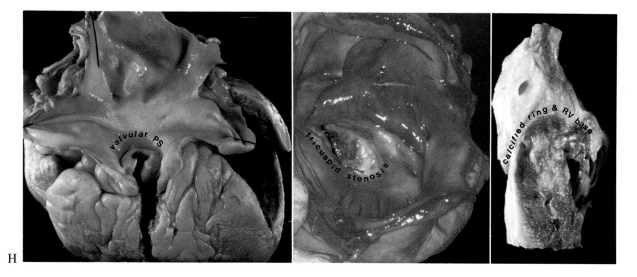

H

Fig. 13-3. *(Continued)* **H,** The patient expired due to inoperable gastric cancer 3 months later. Autopsy revealed congenital valvular PS (left). In the middle are seen a small tricuspid ring and congenital tricuspid stenosis (TS). The calcification extended to the RV base (right).

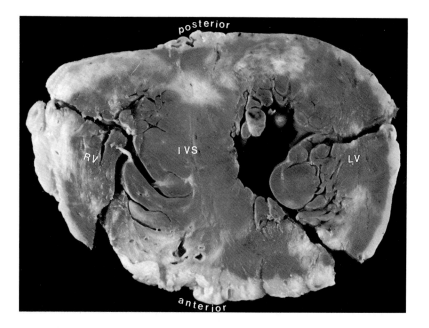

Fig. 13-3. *(Continued)* **I,** The horizontal section of her heart shows a hypertrophied right ventricle, interventricular septum and left ventricle. The RV cavity was markedly decreased in size by the hypertrophied free wall. There were scattered fibroses in the LV free wall with cancer cell invasion. The final diagnoses are: (1) congenital TS, (2) congenital PS with poststenotic dilatation of the main PA, (3) ASD, (4) calcification of the tricuspid ring and the RV base, (5) hypertrophied RV with a small cavity, (6) hypertrophied LV free wall with fibrosis and invasion by cancer cells. In this case, T/F with or without ASD was suspected, but the clinical data were inconclusive. Retrospectively, the patient probably had severe cyanosis during childhood due to a RA to LA shunt which resolved when she developed hypertension.

Chapter 14 Atrial Septal Defect

Pathophysiology and Clinical Clues

Atrial septal defect (ASD) is the most common congenital cardiac lesion among adults. If the defect is located inferiorly and anteriorly, it is an "ostium primum" which is synonymous with an endocardial cushion defect. A defect located in the center of the septum is termed "ostium secundum." A high ASD is called a sinus venosus defect. Patients with ASDs are often asymptomatic and the ASDs are usually discovered incidentally during physical examinations for other reasons. Unless there is coexisting ischemic heart disease and/or hypertension, no dyspnea due to LV failure will be observed. In some cases, PS and anomalous pulmonary venous return and mitral valve prolapse or clefts occur. Because of the pressure gradient between the LA and RA, a LA to RA shunt occurs, resulting in increased pulmonary flow. The intra-atrial shunt is reflected by fixed splitting of the S_2.

The clinical findings in ASD are based on an increase in pulmonary blood flow manifested by:

★★★★ In the ECG diastolic RV overloading is indicated by an rsR′s′ and/or rsR′ patterns in V_1 with right-axis deviation. Associated peaked P waves of RA overloading are often present.

★★★★ Auscultation gives a delayed P_2 with fixed splitting. This P_2 may be transmitted to the cardiac apex indicating an intensified P_2, that may be the result of RV enlargement. There may be a tricuspid inflow murmur and/or tricuspid opening snap caused by an increase in diastolic blood flow through the tricuspid orifice.

★★★★ Chest x-rays show enlargement of the main PA with prominent proximal branches and peripheral pulmonary vessels. Neither the aortic arch nor the LA are prominent, indicating less than normal systemic blood flow compared to the pulmonary circulation.

★★★★ The echo always reveals an enlarged RA and RV, often compressing the interventricular septum (IVS) toward the LV, resulting in a deformed LV. A subxiphoid four-chamber view may disclose the ASD. This is especially true when a contrast echo is used. In an M-mode recording, paradoxical movement of the IVS is often seen caused by the septum moving toward the LV during diastole, which in turn is caused by diastolic overload of the RV.

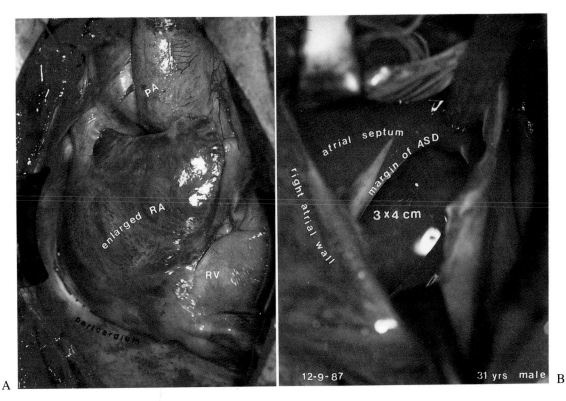

Fig. 14-1. A, The surgical view on the left is from a 31-year-old man with an ASD. An enlarged RA is visible. **B,** On the right, a 3 x 4 cm ASD is shown from the RA side. RV catheterization shows a slightly elevated RA pressure of 9/6, RV 40/10, and PA 36/23 mm Hg. LA pressure was 12/4 and the LV was 99/7 mm Hg.

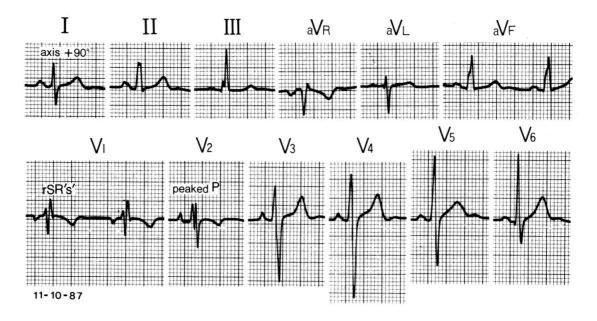

C   11-10-87

Fig. 14-1. *(Continued)* C, A preoperative ECG of the same patient shows a narrow QRS with an axis of +90° with an rSR's' pattern in V₁. This rSR's' pattern is narrow, differs from RBBB, and suggests RV diastolic overloading. For this reason, this should be described as an rSR's' pattern instead of incomplete RBBB. The T waves are inverted only in V₁ and V₂ suggesting a mild diastolic RV overloading. When an rsR' or an rsR's' pattern is observed in ASD, the systolic pressure in the RV is usually less than 45 mm Hg. The RV enlargement is not severe in the present case since there is a qRs in V₆ showing that this lead indicates the LV potential and that apex area is not taken over by the RV.

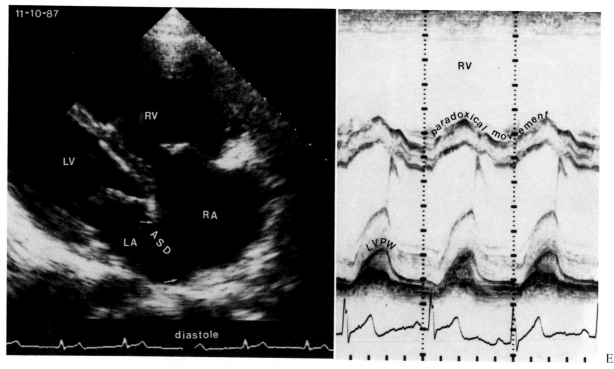

Fig. 14-1. *(Continued)* D, An echo in the subxiphoid four-chamber view of the same patient shows a large ASD (arrows) and enlargement of the RA and RV. E, An M-mode recording shows a large RV with paradoxical movement of the IVS, which is a common finding in ASD because of volume overloading of the RV.

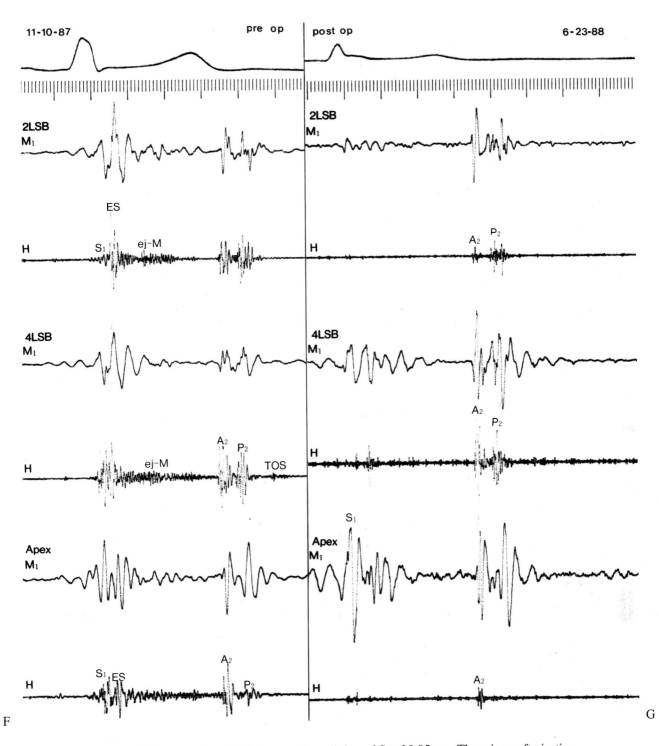

Fig. 14-1. *(Continued)* **F,** Preoperative PCG shows wide splitting of S₂ of 0.05 sec. There is a soft ejection murmur (ej-M) which begins with a loud ejection sound (ES) at the 2LSB, and is transmitted to the 4LSB. A tricuspid opening snap (TOS) is seen at the 4LSB. **G,** About 6 months postoperatively, the PCG shows resolution of the ejection murmur and ejection sound indicating decreased pulmonary flow. However, the S₁ now shows wide splitting at the apex and the previously noted splitting of the S₂ became more marked. RBBB is the cause of this. It is very difficult to explain the RBBB since there was no surgical invasion of the IVS or RV.

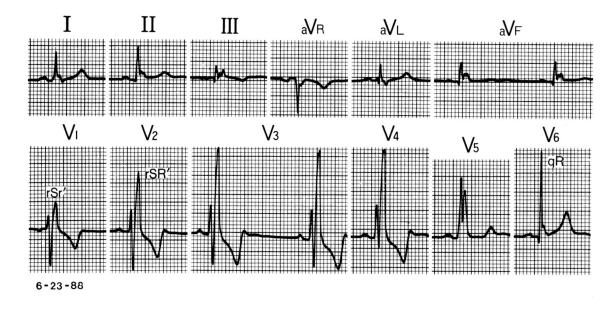

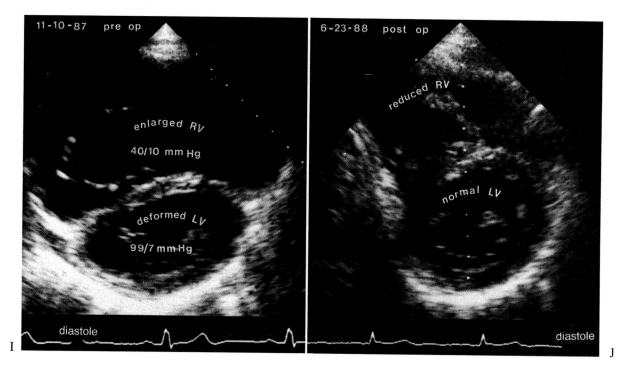

Fig. 14-1. *(Continued)* **H,** Postoperative ECG shows an rSr′ pattern with a wide QRS of 0.12 seconds in V₁, indicating RBBB. Inverted T waves are seen in V₁ to V₄ probably due to the RBBB. The QRS axis is now +45°. There is no evidence to suggest myocardial damage.

Fig. 14-1. *(Continued)* **I,** Preoperative short-axis echos show a deformed LV compressed by an enlarged RV with the IVS almost flat. It is a quite logical assumption that the RV pressure of 40/10 mm Hg cannot compress an LV that has a pressure of 99/7 mm Hg. Therefore, the compression of the LV by the RV is purely due to RV volume overloading. **J,** Six months postoperatively, marked reduction of the RV with normal configuration of the LV can be seen.

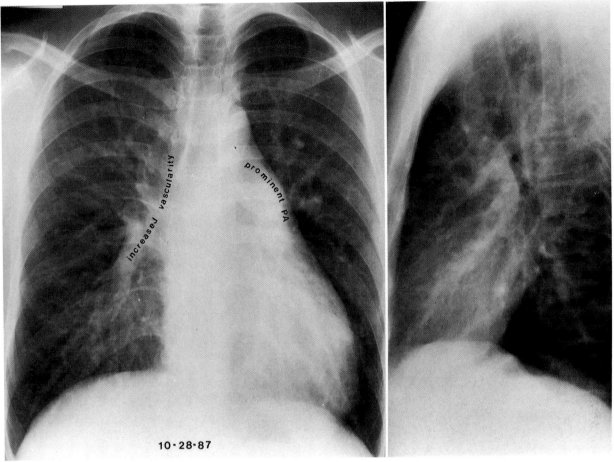

K L

Fig. 14-1. *(Continued)* **K**, Preoperative chest x-rays show a prominent main PA with increased pulmonary vascularity. The aortic arch is normal and there is no evidence of LA enlargement indicating normal or reduced systemic blood flow. The heart is shifted slightly to the left due to a narrow chest, which is often seen in patients with an ASD. **L**, The anterior margin of the heart seems to be enlarged anterosuperiorly.

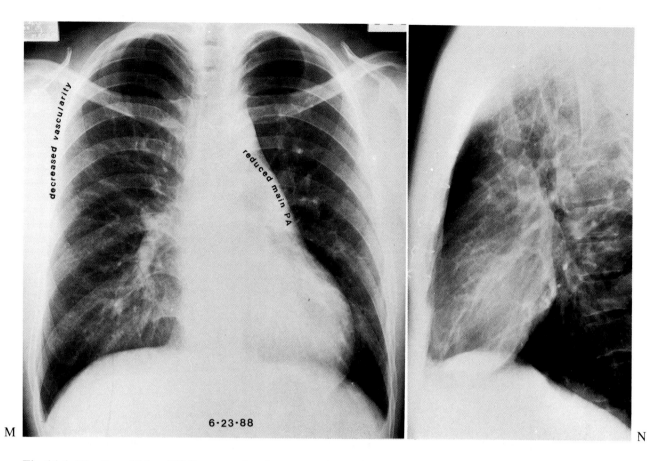

M

N

Fig. 14-1. *(Continued)* **M and N**, Postoperative chest x-rays show a decrease in the size of the main PA segment. Pulmonary vascularity is also less prominent.

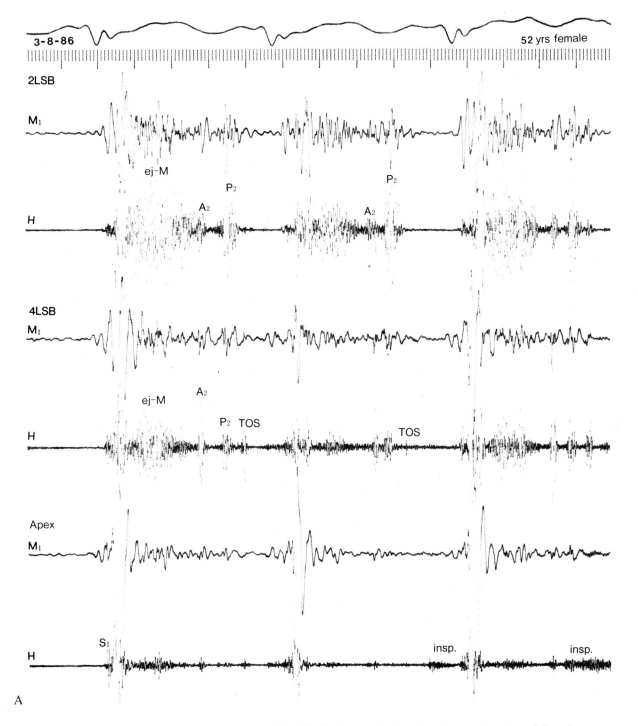

3-8-86   **52** yrs female

2LSB

M_1

ej-M P_2 P_2

A_2 A_2

H

4LSB
M_1

ej-M A_2

P_2 TOS   TOS

H

Apex
M_1

S_1 insp.   insp.

H

A

Fig. 14-2. A, This 52-year-old woman has an ASD. She had several episodes of congestive heart failure but refused surgery and no invasive studies were conducted. Her PCG reveals an ejection murmur (ej-M) loudest at the 2LSB. The ejection murmur varies in intensity with respiration. The S_2 is widely split but not fixed. The P_2 is loud at the base of her heart and is transmitted to the apex, suggesting RV enlargement. There is a probable tricuspid opening snap (TOS) at the 4LSB. The apical tracing of the third cardiac cycle shows some inspiratory (insp.) lung sounds. On auscultation alone, the diagnosis of ASD is difficult since the splitting of S_2 varies.

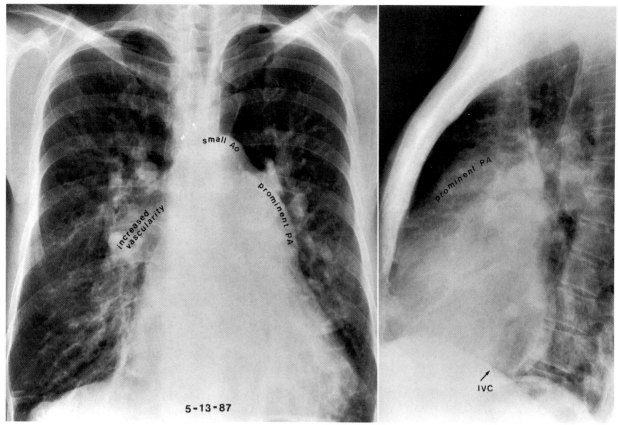

B

5-13-87

C

Fig. 14-2. *(Continued)* **B,** Chest x-rays of this patient show a prominent main PA segment with dilated central pulmonary arteries and increased peripheral vascularity. The cardiac silhouette is also enlarged bilaterally. The aortic arch is small suggesting a relative decrease in the systemic circulation. Small or normal aortic arches and LAs are features of uncomplicated ASDs. **C,** The cardiac silhouette is enlarged anterosuperiorly and posteriorly. This posterior enlargement may be caused by an enlarged right-sided heart displacing the LV posteriorly.

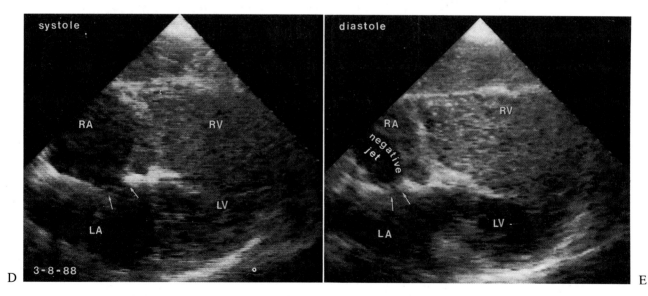

D   3-8-88

E

Fig. 14-2. *(Continued)* **D,** The contrast echoes in the apical four-chamber view appear to show a break in the middle of the atrial septum during both systole and diastole which indicates a probable ASD. **E,** Furthermore, a contrast echo producing a negative jet stream through the ASD during diastole and scattered small particles of microbubbles in the RA confirm the presence of the ASD.

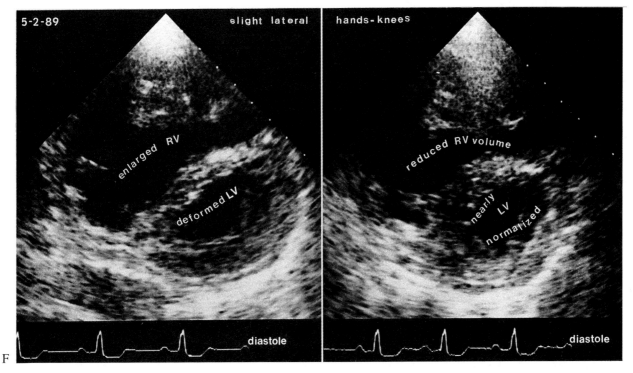

Fig. 14-2. *(Continued)* **F,** Conventional short-axis echo during diastole shows an enlarged RV compressing the LV. **G,** In the recording made in the hands-knees position, the deformed LV became nearly normal in contour. This indicates that the deformed LV in the conventional short-axis recording is caused by large blood volume in the enlarged RV cavity, and not necessarily by increased pressure in the RV. The author believes this is the first demonstration of such a hypothesis.

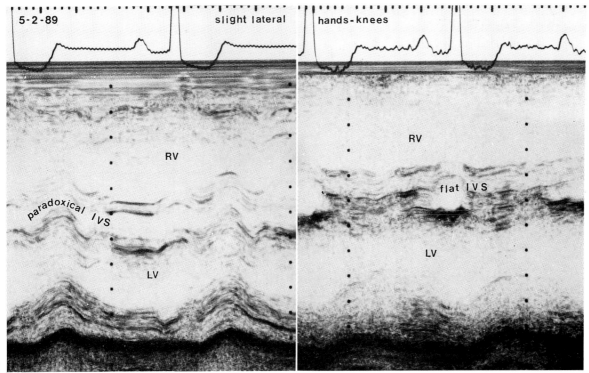

Fig. 14-2. *(Continued)* **H,** M-mode recording shows paradoxical movement of the IVS due to the enlarged RV. **I,** M-mode recording made in the hands-knees position shows a flat but not typically paradoxical septal movement. These findings indicate that the deformed LV in ASDs is due to gravity effect of a large blood volume in the enlarged RV rather than its increased pressure in the RV.

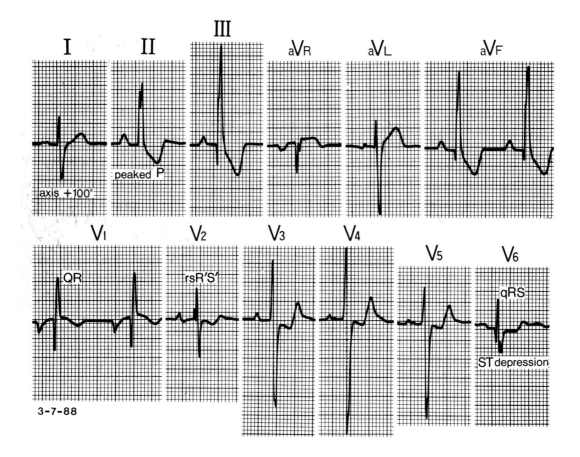

Fig. 14-2. *(Continued)* **J**, ECG of the same patient shows a QRS axis of +100°, and V₁ shows a negative P wave in its early portion with a QR pattern suggesting an enlarged RA. There is an rsR′S′ in V₂ and an S wave in V₅ to V₆ indicating diastolic RV overloading. In uncomplicated ASDs the RV systolic pressure does not rise to more than 45 mm Hg, and an inverted T wave is usually seen only in V₁ to V₃.

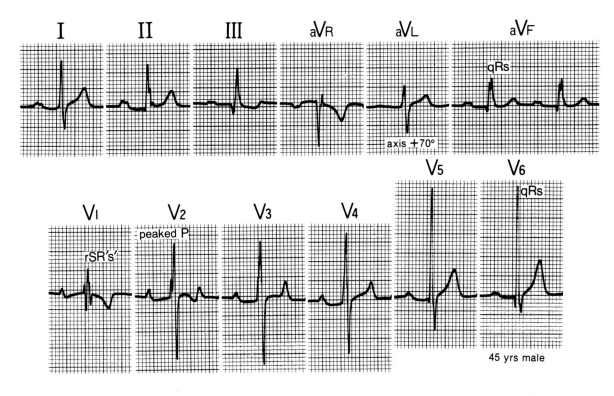

Fig. 14-3. This 45-year-old man has an ASD. His ECG shows a first degree AV block, which is seen in 20 to 30% of ASD patients. V_1 shows an rSR's' pattern. The "dome and dart" or "terminal angular positive T" in V_2 and V_3 is characteristic of ASD. A tall qRs in V_5 and V_6 is a rather common finding in ASD patients with narrow chests, as in the straight back syndrome.

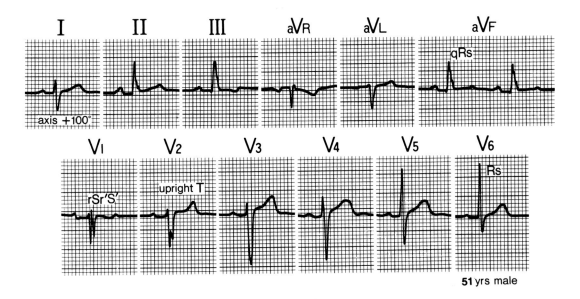

Fig. 14-4. This ECG is from a 51-year-old man with an ASD. It shows a +100° right-axis deviation but without tall or peaked P waves to suggest RA overloading. However, the QRS complex in V_1 is an rSr'S' with embryonic r or a notched S in V_2. A right-axis deviation and an rSr's' and/or a RBBB pattern in V_1 in a patient over age 30 are ECG signs suggestive of an ASD.

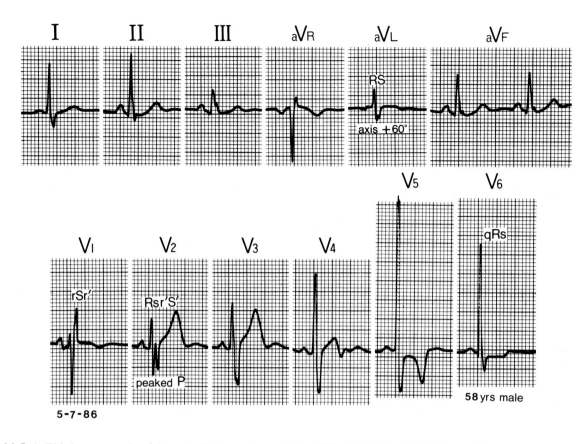

I II III aVR aVL aVF

V1 V2 V3 V4 V5 V6

RS
axis +60°

rSr'

Rsr'S'
peaked P

qRs

58 yrs male

A   5-7-86

Fig. 14-5. A, This is an example of the potential importance of the rsR′ in ASD. This ECG is from a 58-year-old hypertensive man diagnosed as having a hypertrophic cardiomyopathy. A tall QRS complex is seen in leads V_5 and V_6 with ST depression and the inverted T waves are compatible with systolic LV overloading. The QRS complex begins with an initial q wave in V_6 but it has an s wave. It seems rather peculiar to observe an rSr′ in V_1 in systolic LV overloading. In addition, a peaked P wave in V_1 to V_3 cannot be explained by LV overloading alone and suggests bi-ventricular overloading.[*]

[*] An rSr′ is not characteristic of ASD. An ASD is more likely to have rsR′ or rsR′s′ with narrow QRS complexes because a deep S in V_1 suggests LV overload — not a feature of ASD.

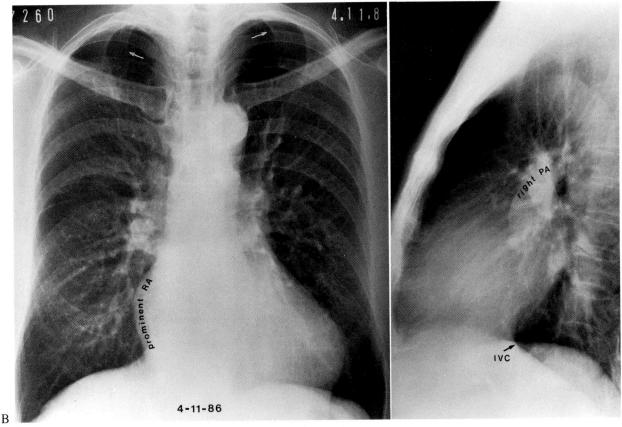

B

C

Fig. 14-5. *(Continued)* Chest x-rays of the same patient suggest emphysema and an elongated Ao. The RA seems to be prominent and there may be prominence of the proximal pulmonary artery branches, but this is not definite. **B,** There is neither a prominent main PA nor increased peripheral pulmonary vascularity to suggest a L to R shunt. There are right and probably left cervical ribs, indicated by arrows. **C,** The right pulmonary artery is prominent but there is no evidence of right-sided cardiac enlargement.

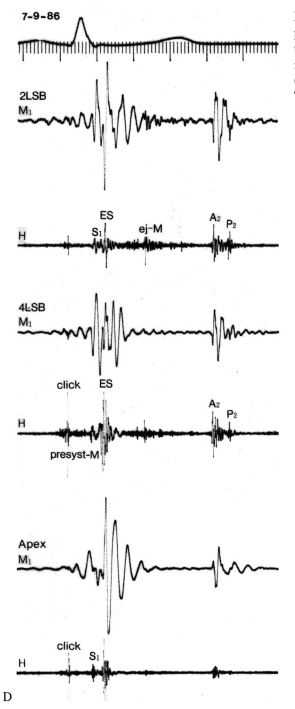

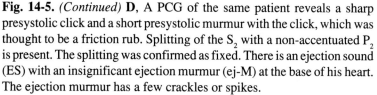

Fig. 14-5. *(Continued)* **D**, A PCG of the same patient reveals a sharp presystolic click and a short presystolic murmur with the click, which was thought to be a friction rub. Splitting of the S_2 with a non-accentuated P_2 is present. The splitting was confirmed as fixed. There is an ejection sound (ES) with an insignificant ejection murmur (ej-M) at the base of his heart. The ejection murmur has a few crackles or spikes.

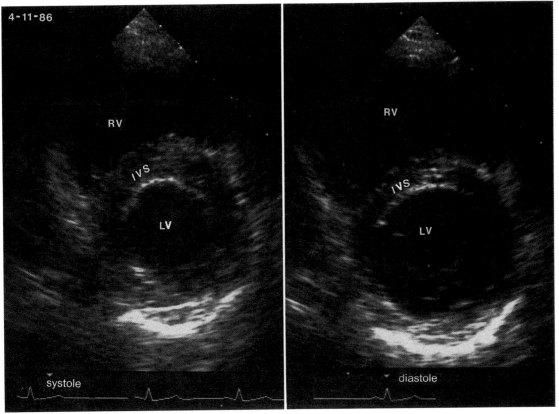

E

Fig. 14-5. *(Continued)* **E,** Short-axis echoes of the same patient seemed to demonstrate an ASD on video tape but cannot be reproduced. The patient had a slightly enlarged RV but the LV appeared to be of normal shape. Finally, a tentative diagnosis of ASD was made, and angiography was performed.

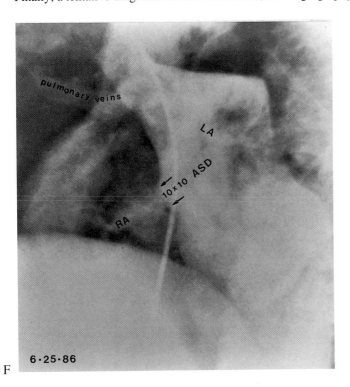

F

Fig. 14-5. *(Continued)* **F,** To our surprise, an angiogram showed a small L to R shunt at atrial level (arrows). Pressures were 7/4 in the RA, 29/8 in the RV, 21/13 in the PA, 9 mm Hg in the pulmonary capillary wedge, and 140/13 in the LV. By angiography, we estimated the size of the ASD (foramen ovale defect) at 10 x 10 mm. There was a 12% oxygen step-up in the RA with an estimated pulmonary blood flow of 7.6 L/min and systemic flow of 4.3 L/min. This case demonstrates the importance of the seemingly unimportant rSr′ complex in V_1. The LV overload is probably due to his long-standing hypertension.

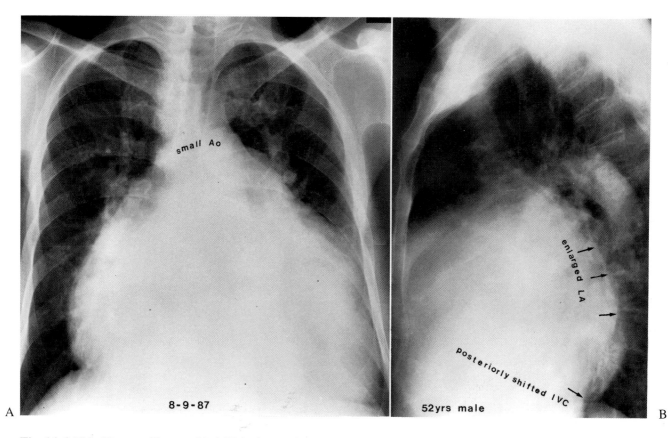

A

8-9-87

small Ao

enlarged LA

posteriorly shifted IVC

52yrs male

B

Fig. 14-6. This 52-year-old man with ASD had several attacks of congestive heart failure but refused to have any invasive diagnostic studies. **A,** His chest x-rays show marked cardiac enlargement which masked pulmonary vascularity, and the aortic arch is relatively small. **B,** An anterosuperiorly dilated right-sided cardiac enlargement displaces the left heart posteriorly as shown by a posteriorly displaced inferior vena cava (IVC) (arrow). The LA seems to be enlarged (arrows).

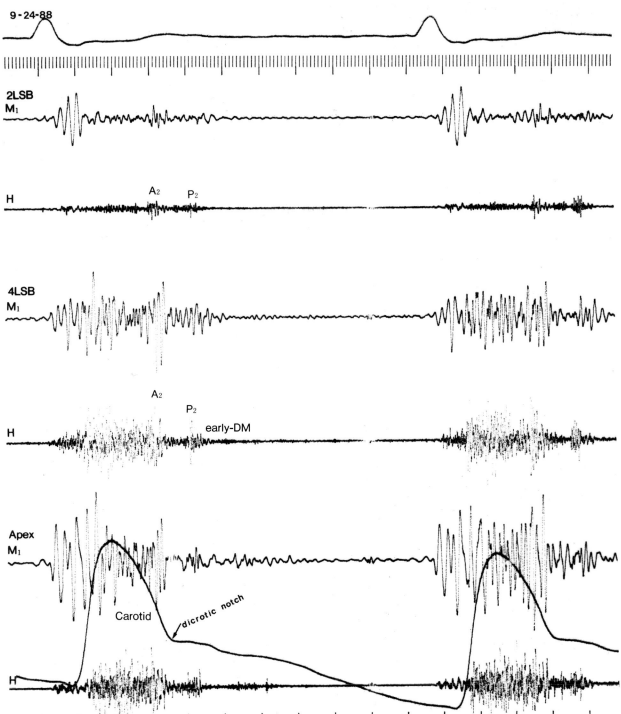

Fig. 14-6. *(Continued)* C, PCG shows wide splitting of S_2 with a soft early diastolic murmur (early-DM) of probable pulmonary regurgitation. A systolic murmur of relatively long duration from the 4LSB to the apex is difficult to explain. Whether it is an ejection murmur or regurgitant murmur is impossible to say especially since the S_1 cannot be defined. However, the location of the murmur's maximum intensity suggests either MR or tricuspid regurgitation.

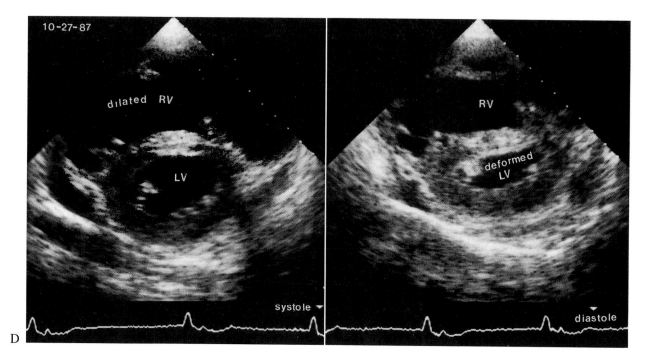

Fig. 14-6. *(Continued)* **D,** Short-axis echoes of the same patient show a deformed LV caused by a volume overloaded RV. There is no enlargement of the LV, confirming that the chest x-ray findings are the result of right-sided cardiac enlargement.

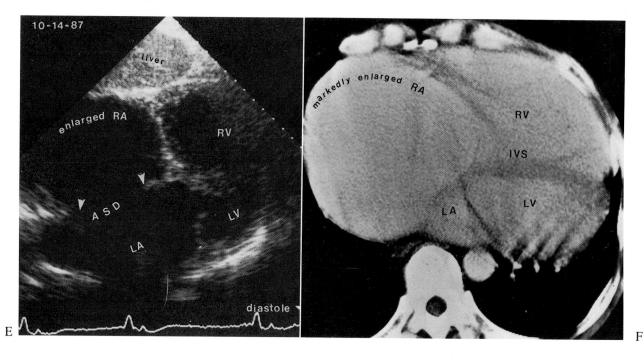

Fig. 14-6. *(Continued)* **E,** An echo in the subxiphoid four-chamber view shows a large ASD (arrowheads). **F,** A cardiac CT section near the AV valves shows marked dilatation of the RA and RV with a relatively small portion of LA and LV. The marked enlargement of the right-sided heart results in a horizontal orientation of the IVS against the anterior chest wall. Normally the IVS is oriented about 45° from the anterior chest wall.

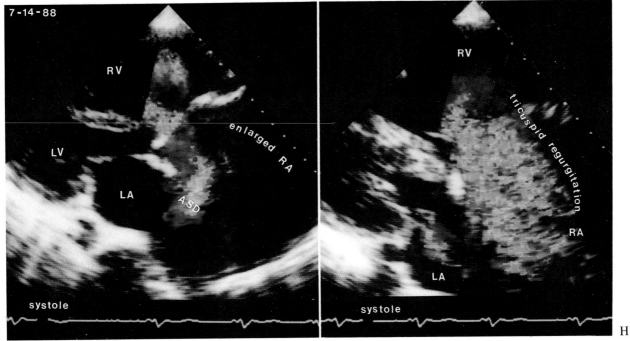

Fig. 14-6. *(Continued)* **G**, The color Doppler echoes of the same patient disclose a left-to-right shunt at atrial level as indicated by the orange flow. **H**, A massive blue-orange color flow indicates a regurgitant flow of tricuspid regurgitation. Minimal MR in the LA is indicated by the blue.

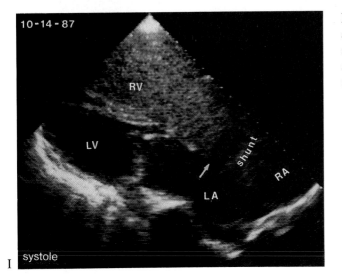

Fig. 14-6. *(Continued)* **I**, When a color Doppler echo is not available, a contrast echo may be helpful. This echo in the subxiphoid four-chamber view shows contrast media in the RA and RV. A negative defect in the RA indicates the left-to-right shunt through the ASD.

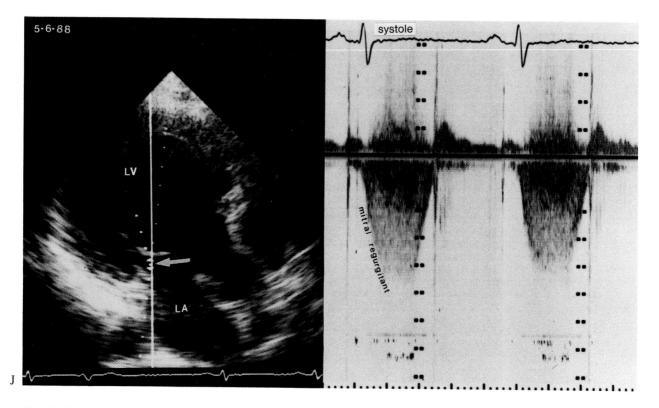

Fig. 14-6. *(Continued)* **J,** A continuous Doppler echo of the same patient shows a regurgitant flow during systole at the mitral valve area indicating MR. An arrow shows the site of sample volume. Thus the regurgitant flow is shown below the base line as a flow away from the transducer.

Chapter 15 Ostium Primum Types of Endocardial Cushion Defect

Pathophysiology and Clinical Clues

During the fetal period the atrial septum descends and joins the ascending interventricular septum to separate both atria and ventricles into left and right sides of the heart. However, when the degree of atrial septal descent is not sufficient, an anteroinferior atrial septal defect occurs which is called ostium primum type of endocardial cushion defect (ECD). This resembles a hole in the lower portion of the wall between 2 chambers with the floor sinking below the wall. Because of the defect in the lower portion of the atrial septum, an atrioventricular or bundle-branch conduction disturbance may result. The anterior division of the left bundle branch is usually involved and produces an anterior divisional block manifested by left-axis deviation. As with an ostium secundum ASD, an ostium primum type of ECD may be overlooked during childhood and may present as a large heart with minimal symptoms in adulthood. A cleft anterior mitral leaflet is common with ECD.

The clinical features of the ECD are as follows:
★★★★ The ECG pattern is identical to that of ASD but also shows left-axis deviation (LAD); in other words, the features are an rsR′s′ in V_1 or typical RBBB with peaked P waves, and often P-R interval prolongation with LAD.
★★★★ The 2D-echo shows both RA and RV dilatation as well as a low atrial septal defect in the subxiphoid four-chamber view.
★★★★ Auscultation reveals fixed splitting of S_2 as seen in any ASD and a mitral regurgitation (MR) murmur when there is a cleft mitral valve.
★★★★ The chest x-ray is also similar to that of any ASD. However, generalized or prominent LV enlargement may be seen when there is a mitral cleft with resultant mitral regurgitation.

The most pertinent diagnostic feature of an ostium primum ECD is angiographic demonstration of the typical goose-neck configuration on the cardiac silhouette. According to S.Kawada, the true meaning of the goose neck sign is unclear. In general, it is a narrowing and elongation of the LV outflow tract. Despite many discussions, there is no definitive answer as to what causes the goose-neck shape. The deformity resembles the neck and breast silhouette of the goose as shown in Figure 15-1A. The aortic root serves as the head of the goose.

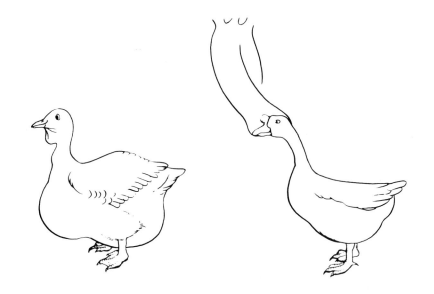

A

Fig. 15-1. A shows a goose and a swan with an Ao. It seems that the typical appearance of a "goose neck" has to have an Ao on its neck.

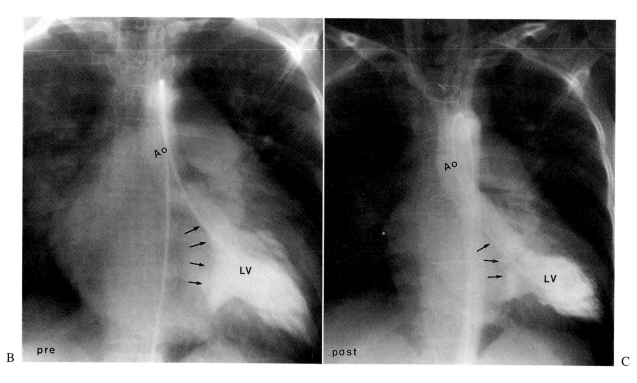

B   pre   post   C

Fig. 15-1. *(Continued)* **B and C**, Pre- and postoperative angiograms of a 31-year-old female with an ostium primum ECD. During diastole in both angiograms a displaced mitral valve causes a scooped or goose neck appearance below the Ao as indicated by arrows. However, without the Ao, the silhouette does not seem to be either a swan or a goose. The postoperative LV angiogram, **C**, shows no remarkable change in its appearance.

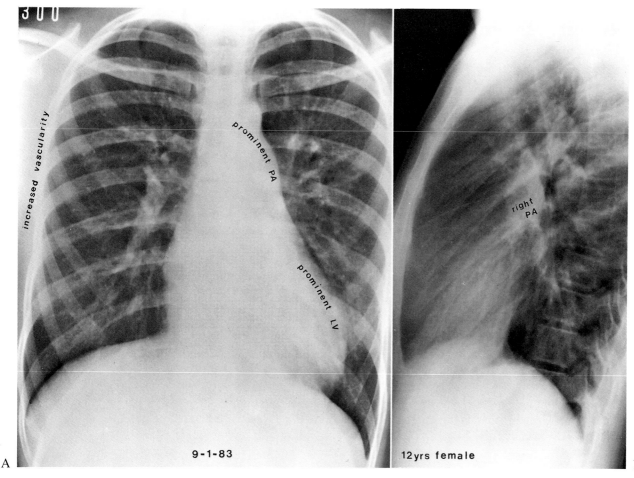

A   9-1-83   12yrs female   B

Fig. 15-2. A and B, Chest x-rays of a 12-year-old school girl who was found to have an abnormal ECG at a physical examination. X-rays show a slightly prominent LV segment with some increased pulmonary vascularity suggesting a left-to-right shunt. The aortic arch is small but the main pulmonary artery segment is slightly enlarged. Therefore, there is a possibility of a VSD but not a PDA. Furthermore, a prominent LV tends to rule out the presence of an ASD.

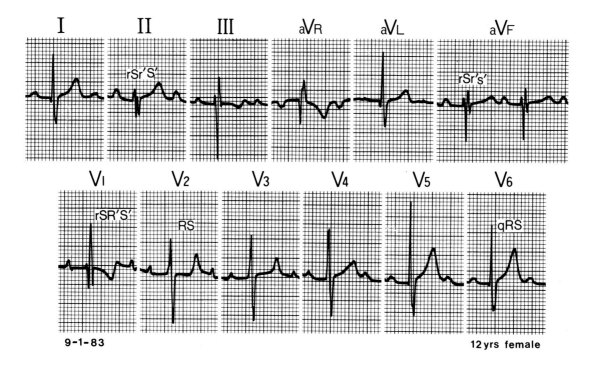

I II III aVR aVL aVF

rSr'S' rSr's'

V1 V2 V3 V4 V5 V6

rSR'S' RS qRS

Fig. 15-2. *(Continued)* C, An ECG of the same patient shows an rSR'S' pattern in V$_1$ with left-axis deviation (LAD) of approximately –45°. There is a first degree AV block. The peaked P waves in V$_1$ and V$_3$ suggest right-sided cardiac overloading. This finding together with LAD is a typical feature of an ECD with an ostium primum defect.

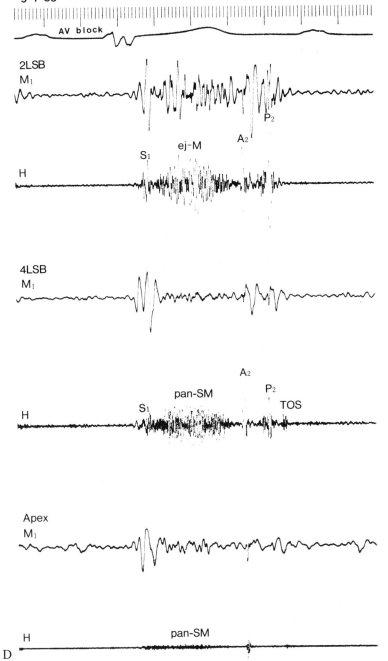

9-1-83

AV block

2LSB
M₁

S₁   ej-M   A₂   P₂

H

4LSB
M₁

A₂
pan-SM   P₂
S₁   TOS

H

Apex
M₁

H   pan-SM

D

Fig. 15-2. *(Continued)* **D**, Her PCG shows an ejection murmur (ej-M) loudest at the 2LSB and transmitted to the apex. The S₂ is widely split, followed by a sharp tricuspid opening snap (TOS) caused by relative tricuspid stenosis.

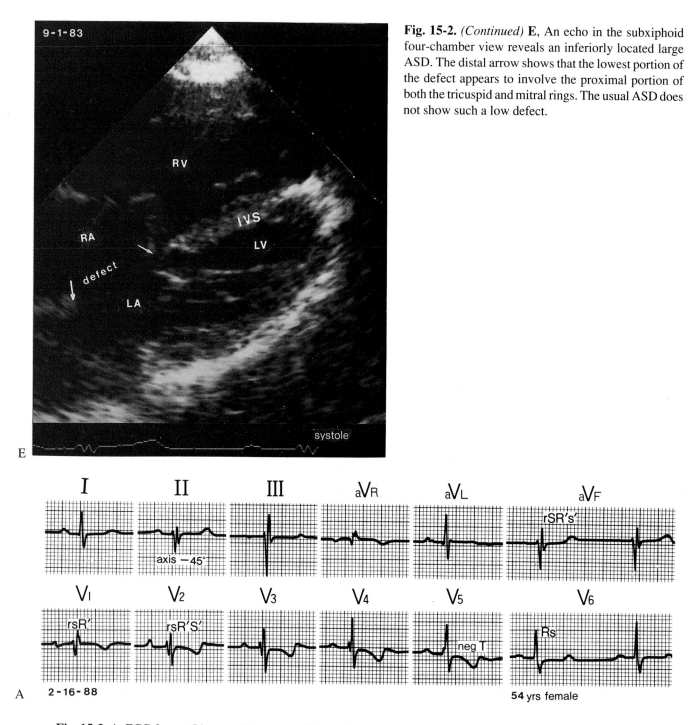

Fig. 15-2. *(Continued)* **E,** An echo in the subxiphoid four-chamber view reveals an inferiorly located large ASD. The distal arrow shows that the lowest portion of the defect appears to involve the proximal portion of both the tricuspid and mitral rings. The usual ASD does not show such a low defect.

Fig. 15-3. A, ECG from a 54-year-old woman with an ostium primum ECD. Since the P wave in aVF is flat, the rhythm may not be sinus. The P-R interval may be slightly prolonged. The QRS axis is nearly −45°, and there is an rsR′ pattern in V_1 with Rs in V_6. The T waves are inverted from V_1 to V_5 suggesting that a large RV is occupying almost the entire anterior portion of the precordium. An rsR′ pattern in V_1 with LAD is a typical feature of ECD.

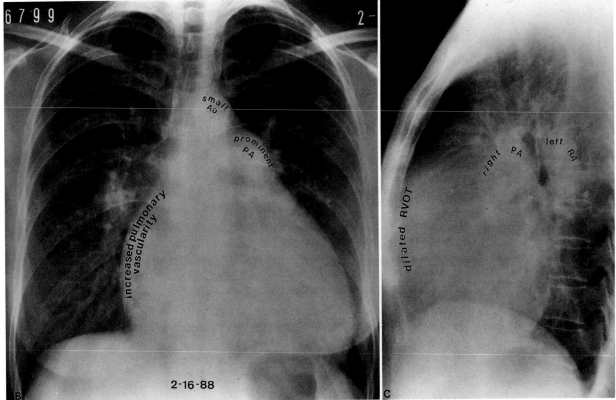

Fig. 15-3. *(Continued)* **B,** The patient's chest x-rays show marked cardiomegaly with increased pulmonary vascularity, indicating a left-to-right shunt. The main PA is prominent and the aortic arch is relatively small which suggests that the shunt is at either the atrial or ventricular level and is not due to a PDA. **C,** An anterosuperiorly dilated right ventricular outflow tract (RVOT) is seen with large left and right pulmonary arteries. The cardiac silhouette is displaced posteriorly by an enlarged right-sided heart.

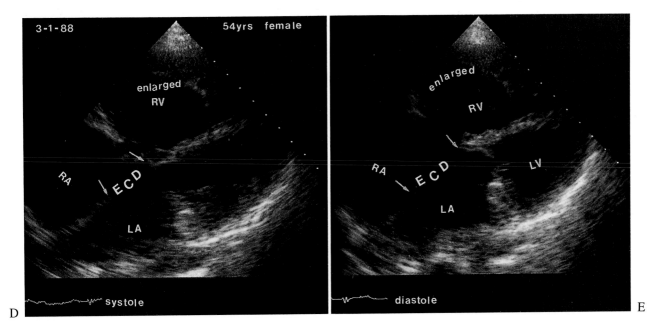

Fig. 15-3. *(Continued)* **D,** Her echoes in the subxiphoid four-chamber view show a large ASD at the inferior region of the interatrial septum which seems to involve the AV valves. **E,** Both RA and RV are dilated but there is no LV enlargement. This confirms that the chest x-ray finding of cardiomegaly is due to right-sided enlargement.

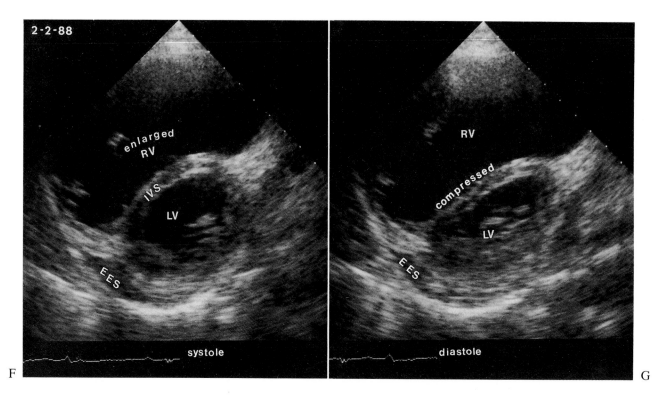

Fig. 15-3. *(Continued)* **F**, Short-axis echoes show a deformed LV compressed by a markedly volume-overloaded RV. **G**, Posterior to the IVS, there is an extra-echo space (EES) which probably represents subepicardial fat.

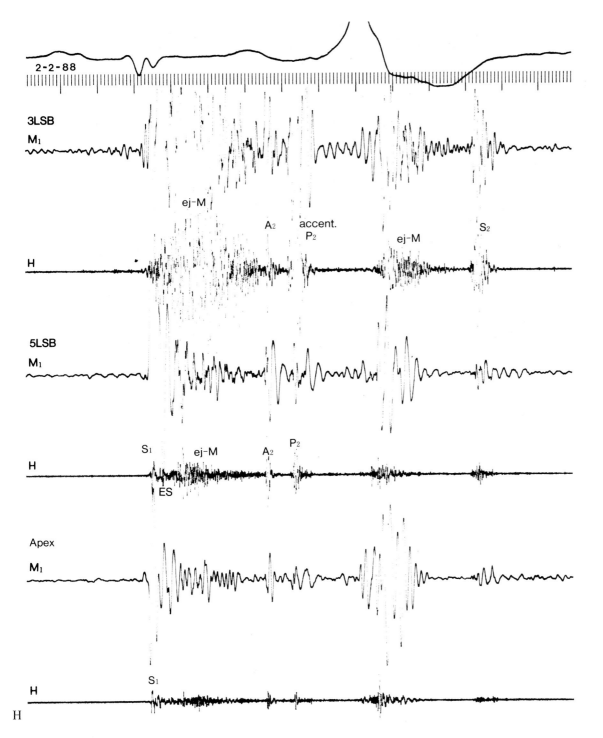

Fig. 15-3. *(Continued)* **H,** PCG of the same patient shows a ventricular extrasystole. The S_2 in the normal beat is widely split with an accentuated P_2. A coarse ejection murmur (ej-M) at the 3LSB is transmitted to the apex. Due to the short diastolic period, the extrasystole produces a soft ejection murmur and the splitting of S_2 is not sharp. The patient has been asymptomatic and refused surgical treatment.

Chapter 16 Ebstein's Anomaly

Pathophysiology and Clinical Clues

Ebstein's anomaly consists of congenital redundancy of the tricuspid valvular tissue with the septal and posterior leaflets displaced into the RV. The downward displacement of the leaflets causes the tricuspid valve to originate from the RV wall instead of the atrioventricular ring. The portion of the RV between the atrioventricular ring and the ectopic origin of the tricuspid valve is termed the "atrialized ventricle." Clinical manifestations vary depending on the degree of the tricuspid valve displacement. In many cases, a coexisting pre-excitation syndrome (W-P-W) often causes supraventricular tachycardia, which may be the first clue to the diagnosis. An RA to LA shunt may occur due to an ASD. However, there may be no symptoms, and the diagnosis may be made incidentally.

The approach to diagnosing Ebstein's anomaly is as follows:

★★★★ A 2D-echo in the four-chamber view often reveals an enlarged RA, downward displacement of the tricuspid valve, and an atrialized RV. Delay in closing the tricuspid valve is seen in M-mode recordings.

★★★★ Chest x-rays show cardiomegaly, especially an enlarged RA and slightly decreased pulmonary vascularity. There is no enlargement of either the aortic arch or the main PA segment.

★★★ The ECG often shows an rsR's′ pattern in V_1, and either narrow or wide QRS complexes with tall peaked P waves. The P-R interval may be prolonged. There may be a W-P-W pre-excitation pattern with or without supraventricular tachycardia.

★★★ Auscultation and/or the PCG may show a right-sided S_3 and S_4 with quadruple rhythm, an S_1 with a loud second component (sail sound), wide splitting of S_2, with a tricuspid opening snap and a tricuspid regurgitation (TR) murmur.

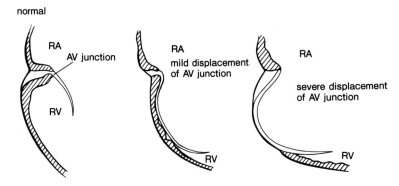

Fig. 16-1. Schematic drawings of Ebstein's anomaly show a normal AV junction, mild or marked displacement of the AV junction with decreased thickness of the RV wall, and an atrialized RV.*

* In cases of severe Ebstein's anomaly, the junction between the atrialized RV and the true RV produces nicking which can be seen either by echo or angiography.

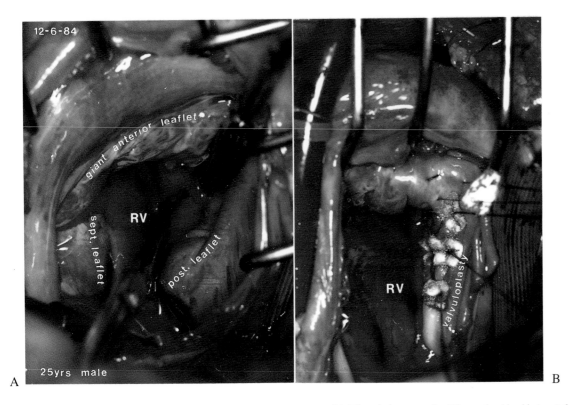

A, 12-6-84, giant anterior leaflet, sept. leaflet, post. leaflet, RV, 25yrs male

B, RV, valvuloplasty

Fig. 16-2. A, Surgical photographs from a 25-year-old man with Ebstein's anomaly. The patient had intractable paroxysmal supraventricular tachycardia (PSVT). **B,** The RA was markedly dilated and the septal and posterior leaflets of the tricuspid valve were displaced into the RV. A large anterior leaflet compensated for the tricuspid valvular dysfunction. After valvuloplasty and resection of an accessory AV bundle (bundle of Kent), the tachycardia resolved.

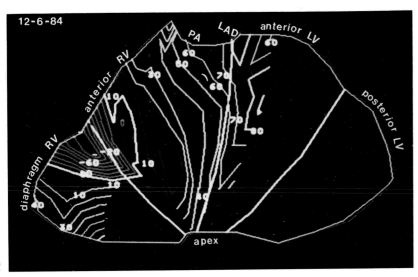

C, 12-6-84, anterior RV, PA, LAD, anterior LV, posterior LV, diaphragm RV, apex

Fig. 16-2. *(Continued)* **C,** Epicardial ECG mapping during surgery showed an early excitation region in the diaphragmatic portion of the RV and part of the anterior RV, shown in blue. This indicates that the accessory bundles are located here.

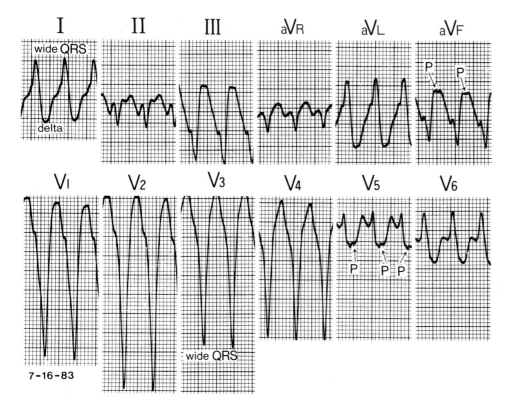

Fig. 16-2. *(Continued)* **D,** An ECG made during his paroxysmal supraventricular tachycardia shows a rate of 188 with a wide QRS complex associated with a delta wave in lead I. Small P waves immediately following each QRS complex are present in leads aV$_F$ and V$_5$, indicating supraventricular tachycardia with atrioventricular pre-excitation rather than a ventricular tachycardia.

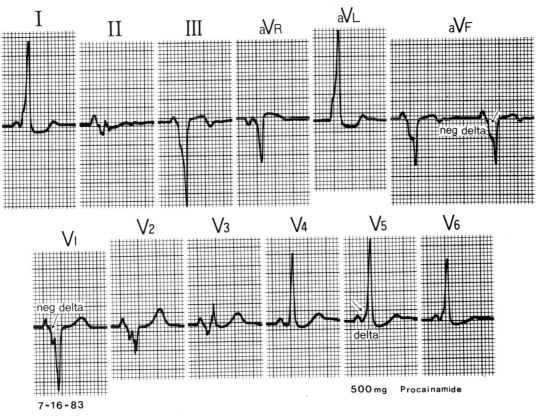

E   7-16-83   500 mg   Procainamide

Fig. 16-2. *(Continued)* **E,** An ECG made after the intravenous administration of 500 mg procainamide shows sinus rhythm with the pre-excitation remaining. The negative delta waves in V_1 and V_2 and positive delta waves in the LV leads suggest an accessory bundle situated anteriorly in the RV as in type C W-P-W.[*]

[*] If the delta wave is anterior but the QRS is posterior so that V_1 has an rS, this is called type B W-P-W.

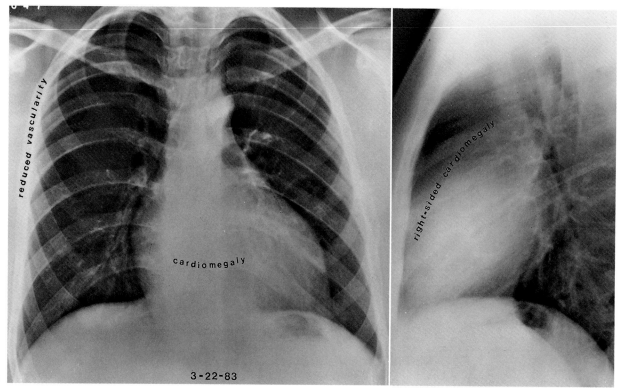

F   3-22-83   G

Fig. 16-2. *(Continued)* **F**, Preoperative chest x-rays show generalized cardiomegaly especially involving the RA. There is decreased pulmonary vascularity. The aortic arch is also small. **G**, The right-sided cardiac enlargement is evident.

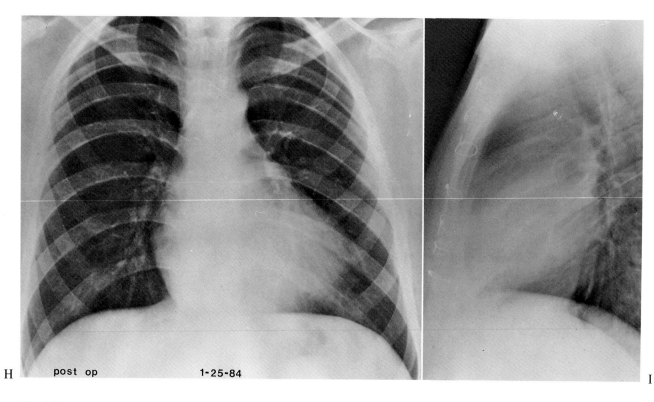

H   post op   1-25-84   I

Fig. 16-2. *(Continued)* **H**, Approximately 6 weeks postoperatively, his chest x-rays show a decrease in the size of the RA and of the entire cardiac silhouette. Pulmonary vascularity remains unchanged. **I**, The left lower cardiac border, however, is unusual in that the apex is elevated and blurred. This may be due to the smaller right-sided heart reduced by valvuloplasty.

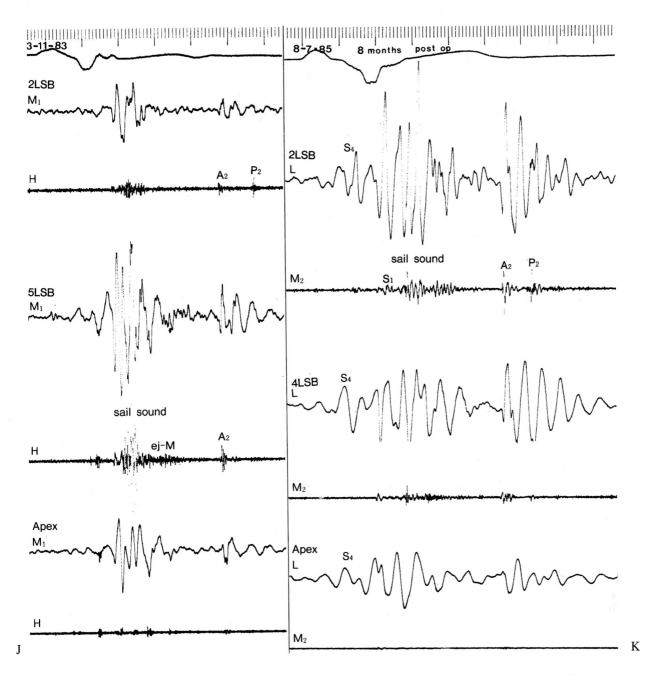

Fig. 16-2. *(Continued)* **J**, Preoperative PCG shows a large sail sound with a soft ejection murmur (ej-M) at the 5LSB. There is no S_3 or S_4, and splitting of S_2 is seen only at the 2LSB. **K**, PCG made 8 months postoperatively shows decreased amplitude of the sail sound at the 4LSB. Narrower splitting of S_2 and a newly appearing S_4 are now seen. Since this S_4 is present from the 2LSB to the 4LSB, a right-sided cardiac origin is suspected.

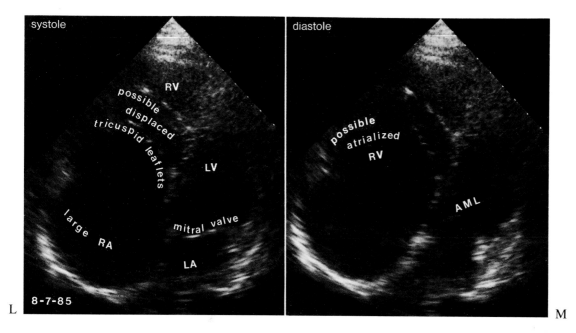

Fig. 16-2. *(Continued)* **L,** Postoperative echoes in the four-chamber view of the same patient show the mitral valve to be closed during systole. The tricuspid valve is still displaced into the RV and its movement is not clearly seen. **M,** In diastole, the mitral valve is open but the displaced tricuspid valve is obscure. During both systole and diastole, a dilated RA and possibly an atrialized RV are seen. The RV appears to be small.

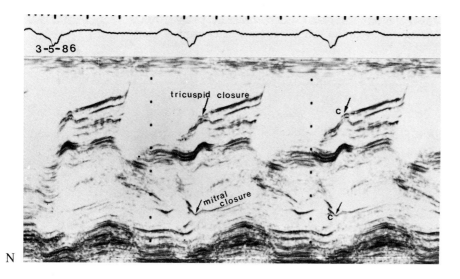

Fig. 16-2. *(Continued)* **N,** A postoperative M-mode echo with simultaneous recording of the tricuspid and mitral valves shows about a 0.04 seconds delay in closure of the tricuspid valve, indicated by the large arrow. Smaller arrows indicate the closure of the mitral valve. This delay of tricuspid closure must have been longer preoperatively, and it produced splitting of S_1 with a loud second component which is termed a "sail sound."

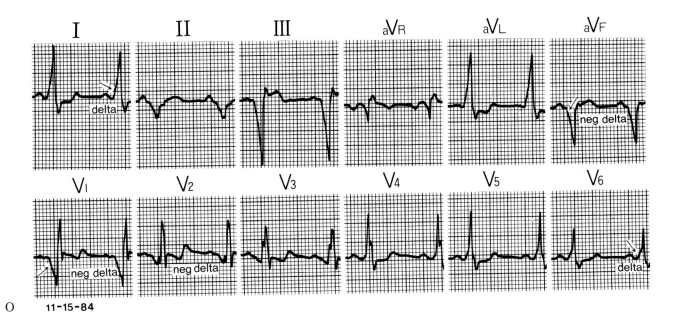

O   11-15-84

Fig. 16-2. *(Continued)* **O**, An ECG made about 3 years postoperatively, shows a W-P-W type atrioventricular pre-excitation which is different from his preoperative ECG. At surgery, epicardial mapping showed early excitation at the diaphragmatic and anterior RV wall. An incision at these sites did not resolve the W-P-W conduction.* The patient has not developed PSVT postoperatively.

* Preoperatively there was a negative delta wave with a negative QRS in V₁, which became terminally positive postoperatively. This suggests that there was another accessory bundle on the LV side. The terminal conduction change is a force proceeding to the right and anteriorly, and it is slow; it is actually a RBBB, which is expected only if the initial accessory pathway is in the LV.

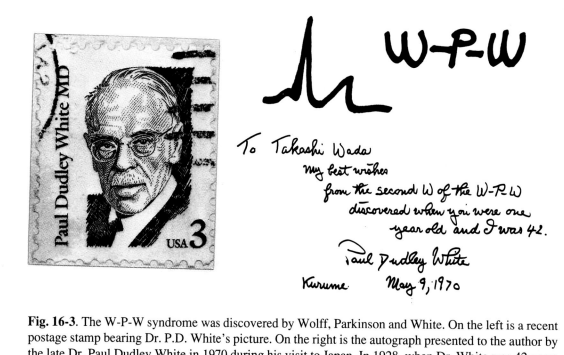

Fig. 16-3. The W-P-W syndrome was discovered by Wolff, Parkinson and White. On the left is a recent postage stamp bearing Dr. P.D. White's picture. On the right is the autograph presented to the author by the late Dr. Paul Dudley White in 1970 during his visit to Japan. In 1928, when Dr. White was 42 years old, the W-P-W syndrome was discovered.

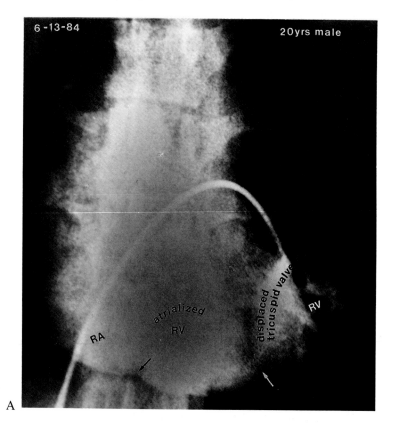

A

Fig. 16-4. A, This angiogram is from a 20-year-old man with Ebstein's anomaly. The tip of the catheter is in the RV where marked trabeculations are observed. Proximal to the RV, there is an indentation indicating the site of a displaced tricuspid valve (white arrow). At the lower margin of the RA, there is another indentation demarcating the AV junction (black arrow). Between the AV junction and the displaced tricuspid valve is the atrialized RV.

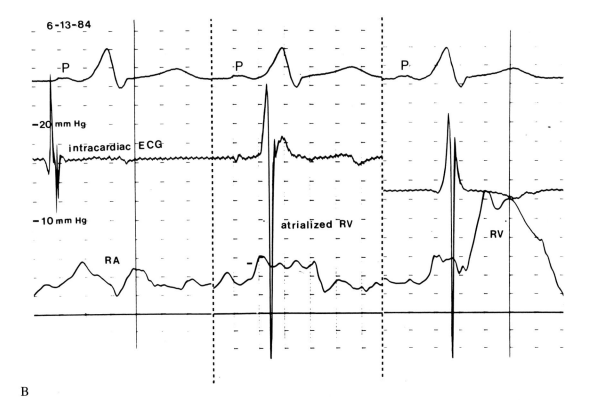

B

Fig. 16-4. *(Continued)* **B,** This is an intracardiac ECG tracing of the same patient. On the left, the intracardiac ECG tracing of the upper portion of the RA coincides with the beginning of the P wave of the conventional ECG indicating atrial activation. In the middle, an intracardiac ECG tracing low in the RA, simultaneous with the QRS complex of the conventional ECG and the pressure curve, shows the atrial tracing which demonstrates atrialized RV activation. On the right, the RV pressure curve is shown, and the peak of the intracardiac tracing is simultaneous with that of the R wave of the conventional ECG.

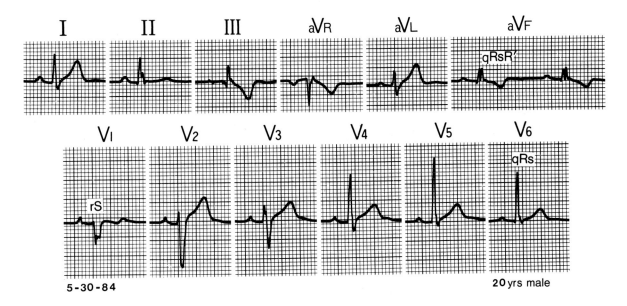

C

Fig. 16-4. *(Continued)* **C,** An ECG tracing of the same patient when he was first referred showed a slightly peaked P in V_1 and V_2 and a negative T in aVF. There is a minor degree of atypical incomplete RBBB pattern. It is atypical because instead of an R' in V_1 there is only a notch on the ascending limb of the S wave.

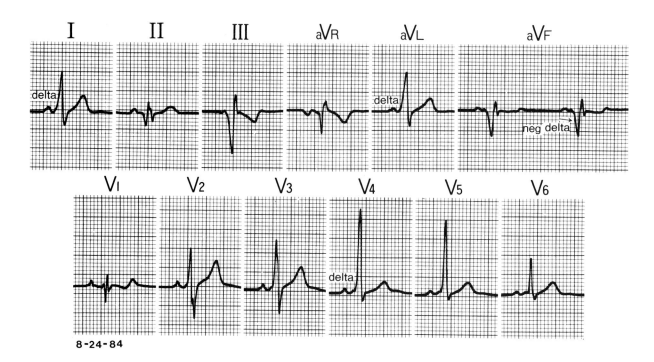

8-24-84

Fig. 16-4. *(Continued)* **D,** During his hospitalization, the patient's ECG showed a W-P-W AV pre-excitation pattern with an rsr's' in V₁. Although a short P-R interval and delta waves are seen, the rsr's' pattern in V₁ is rather unusual for W-P-W conduction. Since the patient had only one episode of PSVT, he is under follow-up observation every 6 months.

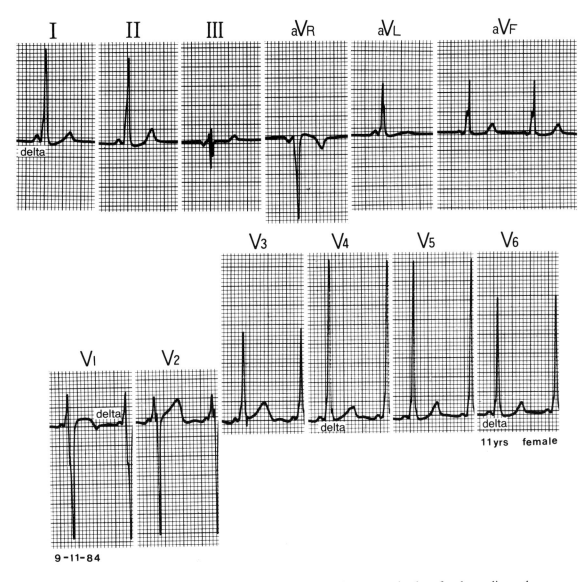

Fig. 16-5. A, This ECG is from an 11-year-old schoolgirl who had frequent episodes of tachycardia, and it shows the W-P-W AV pre-excitation. The delta waves are positive in the RV and LV leads, suggesting that an accessory bundle is in the posterior region of the heart.

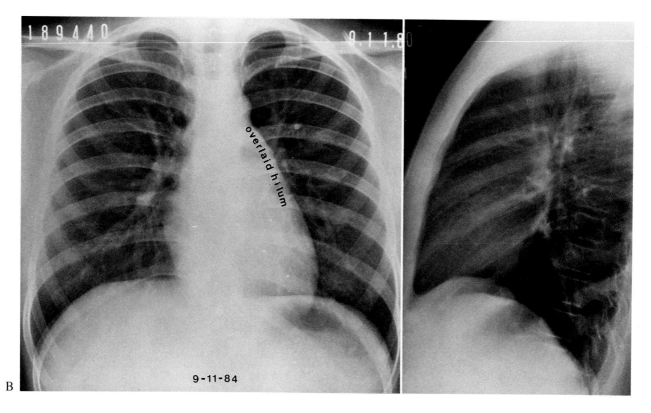

overlaid hilum

9-11-84

B

Fig. 16-5. *(Continued)* **B**, Her chest x-rays show an overlaid hilum so that the main PA is not visible. On the lateral view, the anterior cardiac margin seems to abut more than one third of the sternum, suggesting right-sided cardiac enlargement.

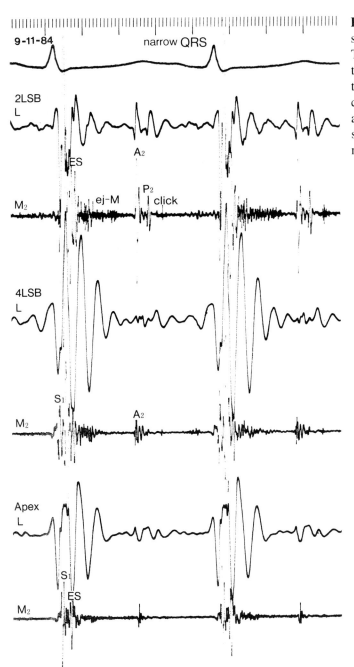

C

Fig. 16-5. *(Continued)* **C**, A PCG shows a prominent ejection sound (ES) followed by a small friction rub-like murmur. There is splitting of S₂ followed by a click which may be a tricuspid opening snap. On the first examination of the patient, the ejection sound was thought to be a sail sound, and considering the findings of the ECG and chest x-rays, Ebstein's anomaly was suspected. When this PCG was made, the ECG showed a normal sinus rhythm, narrow QRS complexes, and normal P waves.

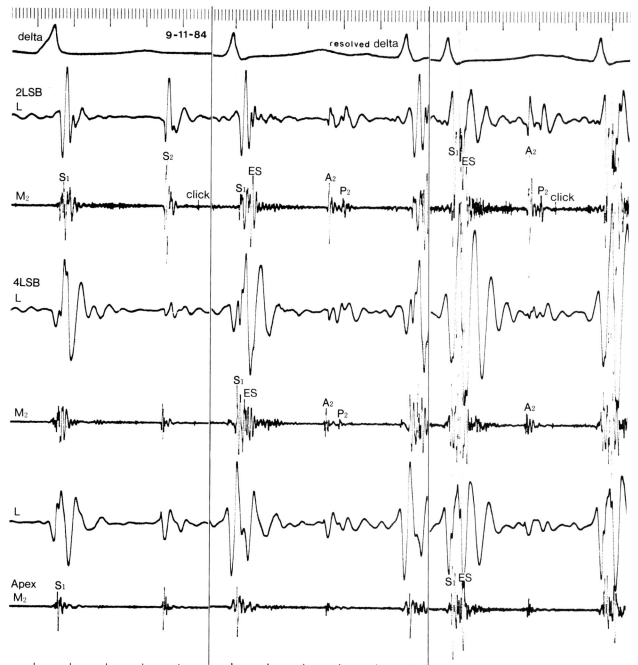

Fig. 16-5. *(Continued)* **D**, On the left, a change in the patient's posture from sitting to lying reproduced the W-P-W AV pre-excitation with normalization of the PCG findings, except for the early diastolic click. In the center, the ECG shows a narrowed QRS complex, the ejection sound (ES), and splitting of S_2. On the right, normalization of the ECG produces a large ejection sound, splitting S_2, and a diastolic click. There is also a systolic friction rub or cardiorespiratory murmur. This patient is a pingpong player and has frequent episodes of tachycardia while picking the ball up off the floor. In addition to the W-P-W syndrome, her chest x-rays suggest right-sided cardiac enlargement. Therefore, Ebstein's anomaly was suspected. Retrospectively, however, her AV pre-excitation could easily be induced by changing her posture from sitting to lying, or by holding her breath. Intensive echo studies did not disclose Ebstein's anomaly.

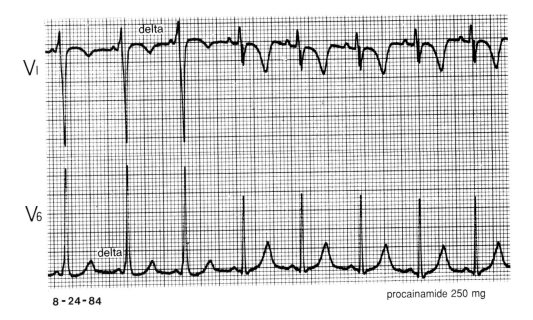

Fig. 16-5. *(Continued)* **E**, When her ECG did not change with changes in her posture, 250 mg procainamide intravenously easily converted her pre-excitation to normal conduction.

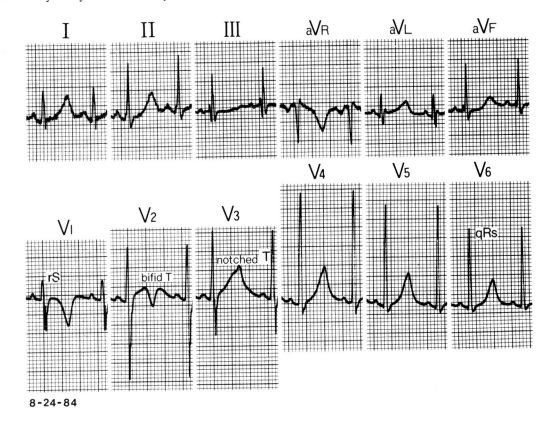

Fig. 16-5. *(Continued)* **F**, Her ECG after resolution of the AV pre-excitation following procainamide shows sinus rhythm with a rate of 100. The T wave is negative in V_1, deeply notched in V_2, and slightly notched in V_3. This is probably due to procainamide effect and is a normal pattern.

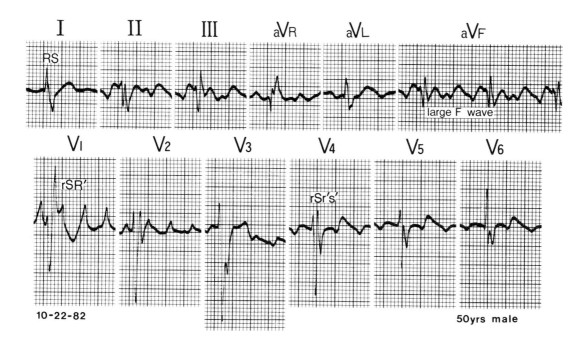

I   II   III   aVR   aVL   aVF

RS

large F wave

V1   V2   V3   V4   V5   V6

rSR'   rSr's'

10-22-82   50yrs male

A

Fig. 16-6. A, This ECG is of a 52-year-old man with Ebstein's anomaly. The patient was referred because of a tachyarrhythmia. There were large amplitude flutter waves in leads aV_F and V_1 which had an rSR' pattern. The QRS axis is indeterminate.

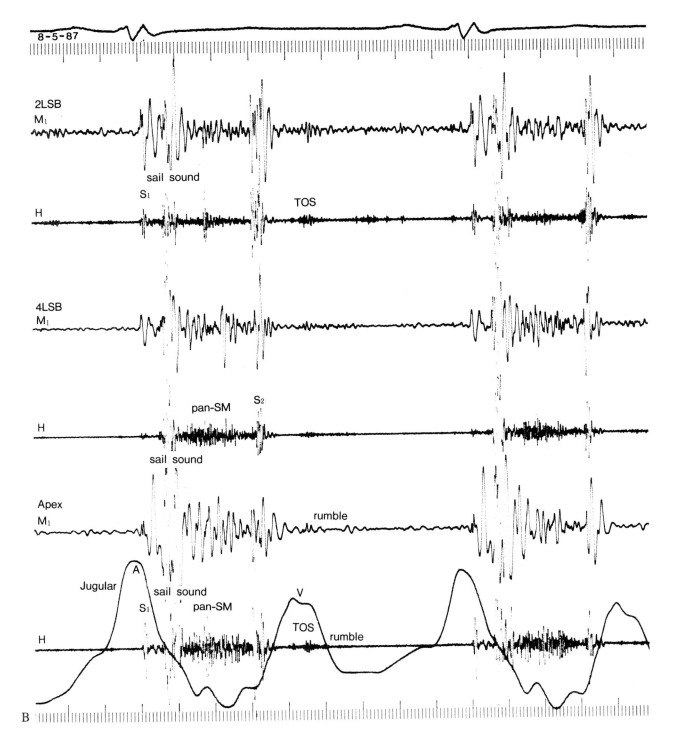

Fig. 16-6. *(Continued)* **B**, A PCG of the same patient shows a loud sail sound with a soft pansystolic murmur (pan-SM) from the cardiac base to the apex. There is also a tricuspid opening snap (TOS) and there may be a soft diastolic rumble. In the jugular tracing, a prominent V wave indicates some tricuspid regurgitation.

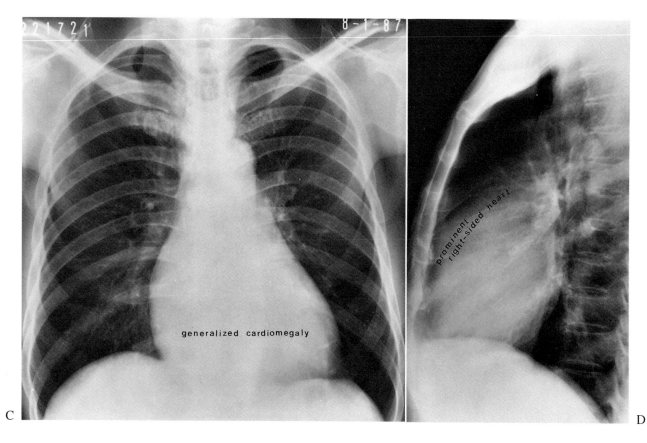

C

D

Fig. 16-6. *(Continued)* **C,** His chest x-rays show moderate generalized cardiomegaly with a dilated RA and relatively reduced pulmonary vascularity. **D,** In the lateral view, there is a prominent silhouette of the right-sided heart. His echo was not conclusive, but his angiogram was typical of Ebstein's anomaly, as indicated by the 2 indentations between the RA and the atrialized RV, and between the latter and the RV.

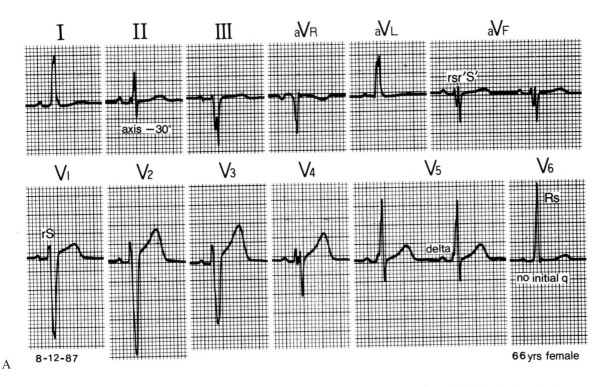

Fig. 16-7. **A**, ECG of a 66-year-old asymptomatic woman with hypertension (160/90). She has had no episodes of tachycardia. Her ECG shows a QRS axis of −30°. There are no septal q waves in the LV leads. A probable delta wave in V_5 suggests AV pre-excitation or an incomplete LBBB pattern.

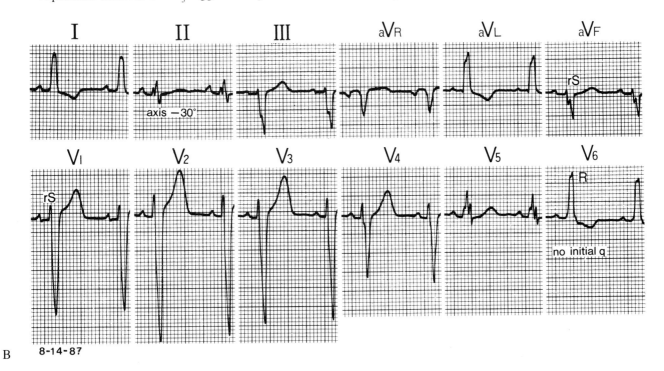

Fig. 16-7. *(Continued)* **B**, Her ECG 2 days later shows slightly broad QRS complexes with a more complete LBBB pattern. The previously noted positive T wave in V_6 is now inverted and the QRS axis remains unchanged.

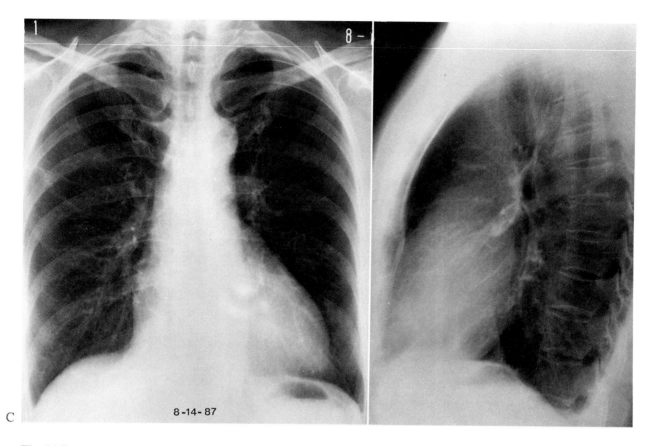

C

Fig. 16-7. *(Continued)* **C,** Chest x-rays of the same patient show a slightly prominent aortic arch (probably due to hypertension) as well as cardiomegaly.

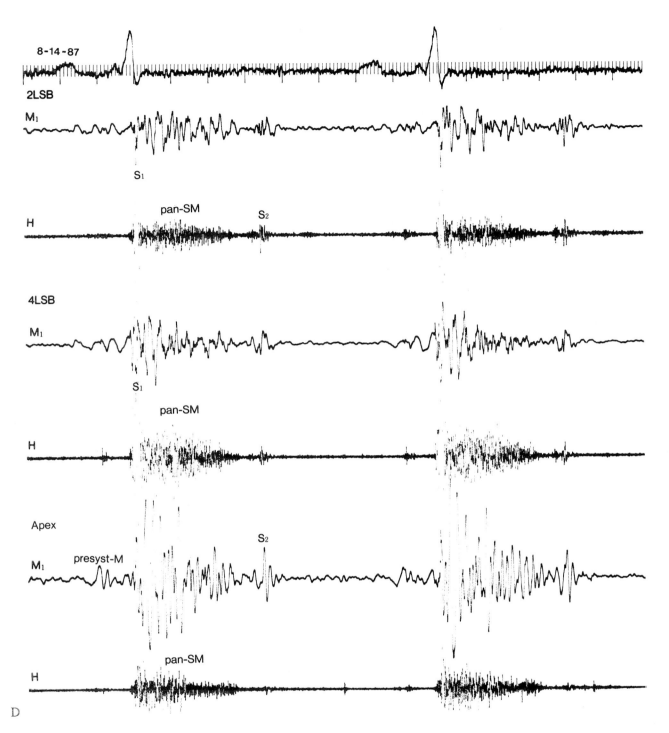

Fig. 16-7. *(Continued)* **D**, Her PCG shows a pansystolic decrescendo murmur (pan-SM) from the base to the apex. There is no sail sound, splitting S$_2$, or tricuspid opening snap. There is, however, a soft presystolic murmur (prest-M) at the apex.

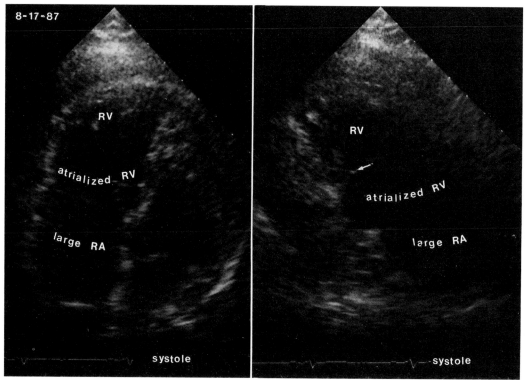

Fig. 16-7. *(Continued)* **E**, The echoes in the subxiphoid view of the same patient show a large RA and the atrialized RV. A muscular protrusion separates the atrialized RV from the RV indicated by an arrow.

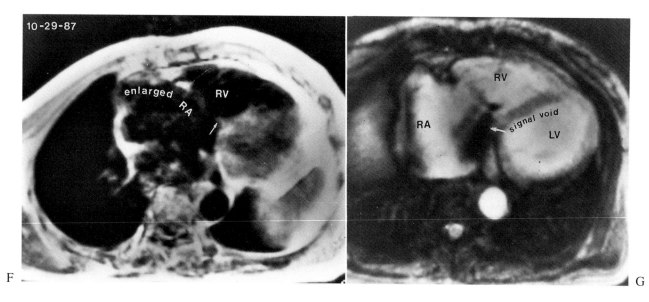

Fig. 16-7. *(Continued)* **F**, MRI confirmed the echo findings. The tricuspid ring is displaced inferiorly, resulting in an atrialized RV. There is abundant subepicardial fat around the heart indicated by a high signal intensity which appears as white. **G**, On the right, a cine MRI shows a large RA and there is a signal void between the RV and RA, suggesting the presence of tricuspid regurgitation. Ebstein's anomaly is thought to be a rare condition, but a careful examination may disclose its presence even with normal chest x-rays, as in this case.

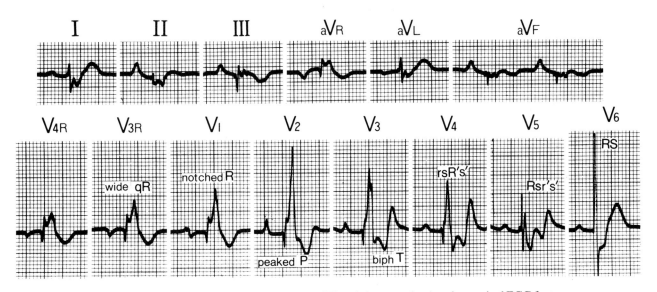

Fig. 16-8. W-P-W pre-excitation is one of the ECG features of Ebstein's anomaly. Another typical ECG feature of this anomaly is a wide rsR′ pattern in V_1 with negative-positive biphasic T waves in the right and mid precordium. This ECG from a 27-year-old man with Ebstein's anomaly shows wide QRS complexes with negative-positive biphasic T waves in V_2 to V_5. There are peaked P waves in leads II, aVF and V_2 and V_3. The QRS complexes in V4R and V_1 are those of qR with a wide notched R wave. The q waves in V4R and V_2 are probably due to the enlarged RA.[*]

[*] A qR or QR in the right precordium suggests that the chest electrode is over a large right atrium.

Chapter 17 Corrected Transposition of the Great Arteries

Pathophysiology and Clinical Clues

Corrected transposition (C/T) is caused by atrioventricular and ventriculoatrial discordance in which the PA arises from a venous ventricle which is a morphological LV. The Ao arises from an arterial systemic ventricle which is a left-sided morphological RV and is located anteriorly. The PA is located posteriorly. Since the A-V valves are actually ventricular structures, the mitral valve is on the right and the tricuspid valve on the left. The inverted left-sided tricuspid valve may become incompetent and produce tricuspid regurgitation (TR) due to the high pressure in the systemic RV. Otherwise, the condition may be overlooked until it is incidentally discovered. In some cases, an associated membranous type of VSD may draw earlier attention to this anomaly.

Approaches to the diagnosis of C/T in adults are as follows:

★★★★ The chest x-ray often shows the ascending Ao as a convex opacity arising from the left cardiac margin and continuing to the aortic arch. The main PA is usually not seen because it is medially displaced behind the Ao. In the lateral projection, the ascending Ao is often seen anteriorly.

★★★★ An ECG shows absence of the septal q wave in leads V_6, with or without a QS pattern in V_1. A deep Q wave with an upright T wave in aVF and left-axis deviation are common.

★★★★ A echo in the four-chamber view shows a right-sided mitral ring which is higher than the tricuspid ring on the left.

★ Auscultatory findings are not characteristic unless there is associated tricuspid regurgitation or other congenital anomalies.

Noninvasive methods are usually sufficient to raise suspicion of C/T; however, angiography, DSA, cardiac CT, and/or MRI are necessary for definitive diagnoses.

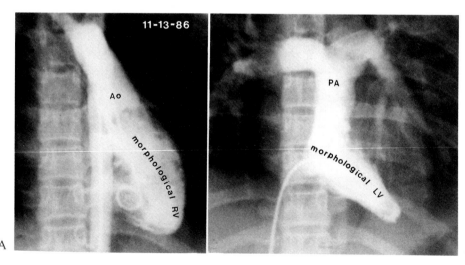

Fig. 17-1. Angiograms from a 13-year-old asymptomatic school girl whose C/T was found during an annual physical examination. **A,** On the left, in the frontal view the Ao arises anteriorly from a trabeculated, left-sided RV. **B,** On the right, in the lateral view a posteriorly-located PA arises from a nontrabeculated, right-sided LV.

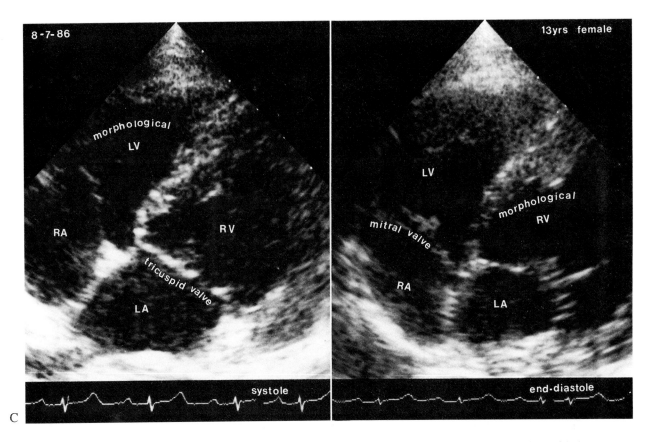

C

Fig. 17-1. *(Continued)* **C,** The echoes in the subcostal four-chamber view of the same patient show a right-sided atrioventricular valve which is higher than that on the left, indicating that the former is the mitral valve. The left-sided RV is identified by its trabeculated endocardium.

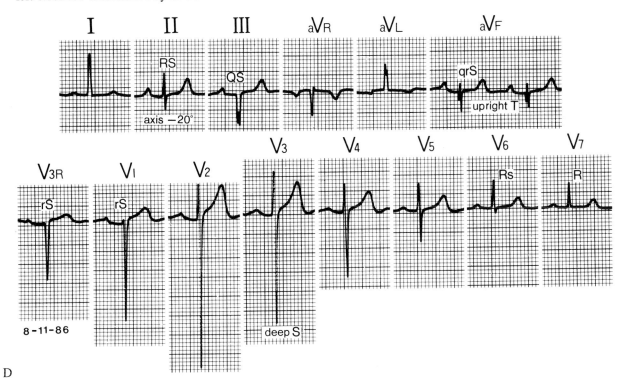

D

Fig. 17-1. *(Continued)* **D,** An ECG of the patient shows a qrS complex in aVF with an upright T wave and a QRS axis of about −20°. Absence of initial septal q waves in I and V_6 indicates abnormal septal activation which occurs from the right-sided LV toward the left-sided RV.[*]

---

[*] In C/T, because of right-to-left septal forces V_1 is expected to show a qrS or QS pattern. However, it is often rS, as in this case, for unknown reasons. However, it may be postulated that an early activation of the right-sided LV free wall causes an rS pattern.

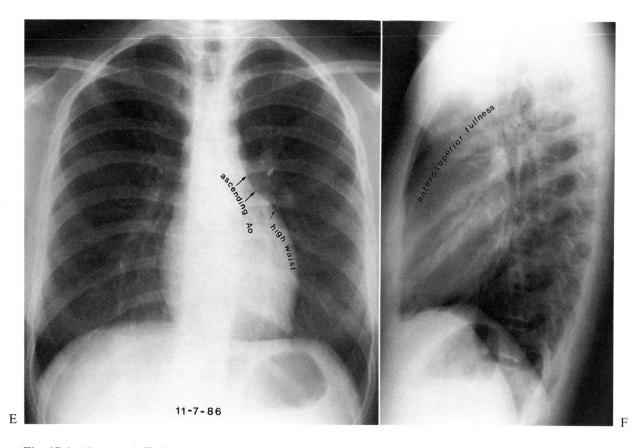

E

F

Fig. 17-1. *(Continued)* **E**, Her chest x-rays show a narrow cardiac base or pedicle. The main PA segment is invisible. The upper portion of the left lower cardiac border is prominent and contiguous with a straight upper cardiac border connecting a left-sided arch, indicating an anterolaterally-located Ao. **F**, In the lateral view, the fullness in the anterosuperior portion of the heart represents the ascending Ao.

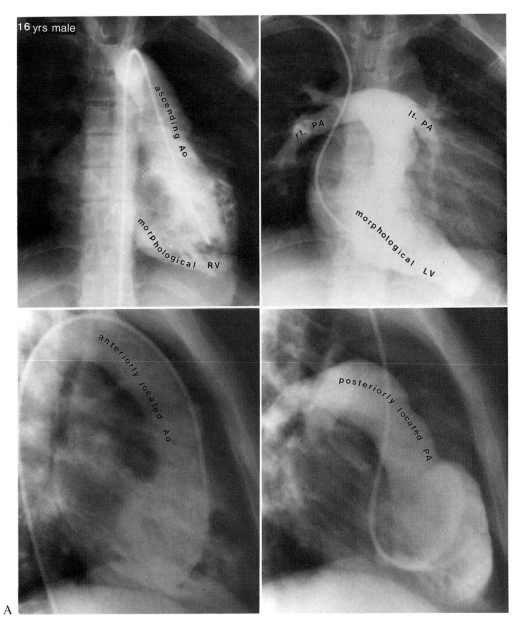

Fig. 17-2. A, Angiograms from a 16-year-old asymptomatic male high school student suspected of having C/T during an annual physical examination. The anterolaterally-located Ao arising from the trabeculated left-sided RV shows on the left. On the right is the posteromedially-located main PA which arises from the right-sided LV.

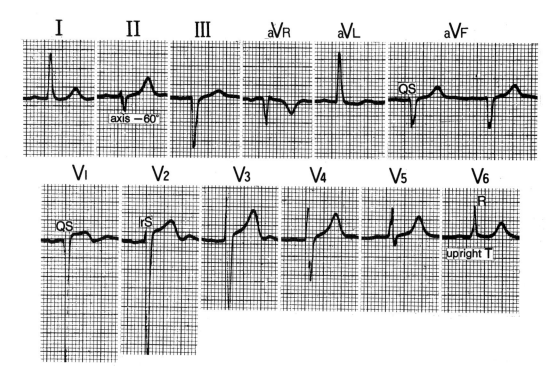

Fig. 17-2. *(Continued)* **B**, His ECG shows about −60° left-axis deviation (LAD) and there is an absence of the septal q wave in leads I and V₆ with upright T waves. A narrow QRS with an upright T wave in V₆ differentiates this from the usual LBBB. There is a QS pattern in V₁.

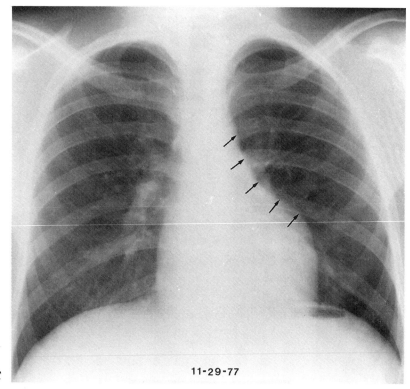

Fig. 17-2. *(Continued)* **C**, Frontal chest x-ray shows the ascending Ao which originates from the left-sided RV as indicated by arrows resulting in an unusual contour with a high waist of the left upper cardiac border.

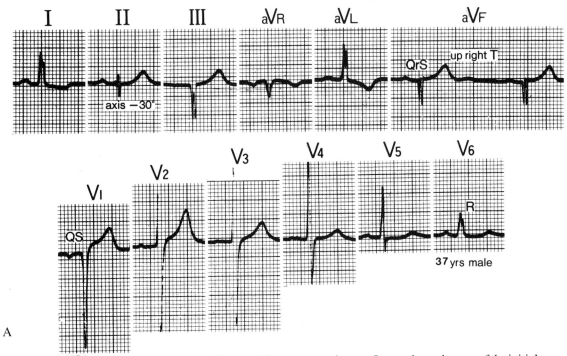

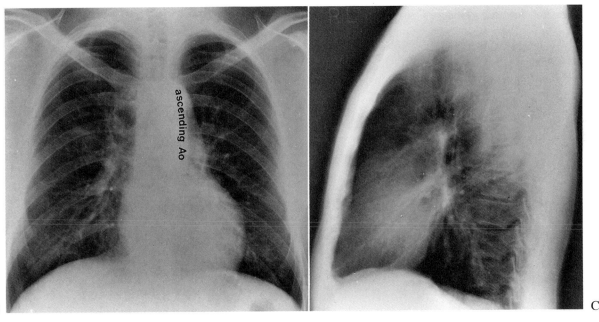

Fig. 17-3. A, This ECG is from a 37-year-old asymptomatic man. It reveals an absence of the initial q wave in leads I and V_6 with an upright T wave in V_6. There is a QS pattern in V_1. The QRS axis is nearly $-30°$. The low amplitude of QRS complex in V_6 in comparison to leads V_4 and V_5 is probably caused by a medially located systemic ventricle and is a common finding in C/T.

Fig. 17-3. *(Continued)* **B,** His chest x-rays show the ascending Ao arising from the left-sided RV. The left hilum is completely hidden by the abnormally positioned ascending Ao and its height is at nearly the same level as that of the right. **C,** In the lateral view, the anteriorly-located Ao is obscure. (Courtesy of S. Ohta, M.D.)

Chapter 18 Pericarditis

Pathophysiology and Clinical Clues

Pericarditis is an infection and/or inflammation of the pericardium. The epicardium, or visceral pericardium, is 5 to 6 μ thick; the parietal pericardium is about 1 mm thick. These 2 layers envelop a potential space termed the pericardial sac; it usually contains 25 to 30 ml of fluid which lubricates the surfaces and prevents friction. Acute pericarditis is most often caused by a virus but the causative virus usually cannot be isolated. Tuberculosis, collagen diseases, uremia, metastasis, myxedema, and aortic dissection may also produce pericarditis. If such pericardial effusions are massive, 2 to 3 L of fluid may accumulate. When a massive effusion develops in a short period of time, cardiac tamponade may result. When tamponade occurs, a paradoxical pulse (an enhanced physiological phenomenon indicated by an abnormal lowering of the blood pressure and pulse pressure during normal inspiration) may occur. In its chronic form, adhesions and calcification of the 2 layers of the pericardium may result in constrictive pericarditis. Pericardial fluid is classified as being a transudate or exudate, and bloody, fibrous, or purulent. Either in massive effusions or in constrictive pericarditis, engorged veins in the neck, an enlarged liver, and ascites may be seen.

Approaches to the diagnosis of pericarditis are as follows:

★★★★ Auscultation reveals friction rubs. In massive pericardial effusion, the heart sounds are distant. In constrictive pericarditis, there is often a loud early S_3 or pericardial knock.

★★★★ The ECG shows ST elevations in all leads except aVR. T waves are upright unless the deeper layers of the myocardium are involved.

★★★ The chest x-ray diagnosis of pericarditis is difficult unless the condition is associated with at least a moderate pericardial effusion. In such cases, cardiac enlargement without increased pulmonary vascularity is observed. Widening of the cardiac base and thickening of the anterior pericardial stripe may be observed. Marked calcification around the cardiac margin is common in constrictive pericarditis especially in the lateral view.

★★★ An erroneous diagnosis of minimal pericardial effusion can be made on echo. The extra echo spaces (EES) in many cases are due to subepicardial fat, especially in elderly persons. Therefore, unless the EES is seen in young persons, the diagnosis of small pericardial effusion by echo is difficult. In massive effusions, an EES is apparent both in the anterior and posterior aspects of the heart, and the heart exhibits a pendular motion.

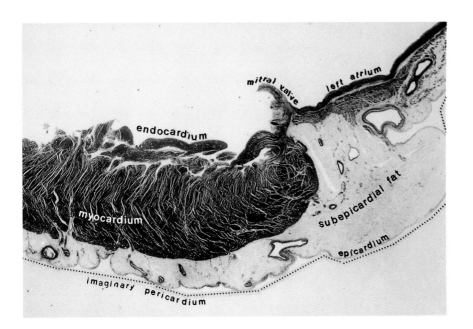

Fig. 18-1. This pathologically normal specimen shows·the relationships of the myocardium, epicardium (visceral pericardium), and parietal pericardium. Between the epicardium and outer surface of the myocardium there is areolar tissue containing abundant fat in which coronary vessels and nerves are located. Between the epicardium and the parietal pericardium (dotted line) is the pericardial sac which is a potential space. Calcifications involve both the epicardium and parietal pericardium, and even the pleura. On echoes, the subepicardial fat has often been misinterpreted as a pericardial effusion.

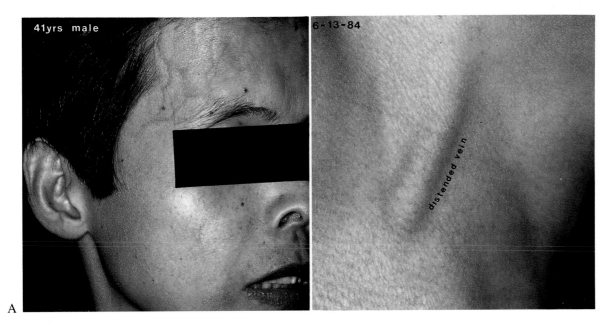

Fig. 18-2. A, Photographs of a 41-year-old man with constrictive pericarditis. The veins on his forehead and neck are engorged. The patient had pulmonary tuberculosis during his teens, he developed ascites and edema of his lower extremities about 10 years prior to admission.

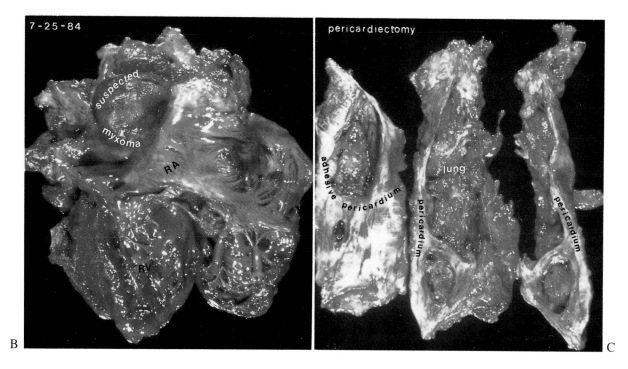

Fig. 18-2. *(Continued)* **B,** Pericardiectomy relieved his venous distension. Unfortunately, however, the patient suddenly expired 2 weeks postoperatively. **B,** A large myxoma-like thrombus was found in the RA on the left. Frontal and lateral aspects of resected specimens on the right, **C,** show fusion of the layers of pericardium with parietal and visceral pleura adherent to the lung tissue. The cause of his death was uncertain.

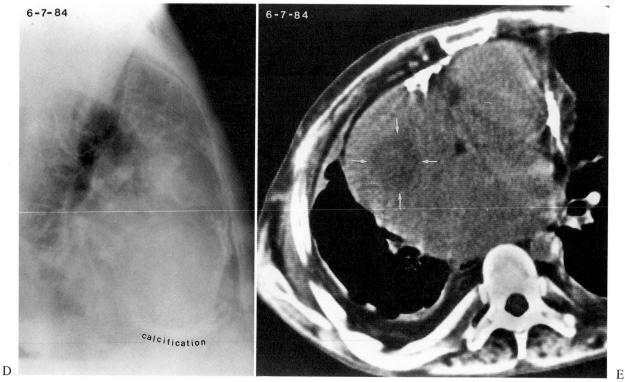

Fig. 18-2. *(Continued)* **D,** A preoperative lateral chest x-ray showed a heavily calcified pericardium anteroinferiorly encasing his heart. **E,** The cardiac CT shows marked calcification as white patches around his heart. The right lung is hypoplastic from long-standing pleurisy and caseous material in the pleural space. This cardiac CT section made at the RA level shows an enlarged RA with a circular low-density zone centrally (arrows). This was interpreted as an artifact but, at autopsy, it was found to be caused by a large thrombus in the RA.

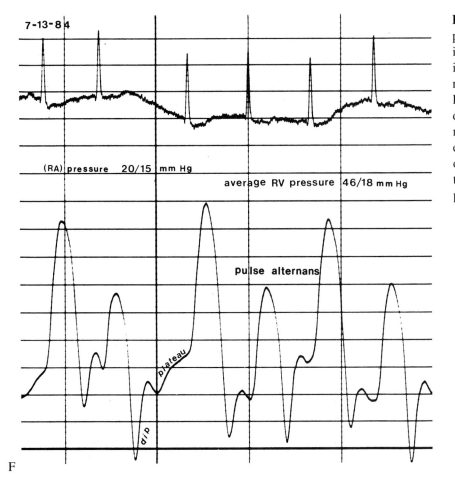

7-13-84

(RA) pressure 20/15 mm Hg

average RV pressure 46/18 mm Hg

pulse alternans

plateau

dip

F

Fig. 18-2. *(Continued)* **F,** A preoperative pressure tracing revealed an RV alternans, indicating that cardiac function was severely impaired. The pressure in the RA was 20/15 mm Hg; in the RV it was 46/18 mm Hg. The RV pressure tracing showed a deep early diastolic dip and plateau indicating marked reduction in the RV distensibility. This early diastolic dip indicates that the RV can only be distended for a very short period of time due to restriction by the constrictive pericarditis.

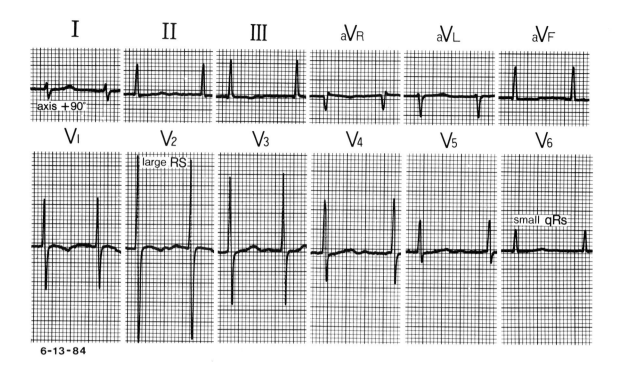

I   II   III   aVR   aVL   aVF

axis +90°

V₁   V₂   V₃   V₄   V₅   V₆

large RS

small qRs

G   6-13-84

Fig. 18-2. *(Continued)* **G,** His preoperative ECG shows atrial fibrillation at a rate of about 80. Extremity leads and V₅ and V₆ show low voltage due to thickening of the pleura, caseous material in the pleural cavity, and displacement of the heart to the right. T waves in V₅ and V₆ are low and may suggest myocardial damage.

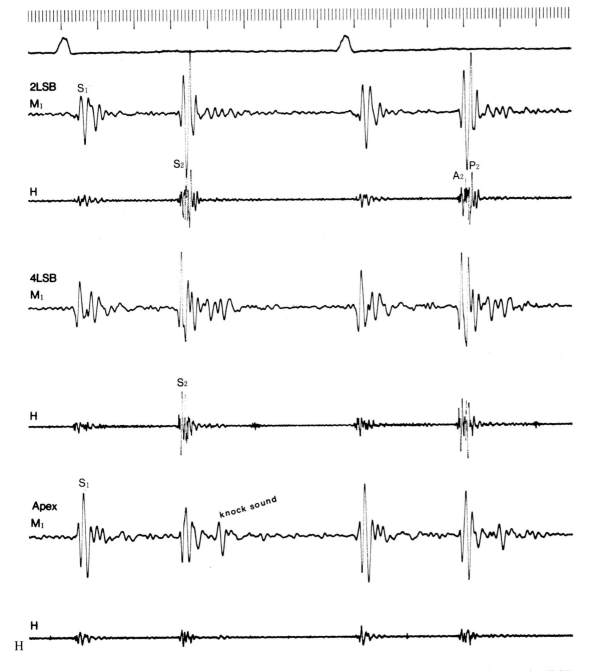

Fig. 18-2. *(Continued)* **H,** His preoperative PCG showed narrow splitting of S_2 on inspiration. At the 4LSB, a low frequency PCG shows an early diastolic sound which may represent a pericardial knock. The P_2 is loud and is transmitted to the apex.

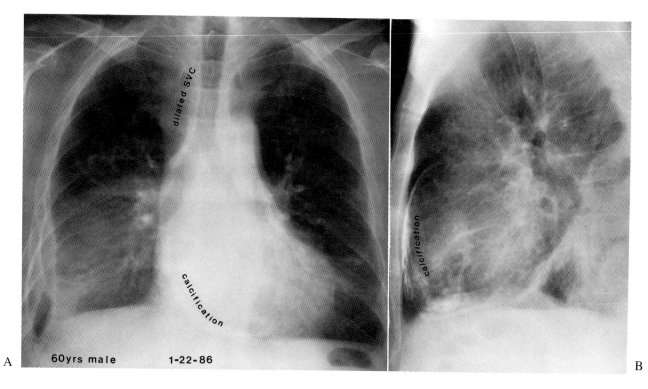

A   **60yrs male   1-22-86**   B

Fig. 18-3. A, These chest x-rays are from a 60-year-old man with constrictive pericarditis. The patient has only gastrointestinal symptoms. His pleural spaces are obliterated bilaterally, and marked calcification of the pericardium encased his heart. **B,** This is better appreciated on the lateral view. Anteriorly, linear calcification is closely attached to more than the lower one-third of the sternum, which indicates right-sided cardiac overloading.

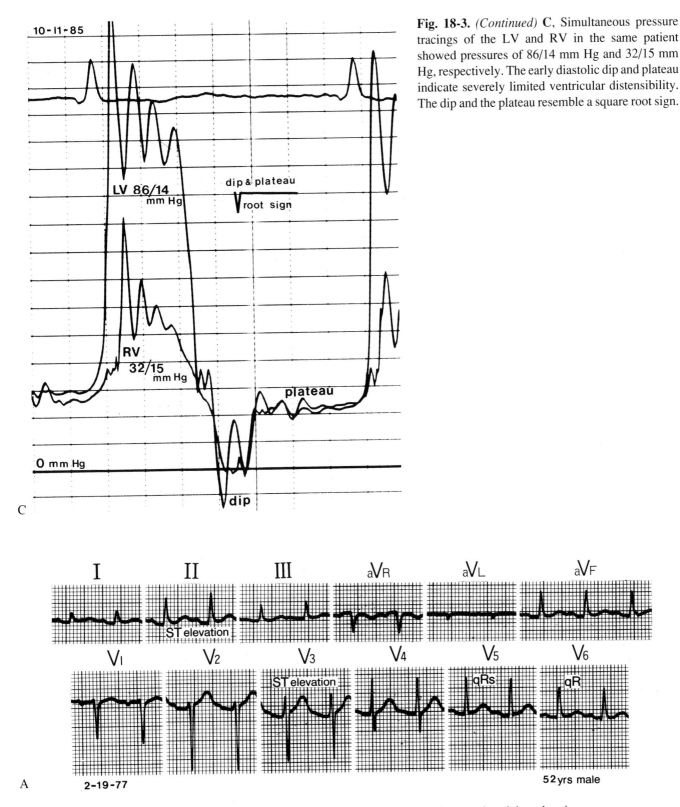

Fig. 18-3. *(Continued)* **C,** Simultaneous pressure tracings of the LV and RV in the same patient showed pressures of 86/14 mm Hg and 32/15 mm Hg, respectively. The early diastolic dip and plateau indicate severely limited ventricular distensibility. The dip and the plateau resemble a square root sign.

Fig. 18-4. A, ECG of a 52-year-old man who complained of high fever and general malaise, showing a generalized ST elevation in all leads except aVR and aVL, indicating pericarditis. The T waves are upright and there is no evidence of myocardial involvement. However, the QRS complexes tend to be low, which suggests the presence of a pericardial effusion.

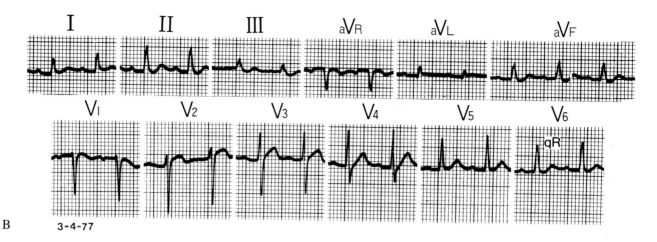

B   3-4-77

Fig. 18-4. *(Continued)* **B**, Despite our advice, the patient did not consent to enter the hospital since he had some important business. During his second visit about 3 weeks later, he was distressed and his ECG showed nearly the same findings except for shortening of the QT interval caused by digitalis.

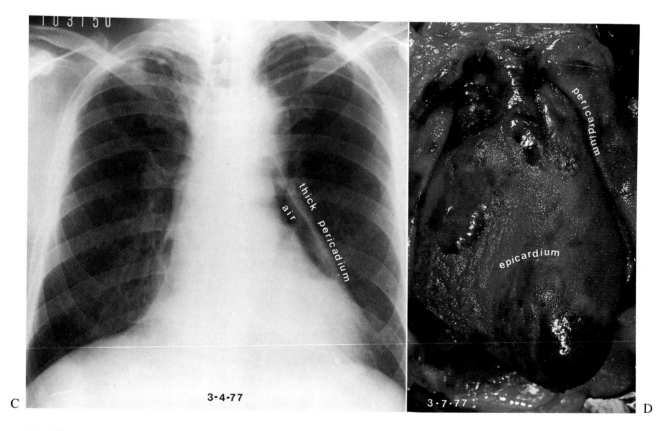

C   3-4-77   3·7·77   D

Fig. 18-4. *(Continued)* **C**, After removal of 800 ml of bloody fluid by pericardiocentesis, the patient's condition improved. The frontal chest x-ray shows thickened pericardium. He expired 3 days later. **D**, At autopsy, the epicardium had a strawberry appearance with some thrombus formation caused by acute tuberculous pericarditis.

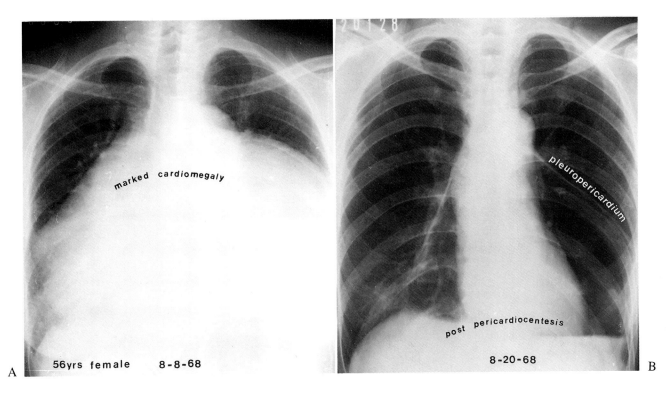

A   **56yrs female   8-8-68**   **8-20-68**   B

Fig. 18-5. A, On the left, frontal chest x-ray of a 56-year-old woman with a long-standing pericardial effusion shows marked enlargement of her cardiac silhouette, which has a water bottle configuration. The patient has hypertension which has been treated by her physician for the past several years. She gradually gained weight, developed edema of her lower extremities, her heart size increased, and she was referred. The patient was not in acute distress, but auscultation disclosed distant heart sounds. Her ECG was of low voltage. By pericardiocentesis, 3 L of tenacious yellowish fluid containing a high concentration of cholesterol were removed. **B,** After pericardiocentesis, air was instilled, and a frontal chest x-ray on the right showed a normal size heart with minimal residual pericardial fluid near the cardiac apex. This is a case of cholesterol pericarditis, which usually runs a benign course.

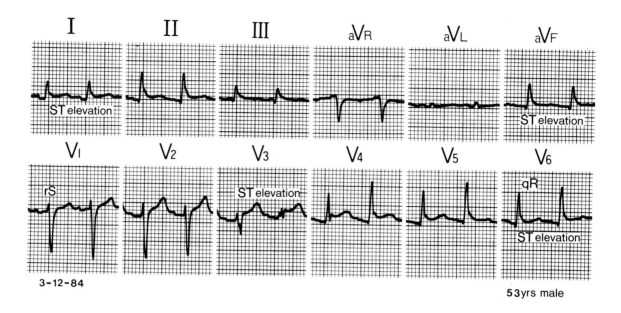

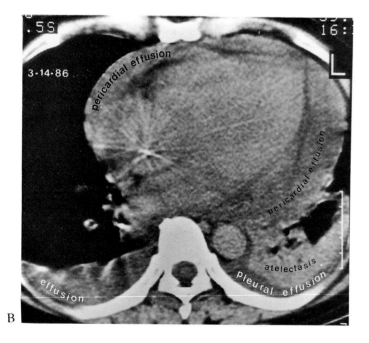

Fig. 18-6. A, This ECG is from a 53-year-old male laborer who had general malaise, fever, and increasing dyspnea. On admission, his ECG showed generalized low voltage with ST elevations in all leads except aV_R, which showed an elevated P-R segment. These are highly characteristic of the ECG in pericarditis.

Fig. 18-6. *(Continued)* **B,** His cardiac CT made 2 days later showed a massive pericardial effusion and pleural effusions bilaterally, with partial atelectasis of his left lung. The CT value was + 20 Hounsfield Units (HU) indicating that the effusion was not blood.

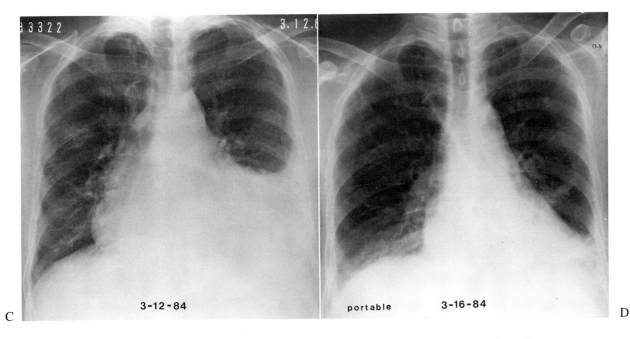

C   3-12-84   portable   3-16-84   D

Fig. 18-6. *(Continued)* **C,** His admission frontal chest x-ray, on the left, showed marked cardiac enlargement with a left pleural effusion. The base of his heart (cardiac pedicle) may be widened. **D,** On the right, a portable anteroposterior projection 4 days after admission shows that his heart size, including the base, had decreased, as did the left pleural effusion, suggesting a diagnosis of pericardial effusion.

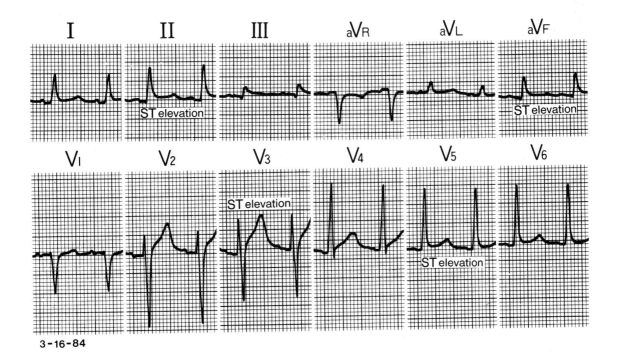

E   3-16-84

Fig. 18-6. *(Continued)* **E,** His ECG on the same day as his second chest x-ray, showed increased amplitude of the QRS and less ST elevation. Unfortunately, the patient discharged himself from the hospital and no follow-up studies were possible.

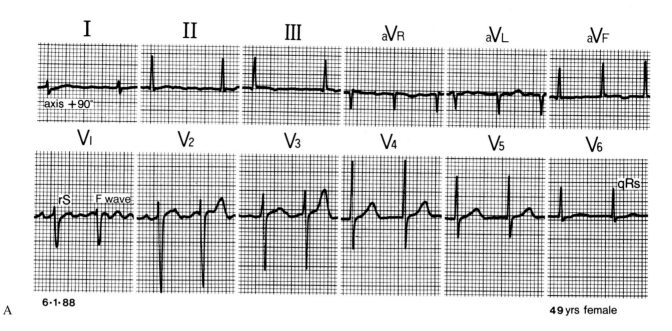

A

6·1·88

49 yrs female

Fig. 18-7. A, This 49-year-old woman complained of edema of her lower extremities. Her ECG shows a generalized low voltage with AF at about 125. There is an rS in V₁ and qRs in V₆, indicating normal septal conduction. Despite low voltage of the QRS complexes, neither ST elevation nor T wave abnormality were present. The ECG diagnosis in this case is difficult, but MS is suspected.

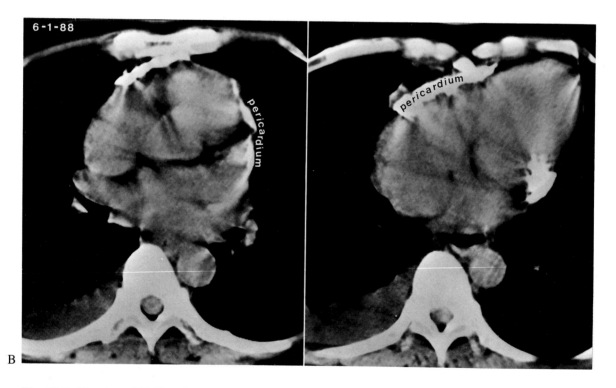

B

Fig. 18-7. *(Continued)* **B,** Her chest x-rays are not conclusive, but cardiac CT shows scattered heavy calcifications around her heart. These are especially prominent at the site of the mitral ring.

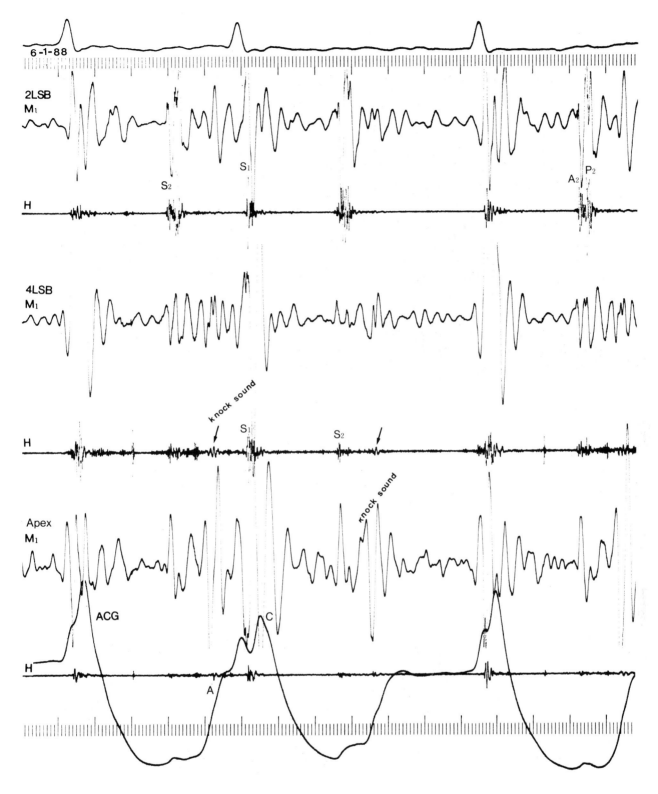

C

Fig. 18-7. *(Continued)* C, Her PCG shows slight splitting of the S_2 with a loud knock sound at the apex. Although the knock sound is of relatively low frequency, on auscultation one may misinterpret it as opening snap (OS). There are click-like sounds in systole, and the high frequency sounds following the S_2 at the 4LSB may represent a friction rub. On a jugular tracing, a tall, bifid, and/or notched wave indicates a C wave. The beginning of the C wave coincides with the first heart sound (S_1).

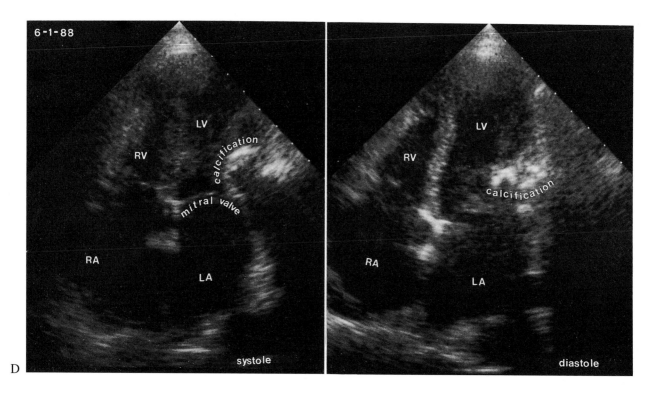

Fig. 18-7. *(Continued)* **D,** The echoes in the apical four-chamber view show heavy calcification of the LV wall just below the mitral valve. This is considered a calcified mitral ring.

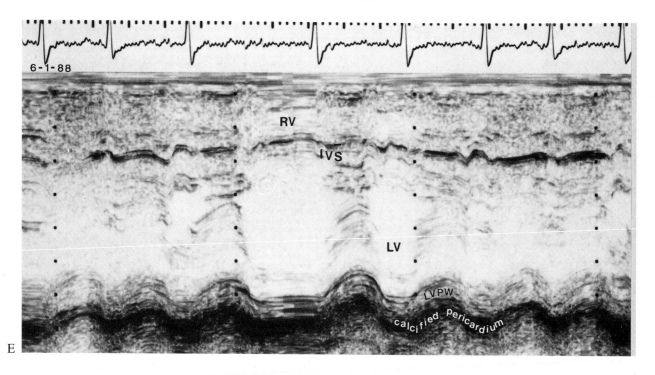

Fig. 18-7. *(Continued)* **E,** An M-mode recording of the same patient also shows a broad band-like echo abutting behind the LVPW, indicating the presence of calcified epicardium-pericardium, and it may include the calcification in the myocardium.

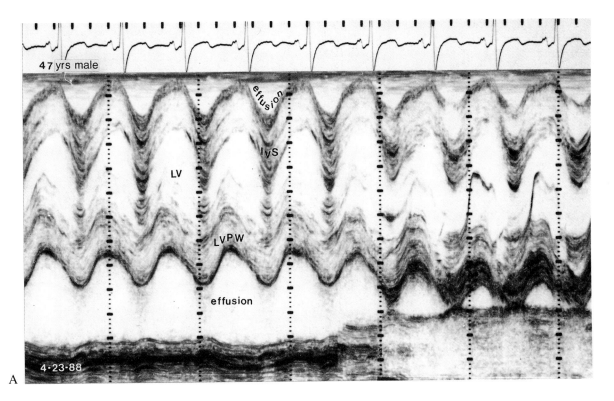

A

Fig. 18-8. A, When a massive pericardial effusion is present, the heart swings in the effusion, resulting in an alternating anterior and posterior movement during systole, termed pendular motion. This M-mode scan from base to apex (right to left) is that of a 47-year-old man with massive pericardial effusion, probably due to metastatic gastric cancer. The LVPW and the RV wall show pendular motion.

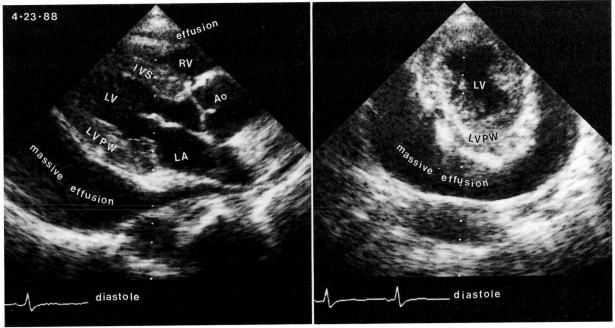

B

Fig. 18-8. *(Continued)* **B,** Both the long- and short-axis echoes show a massive pericardial effusion anterior to the RV and posterior to the LV.

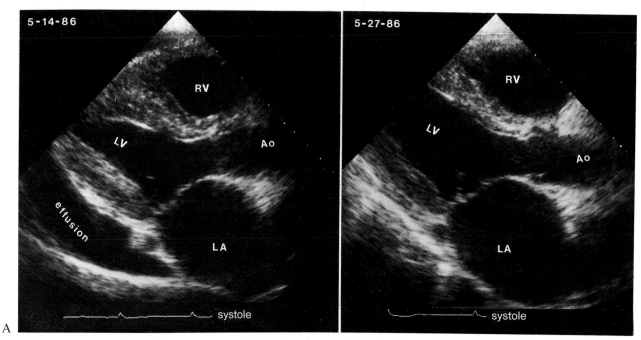

A

B

Fig. 18-9. These long-axis echoes are from a 66-year-old man with an ASD and hypertension. **A,** On the left, a long-axis view 4 weeks after surgery shows a massive pericardial effusion behind the LVPW. The LA was also enlarged from congestive heart failure caused by his hypertension. Compared to the preoperative echo, his RV had become much smaller. It is quite common to see marked pericardial effusions among postoperative patients with a long-standing ASD. It may be that a rapid reduction in size of the enlarged RV and/or malabsorption of effusion by the pericardium plays a role in the accumulation of pericardial effusions. **B,** On the right, a long-axis view made 13 days later shows nearly complete resolution of the pericardial effusion that had caused enlargement of the LV cavity

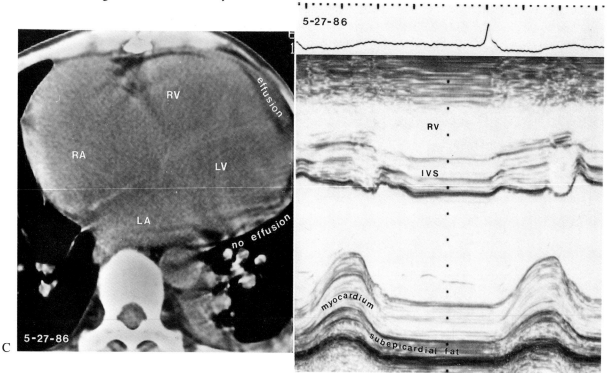

C

D

Fig. 18-9. *(Continued)* **C,** His cardiac CT made the same day shows minimal pericardial fluid anterolaterally but no obvious effusion elsewhere. **D,** An M-mode echo made the same day shows an extra echo space (EES) behind the LVPW apparently due to subepicardial fat rather than to fluid because the pericardial movement is parallel to the LVPW.

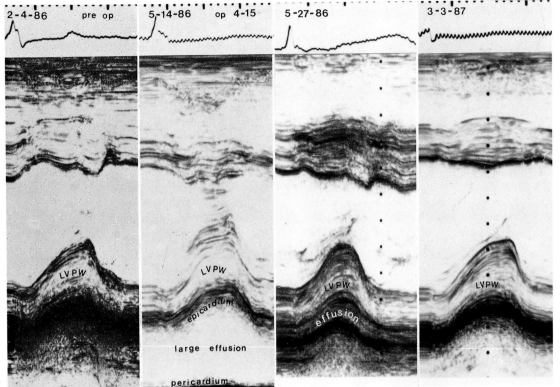

Fig. 18-9. *(Continued)* **E**, This is a serial tracing of M-mode echoes of the same patient. Preoperatively a broad band-like echo behind the LVPW is a fusion echo of the visceral and parietal pericardium. The border zone of this band-like echo and the LVPW are not clearly delineated because of the presence of subepicardial fat. Surgery was performed and an echo 1 month later shows a massive pericardial effusion. The lowest echo is parietal pericardium. A margin of the epicardial echo is not clear for the reason mentioned above. Seven weeks postoperatively, there may be a small pericardial effusion behind the LVPW. However, this is not conclusive, and it may represent the subepicardial fat. Ten months later, the visceral and parietal pericardium show a fusion echo indicating complete resolution of the pericardial effusion.

Chapter 19 Narrow Chest Syndrome

Pathophysiology and Clinical Clues

A short sternovertebral distance, equal to or less than one third the transverse thoracic diameter with or without loss of physiological thoracic spinal curvature may be termed narrow chest syndrome. Pectus excavatum is also included in the narrow chest syndrome. The narrow chest syndrome frequently occurs among those of slender stature. Since the heart is located between the sternum and the thoracic spine, the short sternovertebral diameter may cause displacement of the heart to the left, resulting in a variety of auscultatory findings such as a wide splitting of the S_2, an ejection murmur, and non-ejection clicks, which, at times, make it difficult to differentiate from mitral valve prolapse (MVP) or ASD. Furthermore, the narrow chest syndrome is often associated with other congenital abnormalities, such as the Marfan syndrome, pleuropericardial defects, MVP, and ASD. In spite of marked narrowing of the anteroposterior dimension of the cardiac silhouette on lateral chest films, there may be no specific symptoms.

Clinical findings of the narrow chest syndrome are:

★★★★ Frontal chest x-rays show the posterior portion of the ribs to be oriented horizontally so that the medial and lateral ends are at the same level. The cardiac silhouette is displaced to the left. The lateral view reveals the narrow sternovertebral dimension with or without a straight back and pectus excavatum.

★★★★ Long-axis echoes reveal a shallow aortoseptal angle with a small LV cavity. The M-mode echos show a small LV cavity and the anterior mitral leaflet touches the IVS, resulting in a rounded E point during early diastole. However, the RV cavity is not dilated, as seen in ASD. Coexisting MVP may be commonly observed.

★★★ Auscultation often reveals wide splitting of the S_2, resembling ASD. There may be an ejection murmur, clicks, and friction rub-like murmurs. The friction rub effect may be a cardiorespiratory murmur.*

★★ ECG findings are due to displacement of the heart to the left, which may show a large QRS complex in the LV leads in contrast to a small QRS localized to either V_3 or V_4, possibly due to fibrous tissue beneath the sternum, especially in cases of pectus excavatum.

* A cardiorespiratory murmur is an extracardiac murmur probably produced when the systolic motion of the heart compresses an expanded lung segment. It is high pitched, usually short, and may occur anywhere in systole or early diastole.

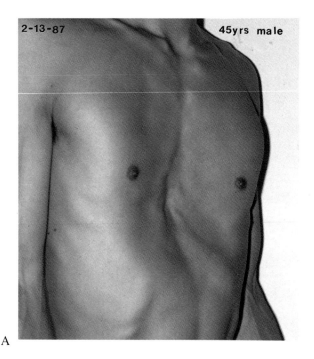

2-13-87   45yrs male

Fig. 19-1. A, This 45-year-old asymptomatic man has a severe pectus excavatum. This photograph was made while he was standing.

A

312   19. Narrow Chest Syndrome

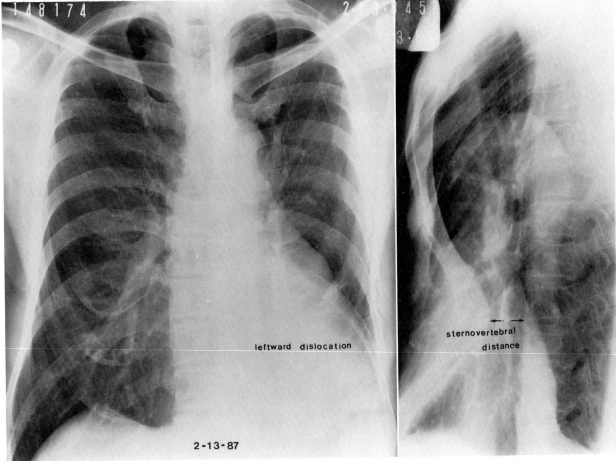

B

C

leftward dislocation

sternovertebral
distance

2-13-87

Fig. 19-1. *(Continued)* **B**, Chest x-rays of the same patient show the posterior aspects of his 3rd to 8th ribs to be horizontally oriented and rather elevated near the lateral margins of his thoracic wall.* In addition, the transverse diameter of his thorax from his 3rd to 8th ribs posteriorly is relatively short. His heart is displaced to the left and the cardiac silhouette is not seen to the right of the sternum. The diaphragm is relatively low, a manifestation of his slender stature. **C**, The lateral view shows a marked pectus excavatum involving the lower one-third of the sternum. The sternovertebral distance is only a few cm; the heart appears to be "sandwiched" between the sternum and the vertebrae, and this has been called a "pancake" heart. The heart is displaced to the left to escape being compressed in the narrow sternovertebral space.

*Horizontally oriented means that the medial and lateral ends of the posterior rib shadows are at the same level.

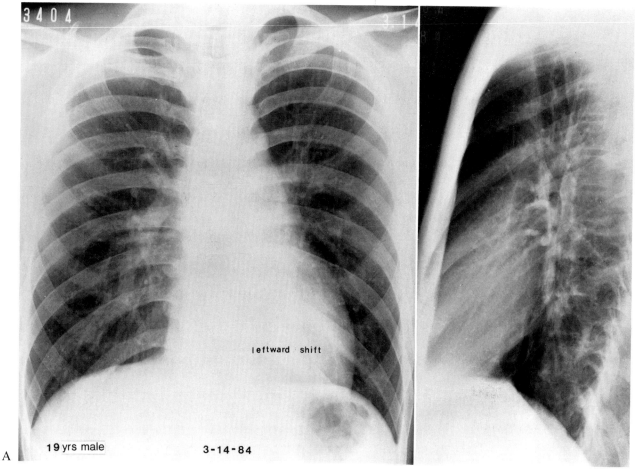

leftward shift

19 yrs male   3-14-84

A

B

Fig. 19-2. A, This is an example of a narrow chest syndrome. The patient is a 19-year-old male student with an abnormal ECG during an annual physical examination. The posterior aspects of his 3rd to 6th ribs are horizontal, but their margins near the thoracic wall are not elevated as in Figure 19-1 B and C. The cardiac silhouette is slightly displaced to the left and is not visible to the right of the sternum. **B,** The lateral view shows a narrow sternovertebral space caused by a straight thoracic spine. The sternovertebral distance on the lateral view should be greater than one-third of the transverse thoracic diameter on the frontal chest x-ray.

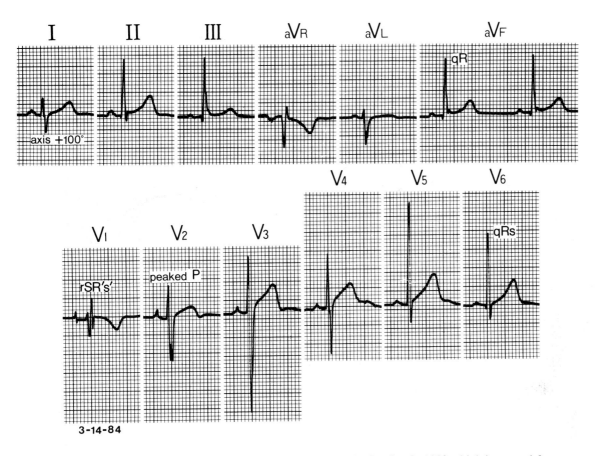

Fig. 19-2. *(Continued)* **C,** An ECG of the same patient shows a QRS axis of +100° which is normal for this age group. The P waves in V_1 and V_2 are somewhat peaked. The QRS in V_1 shows an rSR's' configuration which may suggest diastolic RV overloading. However, with absence of a marked right-axis deviation, RV overloading cannot be diagnosed with confidence. Lead aVR shows a Qr pattern indicating that the terminal QRS force is moving toward the upper portion of the RV, probably up the crista supraventricularis.

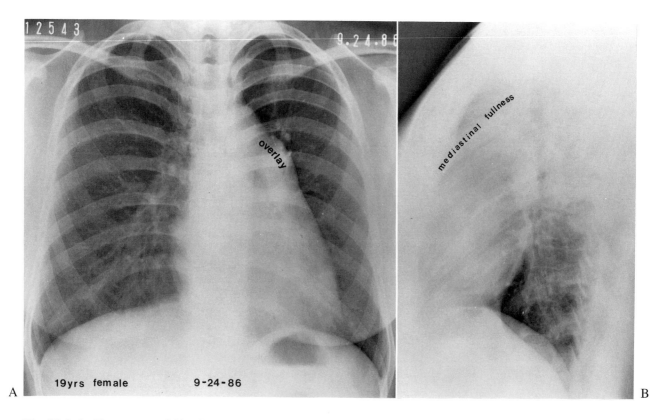

A   B

Fig. 19-3. A, Chest x-rays of this 19-year-old female student were found to be abnormal at her annual physical examination. The frontal chest view shows that the left hilum is overlaid by a central shadow. Her main PA seems to be enlarged, and the posterior aspects of her 3rd to 6th ribs are oriented horizontally suggesting the narrow chest syndrome. **B**, On the lateral view, the superior portion of her cardiac silhouette shows mediastinal fullness suggesting an anterior mediastinal mass. Her thoracic spine is straight; the sternovertebral distance is less than normal.

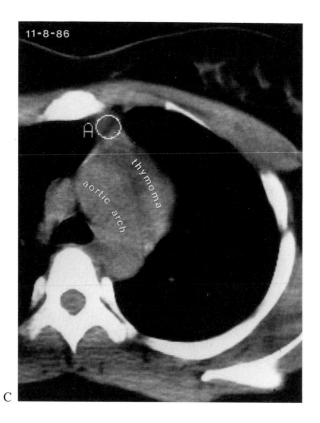

Fig. 19-3. *(Continued)* **C**, A cardiac CT section at the level of the aortic arch shows an opacity along the lateral margin of the Ao indicative of thymoma. This thymoma is the cause of hilar overlay on the frontal projection.

C

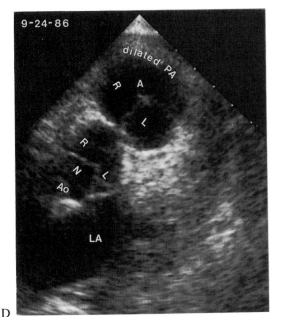

Fig. 19-3. *(Continued)* **D**, Her short-axis echo of the Ao made during diastole shows the Ao to be normal with a right cusp (R), left cusp (L) and a noncoronary cusp (N). Anterior to the Ao, a dilated right ventricular outflow tract (RVOT) and PA are visualized with an anterior (A), right (R) and left cusp (L). Posterior to the Ao, a normal size LA is observed.

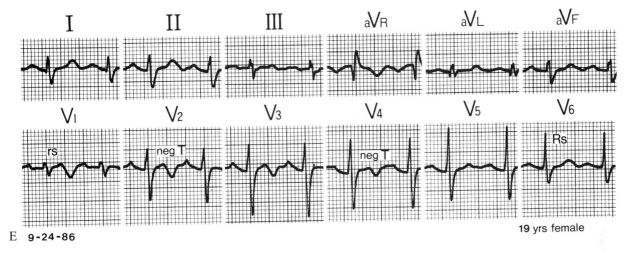

Fig. 19-3. *(Continued)* **E**, There is S$_{I, II, III}$ pattern making an indeterminate axis which is common among young slender patients or those with emphysema. The T waves are negative in leads V$_1$ to V$_4$ which suggests RV overloading, but, in a young person, it may be a normal variant known as a juvenile T pattern.

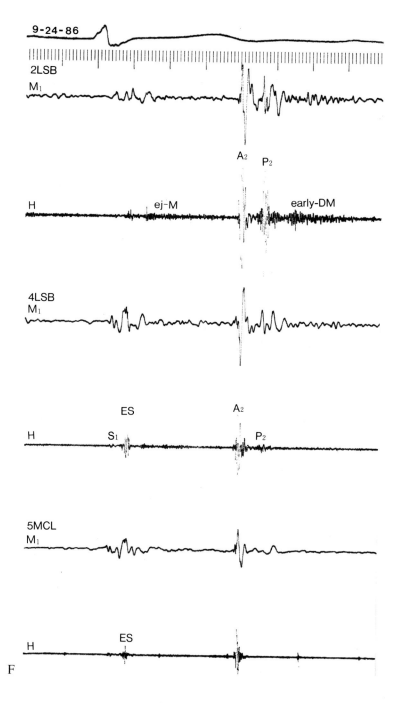

Fig. 19-3. *(Continued)* **F,** The PCG reveals wide splitting of the S$_2$. Since the second component is not transmitted well to the apex, the P$_2$ is not louder than normal. An early diastolic murmur (early DM) of short duration is present, and begins with the P$_2$ indicating a pulmonary regurgitant (PR) murmur. A slight ejection murmur (ej-M) is recorded at the 2LSB. The clinical findings are compatible with a diagnosis of PR, probably caused by idiopathic dilatation of the main PA.

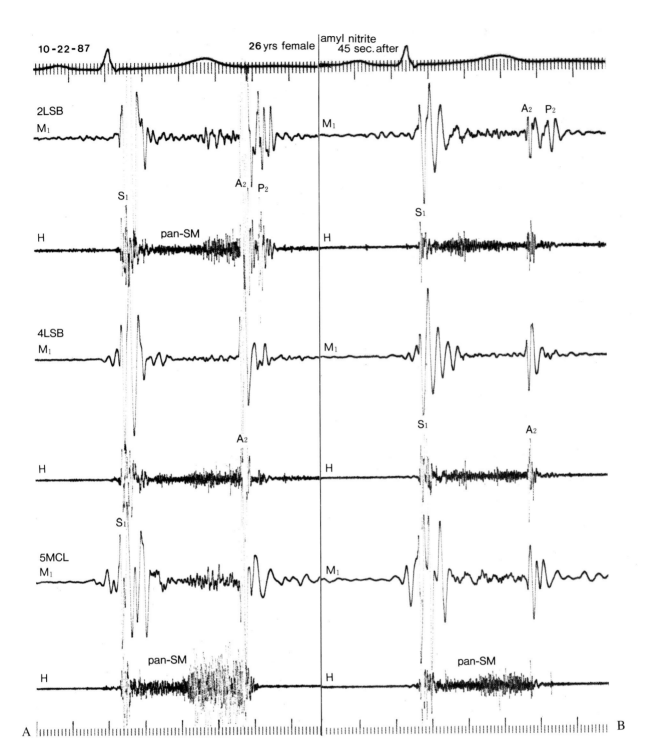

Fig. 19-4. A, This 26-year-old asymptomatic female student was referred because of a previously undisclosed heart murmur. Auscultation showed slight splitting of the S_2. There is a pansystolic murmur (pan-SM) with late systolic accentuation from her base to her apex. **B,** After amyl nitrite inhalation on the right, both the intensity and shape of the pansystolic murmur varied. The reduction of the murmur is caused by the fall in blood pressure which causes an increased systemic flow which in turn causes a decrease in regurgitant flow, a characteristic of systolic regurgitant murmurs.

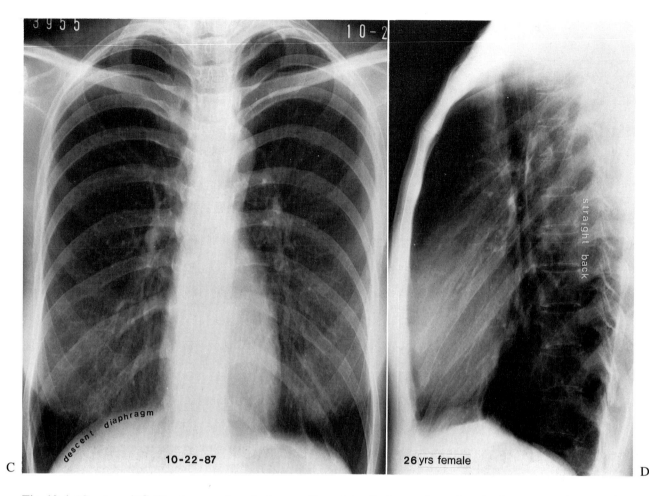

C   10-22-87   26 yrs female   D

Fig. 19-4. *(Continued)* **C**, Chest x-rays show the low position of the diaphragm due to her slender stature. The posterior portions of the 3rd to 7th ribs are horizontally oriented but their margins near the thoracic wall are not elevated as in Figure 19-1B. There is no shift of the cardiac silhouette to the left. **D**, In the lateral view, her sternovertebral distance remains normal despite her straight back.

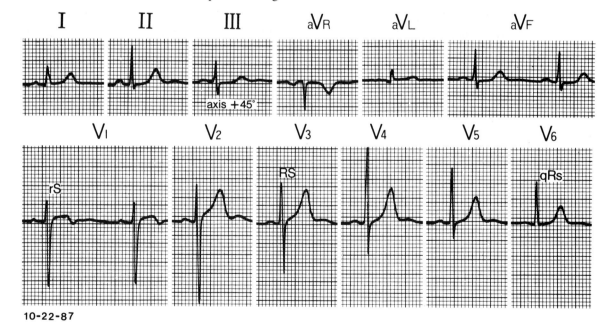

E   10-22-87

Fig. 19-4. *(Continued)* **E**, An ECG of the same patient is normal and shows a QRS axis of about +45° (III is slightly positive).

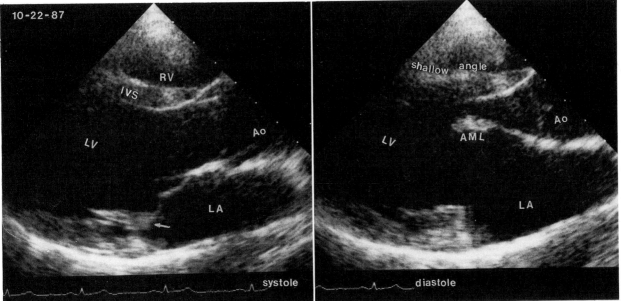

F

Fig. 19-4. *(Continued)* **F,** The long-axis echoes show a shallow aortoseptal angle during both systole and diastole, indicative of the narrow chest syndrome. There may be slight MVP during systole, as indicated by an arrow. The anterior mitral leaflet (AML) is wide open during diastole and nearly touching the IVS, a characteristic of the redundant AML tissue seen with MVP and the narrow chest syndrome.

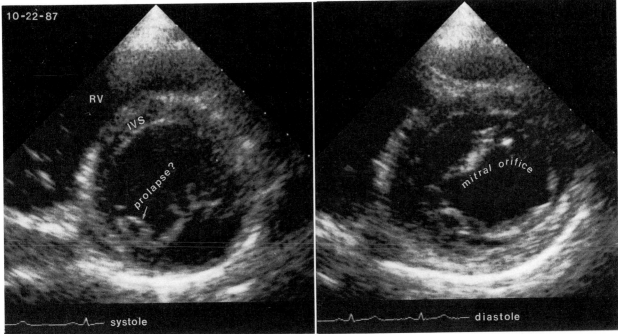

G

Fig. 19-4. *(Continued)* **G,** The short-axis echoes reveal a protrusion of the anterolateral scallop of the posterior leaflet during systole which suggests MVP. The mitral valve is widely open during diastole. The LV cavity appears to be enlarged, which may be caused by LV overloading from the MR.

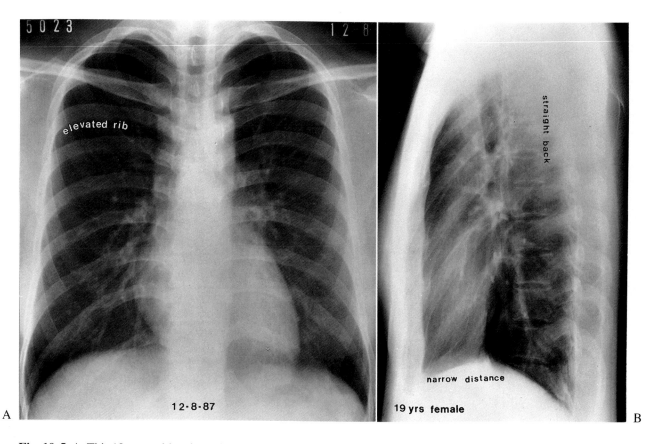

Fig. 19-5. A, This 19-year-old male student was referred with a diagnosis of straight back syndrome. His chest x-rays show horizontally-oriented posterior aspects of his ribs whose margins near the thoracic wall are elevated, a common feature of the narrow chest syndrome. However, the cardiac silhouette is not shifted to the left. **B**, On the lateral view, his thoracic spine is straight and the sternovertebral distance is less than one-third the transverse diameter of his thorax.

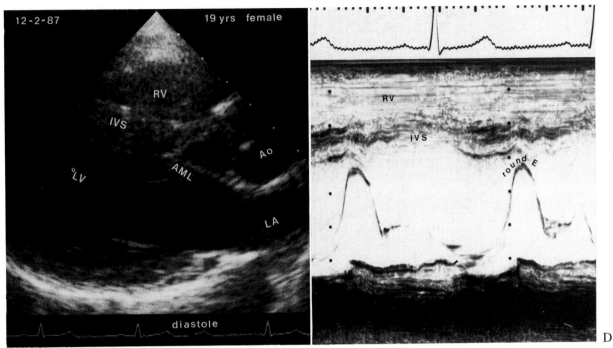

Fig. 19-5. *(Continued)* C, A long-axis echo shows a shallow aortoseptal angle. The anterior mitral leaflet (AML) is widely opened and is nearly touching the IVS. **D,** On the right, an M-mode recording shows a rounded E point and its peak is nearly touching the IVS. This is a common feature in the narrow chest syndrome since a narrow sternovertebral distance results in a shallow aortoseptal angle which, in turn, causes a narrow left ventricular outflow tract (LVOT).

Chapter 20 Pleuropericardial Defects

Pathophysiology and Clinical Clues

A pleuropericardial defect is usually termed a pericardial defect. The parietal pleura and parietal pericardium are each composed of a single layer of tissue, and they can easily be separated from each other. In a pleuropericardial defect, the pleuropericardium is usually absent on the left side because there is hypoplasia of the left common cardiac vein (Cuvier's duct) during fetal life which results in poor nutrition to the pleuropericardium on the left side. Pleuropericardial defects have been classified as complete or partial. In spite of the term "complete absence," there is usually residual pleuropericardium through which a large portion of the heart protrudes, which may produce a fatal herniation of the heart. Therefore, the term "complete absence" should be avoided. The author has recommended the use of "extensive" and "localized" or "partial" pleuropericardial defects.

This congenital anomaly is said to be rare, but this is mainly due to lack of recognition. Extensive absence of the left pleuropericardium results in displacement of the heart to the left from loss of supporting tissue. The heart exhibits vigorous motion and may produce palpitation during exertion and/or in the left lateral decubitus position. The diagnosis of pleuropericardial defect is made difficult by its frequent association with the narrow chest syndrome and/or ASD, and it is often detected only at surgery or autopsy. When the defect is localized or partial, there may be no associated symptoms unless it produces a hazardous herniation of the left atrial appendage.

Approaches to the diagnosis of pleuropericardial defects are as follows:

★★★★ The frontal chest x-ray shows no cardiac margin to the right of the spine because of marked shift of the heart to the left. The angulations of the Ao and PA are sharp because of the absence of the pleuropericardium. In the left lateral decubitus position, the heart approaches the left chest wall. Incidental fluoroscopic examination for an upper GI series often reveals vigorous motion of the heart.

★★★★ ECG usually shows a very small rsr' pattern in V_1 and a very large QRS in V_5 and V_6. Right-axis deviation and a transitional zone to the left are often noted.

★★★★ The echo shows vigorous cardiac motion, especially the LV free wall, with paradoxical movements of the septum on M-mode recording. An enlarged RV with marked clockwise rotation is commonly in the short-axis views.

★★ Friction rubs or cardiorespiratory murmurs may be present.

In the past, an artificial pneumothorax on the left was the only definitive method of diagnosing the condition without surgery. Nowadays, cardiac CT and/or MRI can easily demonstrate the absence of pleuropericardium.

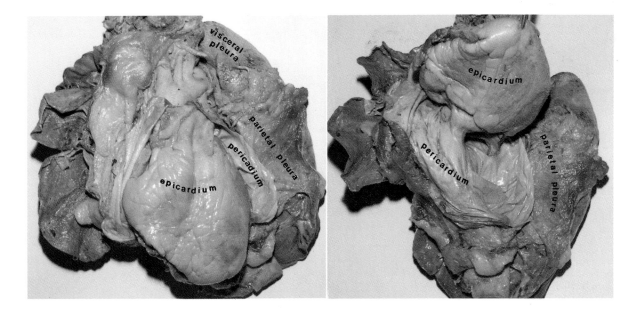

Fig. 20-1. This autopsy specimen of the normal heart and lung illustrates the relationships between the pericardium and the parietal pleura. Behind the sternum, the heart is covered only by pericardium; however, its lateral aspects are surrounded by pericardium and parietal pleura which comprise an apparent single sheet, but actually consist of 2 layers. In a pleuropericardial defect, these 2 layers of tissues are absent and the heart is devoid of surrounding elastic supporting tissues.

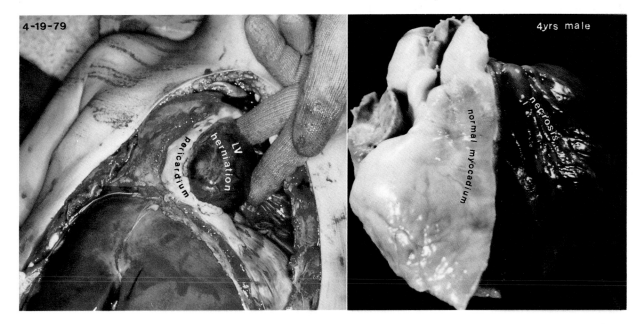

Fig. 20-2. This 4-year-old boy had an extensive left pleuropericardial defect and died of myocardial necrosis following a chest contusion. The patient had experienced occasional vague chest pain but did not seek medical attention. While playing with his sister, he struck his chest with his own fist and developed acute chest pain and cyanosis. He died several hours after he arrived at the hospital emergency room. His ECG after the accident showed marked ST elevations in leads II, III and aV$_F$, simulating an inferior myocardial infarction. **A**, The autopsy photograph on the left shows an extensive pleuropericardial defect through which a portion of the LV was forced out and became necrotized. **B**, On the right is a posterior view of the dark necrotized LV. The defect was 55 × 45 mm with thickened margins indicating that repeated protrusions of the LV might have caused his symptoms. This is certainly an extensive pleuropericardial defect but not a complete absence of the pleuropericardium. There have been at least 3 reports of such cases where death was caused by pleuropericardial defects. (Courtesy of R. Saitoh, M.D.)

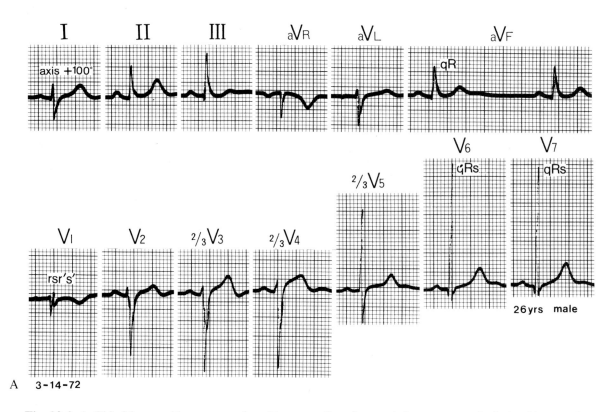

I   II   III   aVR   aVL   aVF

axis +100°   qR

V₁   V₂   ²/₃V₃   ²/₃V₄   ²/₃V₅   V₆   V₇

rsr's'   qRs   qRs

26yrs   male

A   3-14-72

Fig. 20-3. A, This 26-year-old man was referred because of an abnormal chest x-ray made during his annual physical examination. He occasionally complained of exertional palpitation and pleuritic chest pain. His initial ECG shows right-axis deviation of +100° with a very small rsr's' in V₁ and a very large qRs in V₆. The transitional zone is between V₄ and V₅ due to slight clockwise rotation. These findings are typical of an extensive left pleuropericardial defect.

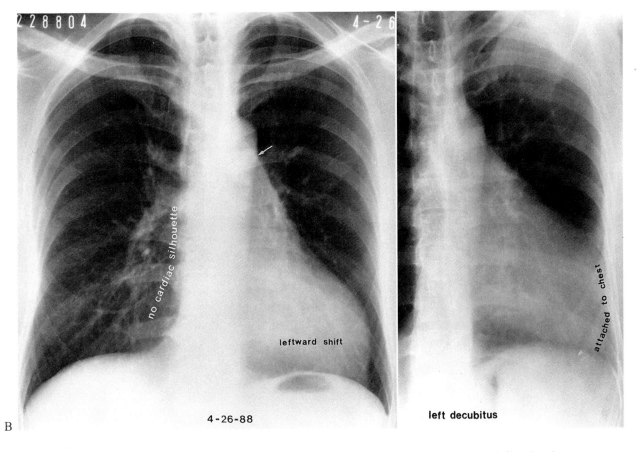

Fig. 20-3. *(Continued)* **B**, Chest x-rays 16 years later show a shift of the cardiac silhouette to the left so that there is no visible cardiac margin to the right of the thoracic spine. This has been unchanged since the initial chest x-ray. The left mid-cardiac border is straight and the LV segment appears to be enlarged. **C**, The left lateral decubitus position results in a further shift of the heart which contacts the chest wall, a very common feature of extensive pleuropericardial defect, due to extensive loss of supporting tissue.

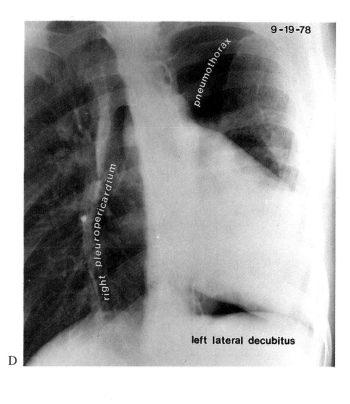

Fig. 20-3. *(Continued)* **D,** This artificial pneumothorax shows air passed from the left pleural space to the pericardial sac via the defect to produce an image of the right pleuropericardium.

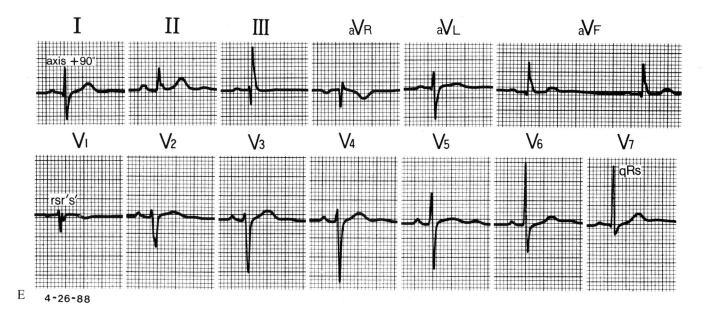

Fig. 20-3. *(Continued)* **E,** During the next 10 years, there was a gradual reduction of the QRS complex and his symptoms as well. His ECG has an rsr's' in V$_1$ as before. The QRS complexes in V$_2$ to V$_6$ are markedly reduced in amplitude, probably from adhesions to the lung and/or the thoracic wall.

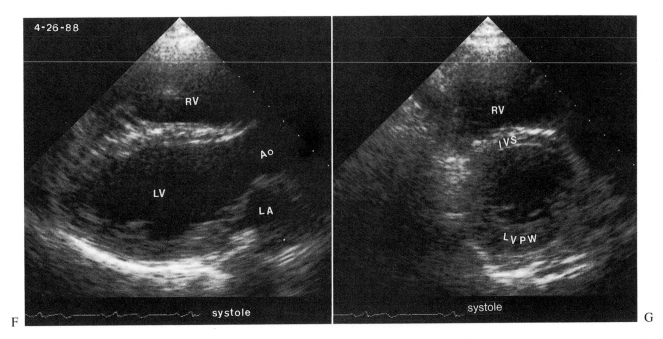

Fig. 20-3. *(Continued)* **F**, On the left, a long-axis echo shows a dilated LV and a small LA. The aortoseptal angle is shallow, indicating either an enlarged RV or narrow chest syndrome. The RV appears to be dilated in this long-axis view and this RV dilatation, together with the narrow chest, compresses the LA. **G**, On the right, a short-axis view shows a dilated RV which is located anteriorly, indicating clockwise rotation.

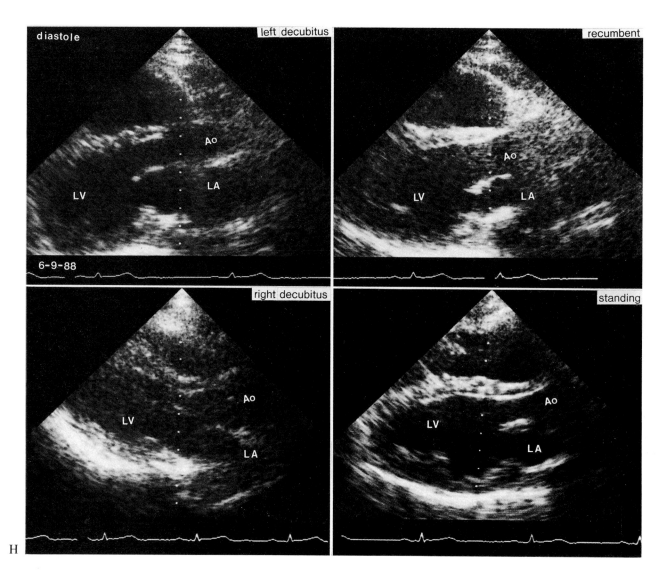

Fig. 20-3. *(Continued)* **H**, These 4 different long-axis echoes of the same patient were made during diastole. In the left lateral decubitus, the LV shifts inferoposteriorly. In the right lateral decubitus, the entire image appears to be normal. In the recumbent position, the RV is dilated and the dilated LV shifts inferoposteriorly. In the standing position, both the RV and LV appear to be normal in size. These findings indicate that marked variations occur in the sizes of LV and/or RV in cases of pleuropericardial defects. The most severe change occurs in the left lateral decubitus position; the patient usually avoids this posture because it produces palpitation.

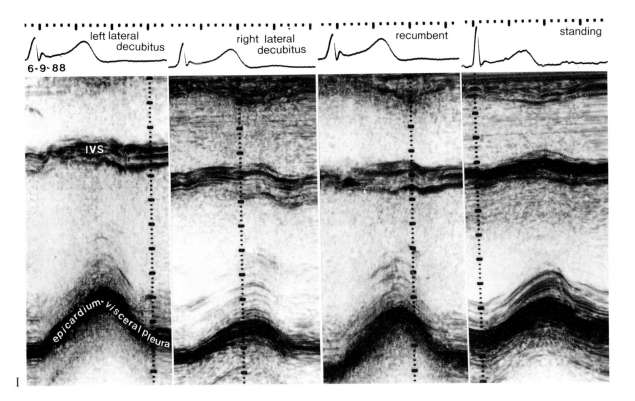

left lateral decubitus

right lateral decubitus

recumbent

standing

6-9-88

IVS

epicardium-visceral pleura

I

Fig. 20-3. *(Continued)* **I,** The M-mode recordings made the same day as the echoes show both the IVS and LV movements. The left lateral decubitus position shows a dilated LV having vigorous movement: movement of the IVS is paradoxical. The right lateral decubitus position shows a nearly normal size and movement of the LV; the IVS movement is paradoxical. In the recumbent position, the LV movement is relatively marked with little movement of the IVS. On standing, the IVS shows paradoxical movement and the LV movement is unremarkable. These again show that the left lateral decubitus position can produce the most vigorous movements of the LV.

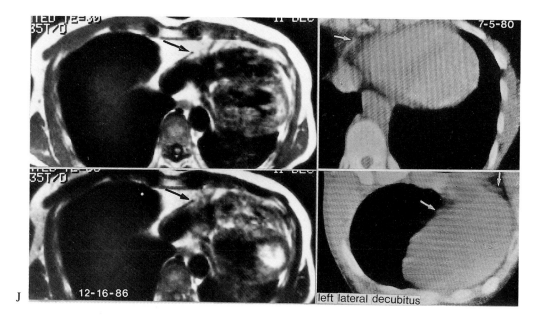

Fig. 20-3. *(Continued)* **J,** In earlier times, an artificial pneumothorax on the left was the diagnostic procedure. Today a noninvasive procedure, such as cardiac CT and/or MRI, is enough to diagnose a pleuropericardial defect. On the left, an MRI of the same patient shows an abrupt disruption of the epicardium-pericardium around the left side of the heart (black arrow). Anterior to the pleuropericardium is pericardial fat shown by the high frequency signal as white. Likewise, posterior to the pleuropericardium white indicates subepicardial fat. On the right, a cardiac CT section near the mitral ring shows that the entire heart is shifted posterolaterally and nearly attached to the chest wall, especially in the left lateral decubitus position. This indicates a loss of supporting tissue around the left side of the heart. A white arrow indicates abrupt disruption of the entire left pleuropericardium. In this case, the pleuropericardial defect is very extensive and shows nearly complete absence of pleuropericardium.

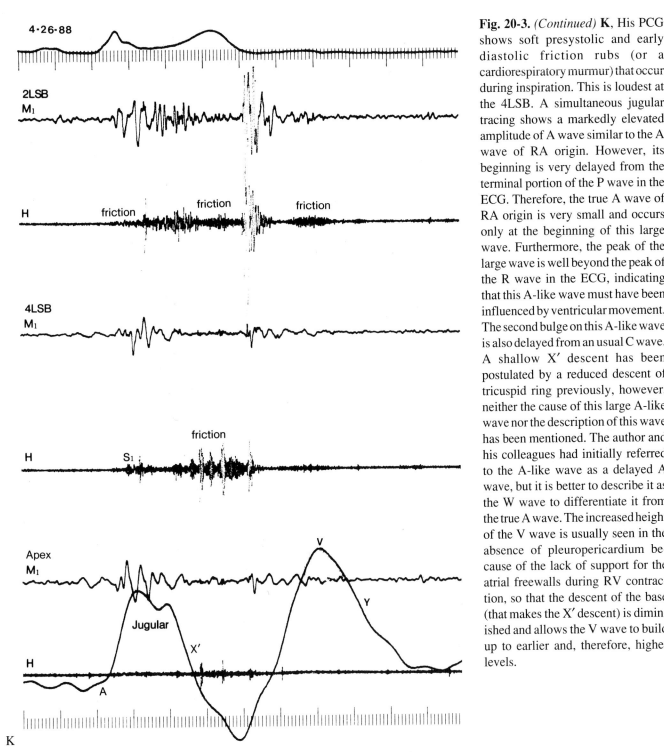

Fig. 20-3. *(Continued)* **K**, His PCG shows soft presystolic and early diastolic friction rubs (or a cardiorespiratory murmur) that occur during inspiration. This is loudest at the 4LSB. A simultaneous jugular tracing shows a markedly elevated amplitude of A wave similar to the A wave of RA origin. However, its beginning is very delayed from the terminal portion of the P wave in the ECG. Therefore, the true A wave of RA origin is very small and occurs only at the beginning of this large wave. Furthermore, the peak of the large wave is well beyond the peak of the R wave in the ECG, indicating that this A-like wave must have been influenced by ventricular movement. The second bulge on this A-like wave is also delayed from an usual C wave. A shallow X' descent has been postulated by a reduced descent of tricuspid ring previously, however, neither the cause of this large A-like wave nor the description of this wave has been mentioned. The author and his colleagues had initially referred to the A-like wave as a delayed A wave, but it is better to describe it as the W wave to differentiate it from the true A wave. The increased height of the V wave is usually seen in the absence of pleuropericardium because of the lack of support for the atrial freewalls during RV contraction, so that the descent of the base (that makes the X' descent) is diminished and allows the V wave to build up to earlier and, therefore, higher levels.

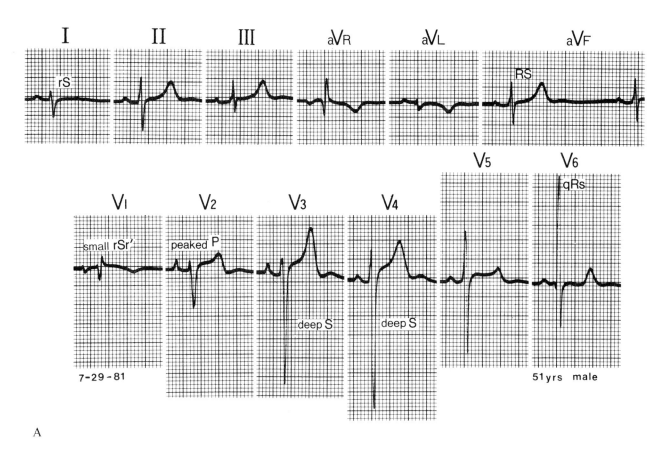

Fig. 20-4. A, This ECG of a 51-year-old man with an extensive left pleuropericardial defect shows a small rSr′ in V$_1$ and a large qRS in V$_6$. The transitional zone is between V$_5$ and V$_6$ indicating a posterior QRS, probably caused by marked clockwise rotation of the heart. The QRS axis is indeterminate.

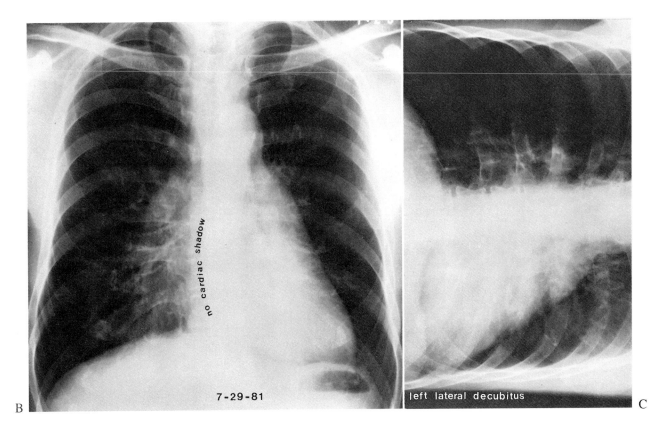

B, His chest x-rays reveal a leftward shift of his heart, and no cardiac margin is visible to the right of the thoracic spine. The Ao-PA angulation is sharp. C, The left lateral decubitus position produces further displacement of the heart to the left so that the cardiac margin is near the chest wall.

Fig. 20-4. *(Continued)* **B**, His chest x-rays reveal a leftward shift of his heart, and no cardiac margin is visible to the right of the thoracic spine. The Ao-PA angulation is sharp. **C**, The left lateral decubitus position produces further displacement of the heart to the left so that the cardiac margin is near the chest wall.

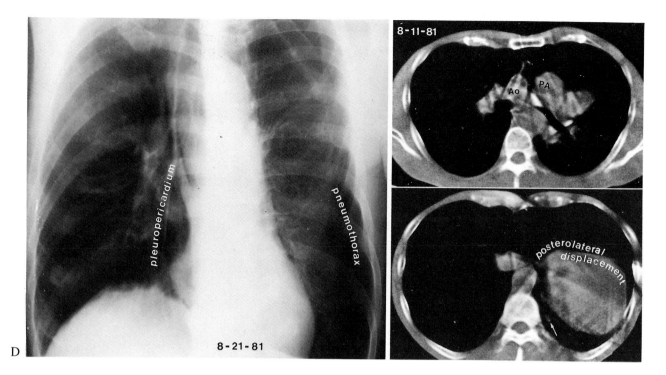

Fig. 20-4. *(Continued)* **D**, On the left, a left pneumothorax visualizes his right pleuropericardium. On the right top, his cardiac CT shows a widely separated Ao and PA which normally should be closely attached to each other because of overlapping pleuropericardium. Right bottom, a cardiac CT section near the mitral ring shows marked posterolateral displacement of his heart. Such a marked displacement suggests some twisting of his coronary arteries; however, his exercise ECG was not remarkable. Since he refused surgery, the extent of the defect could not be determined. The arrow may indicate a trace of pericardium, but there is no pericardium elsewhere. Therefore, the pleuropericardial defect in this case is nearly complete.

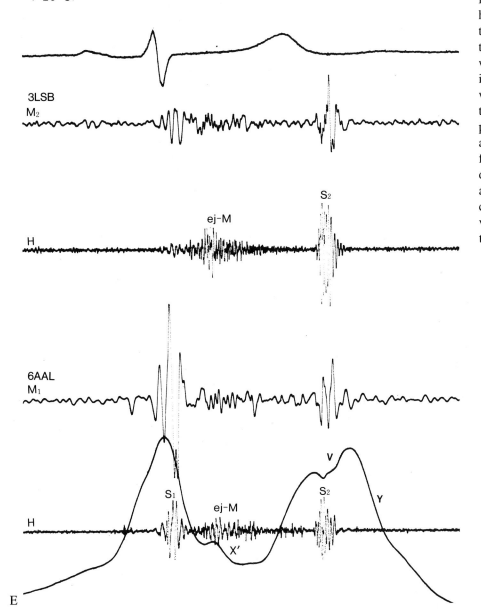

7-29-81

3LSB
M₂

H

ej-M

S₂

6AAL
M₁

H

S₁   ej-M   X'   S₂   V   Y

E

Fig. 20-4. *(Continued)* **E**, His PCG shows an ejection murmur (ej-M) from the 3LSB to the 6AAL where his apex is located. The splitting of the S₂ is very narrow. A jugular tracing shows a high A-like wave (W wave); however, its peak nearly coincides with the first heart sound (S₁) which indicates that this wave is not the true A wave caused by the elevated pressure in the RA. The V wave is tall and is preceded by a bulge, as is frequently seen in pleuropericardial defects. The nature of this S wave is also not clear. The tall V wave indicates either tricuspid regurgitation or vigorous action of the LV transmitted to the right heart chambers.

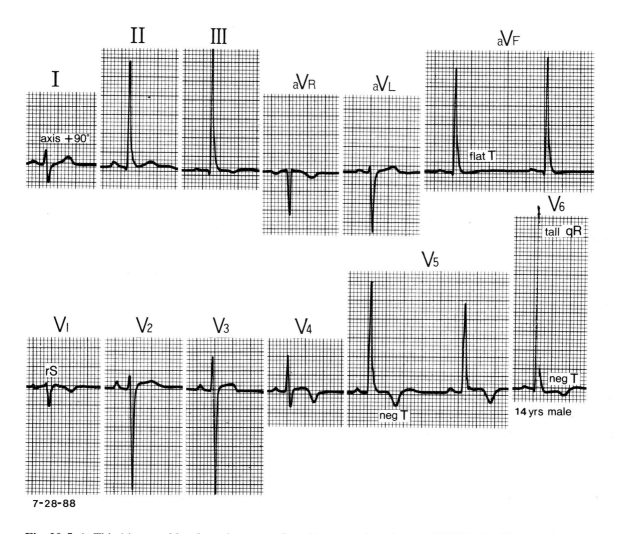

A   7-28-88

Fig. 20-5. A, This 14-year-old male student was referred because of an abnormal ECG during his annual physical examination. He was never told he had a cardiac murmur. He was asymptomatic and participated actively in sports. His ECG shows a QRS axis of about +90°. There is a small rS in V_1 and a very large qR in V_6. The rSr' pattern in V_1, usually seen in left pleuropericardial defects, is not present. In addition, the T wave is inverted in V_4 to V_6, which is very unusual for a pleuropericardial defect.

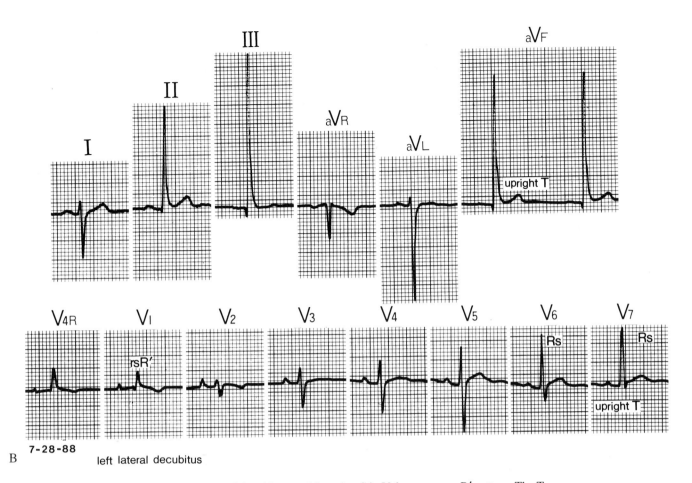

I II III aVR aVL aVF

upright T

V4R V1 V2 V3 V4 V5 V6 V7

rsR′ Rs Rs

upright T

7-28-88
B   left lateral decubitus

Fig. 20-5. *(Continued)* **B,** In the left lateral decubitus position, the rS in V$_1$ became an rsR′ pattern. The T waves also became positive in V$_4$ to V$_6$ with marked reduction in the QRS amplitude. In normals, the left lateral decubitus position usually produces increased amplitude of the QRS in V$_5$ and V$_6$ since the heart comes closer to the chest wall. In left pleuropericardial defects, however, they decrease because the heart may have tilted posteriorly, resulting in an increase in the distance between it and the chest wall. The negative T wave in the LV leads which became positive in the left lateral decubitus position is the author's first such experience with a left pleuropericardial defect. The inverted T waves in the left precordial leads can be explained by the fact that the epicardium abuts the visceral pleura resulting in a repolarization change. In the left lateral decubitus position the LV may be tilted posteriorly and fall away from the visceral pleura.

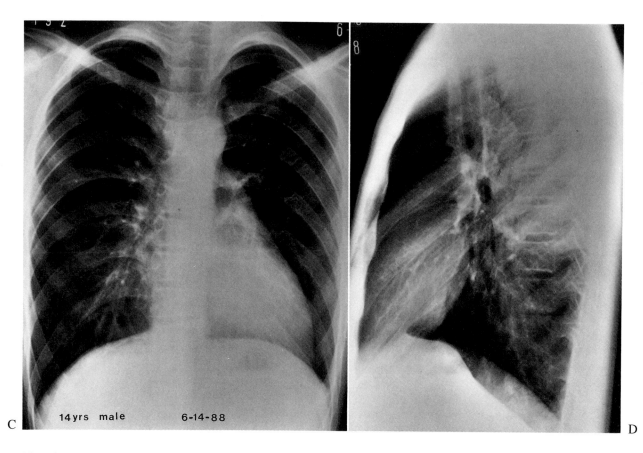

C   D

Fig. 20-5. *(Continued)* **C**, His chest x-rays show typical features of left pleuropericardial defect, i.e., shift of the heart to the left and a sharp Ao-PA angulation. **D**, In the lateral view, there is no evidence of either a narrow chest or LV enlargement.

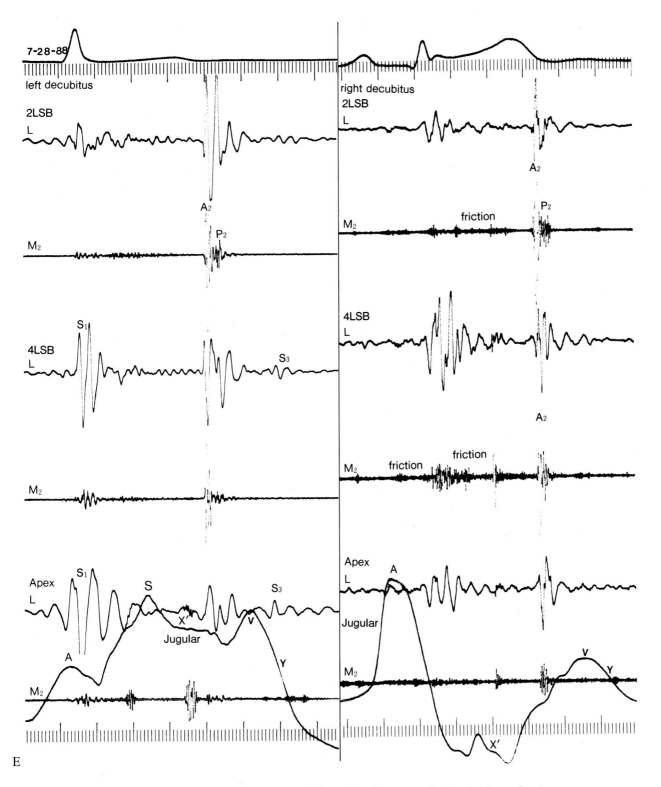

Fig. 20-5. *(Continued)* **E,** His PCGs show only an insignificant S₃ and narrow splitting of S₂ but a simultaneous jugular tracing shows a small X′ descent and a prominent V wave. The upstroke of the A wave is normal but small. The cause of the prominent V wave has already been discussed. In the right lateral decubitus position, friction rubs or cardiorespiratory murmurs occurred in systole and diastole. The jugular tracing changes to show a relatively elevated A wave occurring simultaneously with the terminal portion of the P wave in the ECG. Its peak occurs before the R wave, indicating a usual A wave. Since his 24 hour Holter ECG showed transient ST elevations and depressions, coronary blood flow may be affected by the marked shift of his heart; the patient is scheduled for surgical correction.

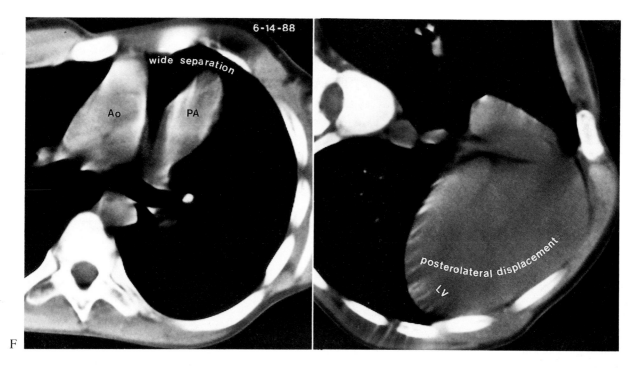

Fig. 20-5. *(Continued)* **F**, Cardiac CT of the same patient shows wide separation of the Ao and PA on the left because of an extensive absence of the left pleuropericardium. A left lateral decubitus projection demonstrates a marked lateral displacement of his heart which contacts the chest wall. There is no trace of pericardium.

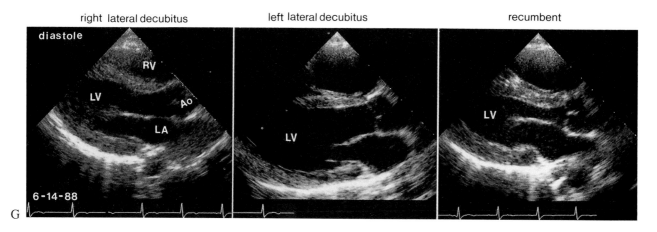

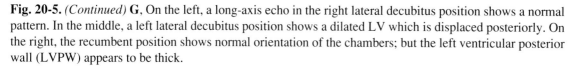

Fig. 20-5. *(Continued)* **G**, On the left, a long-axis echo in the right lateral decubitus position shows a normal pattern. In the middle, a left lateral decubitus position shows a dilated LV which is displaced posteriorly. On the right, the recumbent position shows normal orientation of the chambers; but the left ventricular posterior wall (LVPW) appears to be thick.

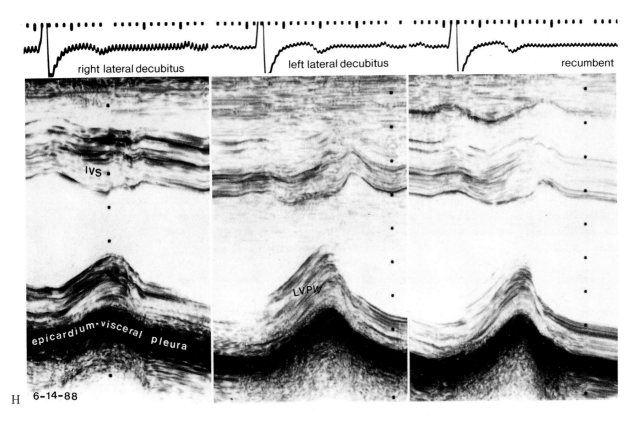

right lateral decubitus   left lateral decubitus   recumbent

IVS

LVPW

epicardium·visceral pleura

H   6-14-88

Fig. 20-5. *(Continued)* **H**, M-mode recordings of the same patient show normal movements of the LV and IVS in the right lateral decubitus position. There is, however, a very broad band-like echo which is probably a fusion echo of the epicardium and pleura. In the middle, an M-mode echo made in the left lateral decubitus position shows vigorous movement of the LV with paradoxical movement of the IVS. On the right, an M-mode recording in the recumbent position appears similar to that in the left lateral decubitus position. The author wishes to emphasize that a fusion echo of the epicardium, the visceral pleura, and possible parietal pleura with lung tissue can produce a broad band-like echo.

Chapter 21 Mitral Stenosis and Regurgitation

Pathophysiology and Clinical Clues

Rheumatic mitral valvular disease refers to mitral stenosis (MS) and mitral regurgitation (MR). MS is often concomitantly associated with MR. Even where the destruction of the mitral valve is severe and MR is dominant, fusion of the commissures and/or the chordae tendineae may cause associated MS. However, ruptured chordae, elongation of the chordae tendineae in the presence of mitral valve prolapse (MVP) or papillary muscle dysfunction from IHD or an enlarged LV from any cause may produce pure MR without MS. Remember that MS or MR commonly accompanies rheumatic aortic valvular disease.

The clinical approach to diagnosing mitral valvular disease is as follows:

★★★★ The echo identifies enlargement of the LA, limited movement of the mitral valve, valvular calcification, the presence of vegetations, and the flail leaflet of ruptured chordae tendineae.

★★★ Auscultation in MS reveals an accentuated S_1, an opening snap of the mitral valve, and a diastolic rumble. When MR is predominant, there may be a diminished S_1 and splitting of S_2 with a loud plateau pansystolic murmur at the apex.

★★★ The chest x-ray may show enlargement of the LA as indicated by a double density along the right cardiac border and/or elevation of the left mainstem bronchus. Abnormal distribution of the pulmonary vasculature is evidence of passive congestion.[*]

★★★ The ECG features of rheumatic mitral valvular disease are atrial fibrillation and, in the presence of MS, low voltage in leads I and V_1 with RV overloading as indicated by right-axis deviation. In MS in normal sinus rhythm, P waves may show both right and left atrial overloading. When the dominant lesion is MR, a diastolic LV overloading may occur.

[*] In cases of predominant MS, the aortic arch is not prominent and dilatation of the main PA is seen which may make differentiation from ASD difficult.

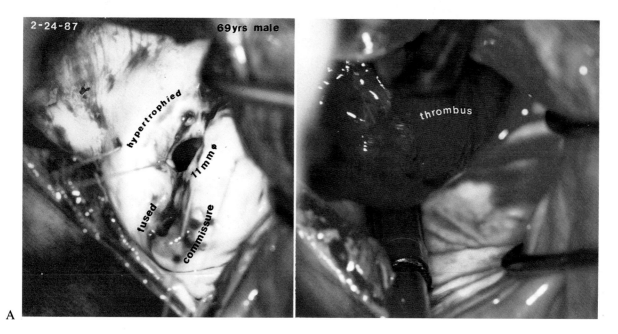

A

Fig. 21-1. A, These surgical specimens are from a 69-year-old man with recurrent orthopnea of 10 years duration. Combined valvular disease was verified and mitral valve replacement was performed. The mitral orifice was about 11 mm in diameter, with a thickened valve and fusion of the commissures. A large thrombus measuring 3 × 4 cm was attached to the posterior wall of the LA.

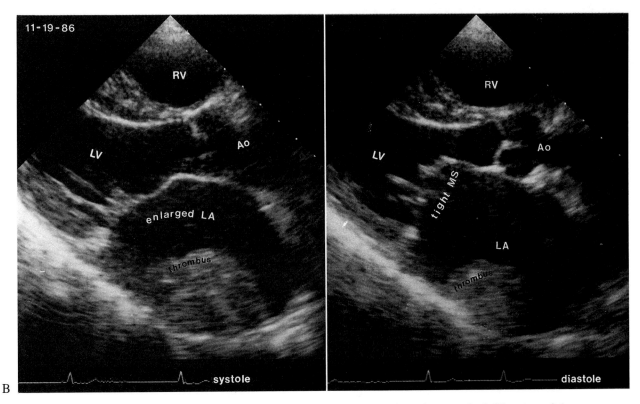

B

Fig. 21-1. *(Continued)* **B,** Preoperative long-axis echoes of the same patient show marked dilatation of the LA with a large thrombus on the posterior wall of the LA. The aortic valve is partially domed and its movements are limited to the same degree as those of the mitral valve.

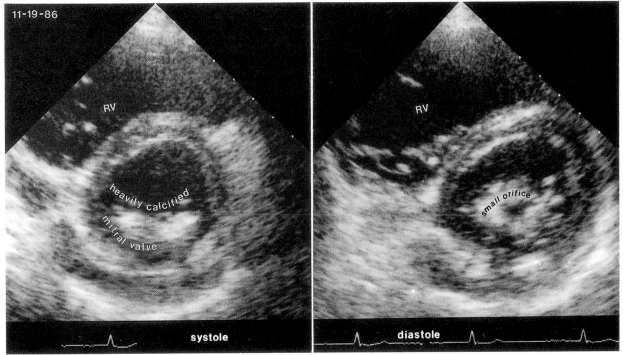

C

Fig. 21-1. *(Continued)* **C,** Short-axis echoes clearly show calcification of the mitral valve with a small orifice during diastole. Normally, the LV is circular in shape; however, during diastole it is deformed by an enlarged RV which is not apparent in the long axis view. This is assumed to be caused by volume overloading of the RV and not to an elevated pressure in the RV since it was 35/8 mm Hg.

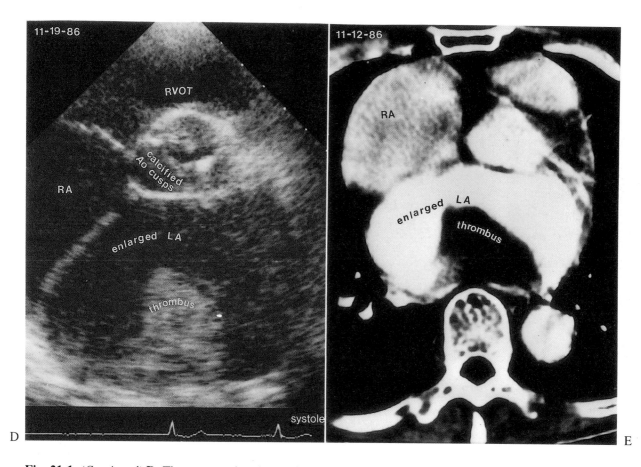

Fig. 21-1. *(Continued)* **D**, The preoperative short-axis echo of the Ao shows a calcified aortic valve with a severely limited orifice during systole. Behind the Ao is a huge LA containing a large thrombus. **E**, On the right, a cardiac CT section at the level of the LA verifies the findings of the echo.

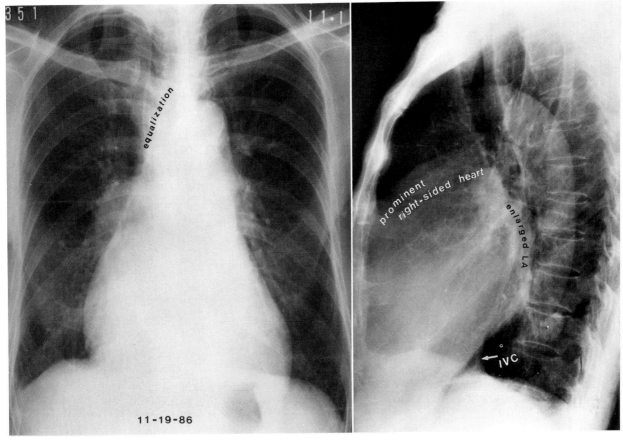

Fig. 21-1. *(Continued)* **F,** His chest x-rays show a rather normal aortic arch except for linear calcification. There is a questionable double density of an enlarged LA. The pulmonary peripheral vascularity is about the same in the upper and lower lung fields on the right, indicating equalization. This suggests the presence of passive congestion. **G,** In the lateral view there is an enlarged LA; the heart contacts more than one third of the sternum, suggesting right-sided cardiac enlargement.

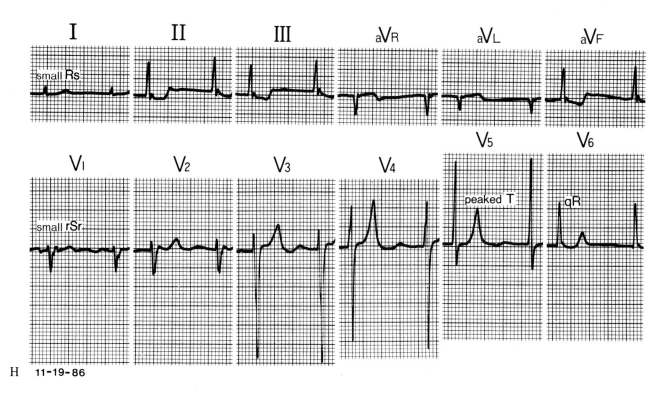

Fig. 21-1. *(Continued)* **H,** His ECG shows AF at a rate of about 75 and voltage is low in leads I and V$_1$, a common feature in MS. In spite of receiving digitalis, peaked T waves in V$_4$ and V$_5$ suggest diastolic LV overloading, possibly from AR and/or MR.

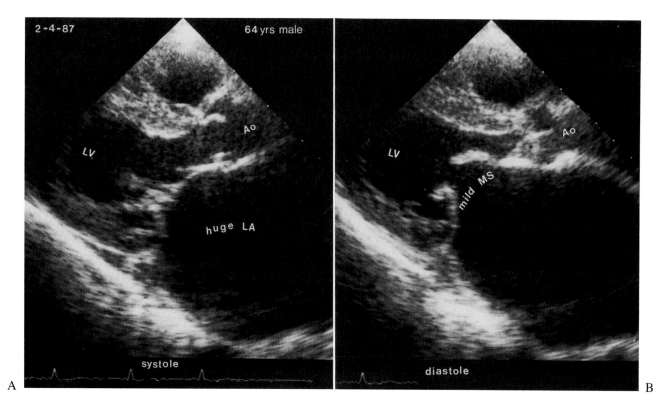

Fig. 21-2. A, This 64-year-old man has MR. The long-axis echoes show a huge LA. There may be protrusion of the posterior leaflet toward the LA during systole, but in diastole, **B,** its opening is limited by both the anterior and posterior mitral leaflets. There is also limited aortic valvular opening with doming during systole.

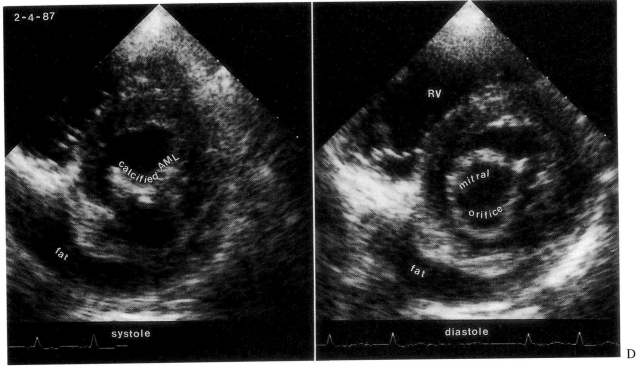

C   D

Fig. 21-2. *(Continued)* **C,** The short-axis echoes show a calcified mitral valve during systole. **D,** During diastole, movement of the mitral valve is sufficient to produce a fairly large orifice which could not be appreciated from the long-axis view. The RV is not dilated and the LV remains normal or slightly dilated, so that MR is dominant with minimal MS. Behind the left ventricular posterior wall (LVPW) there is an extra echo space (EES) which most likely represents a subepicardial fat layer in the atrioventricular sulcus.

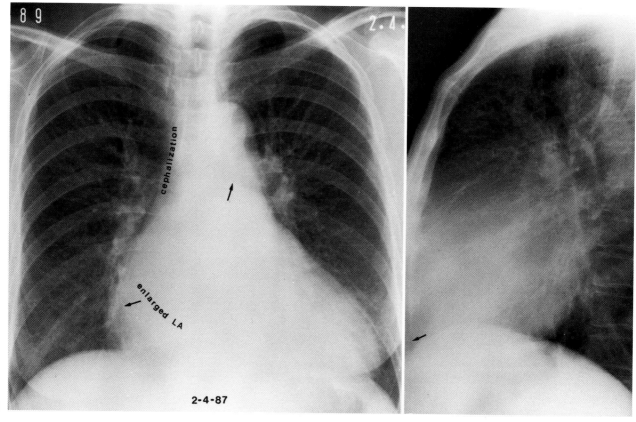

E   F

Fig. 21-2. *(Continued)* **E,** His chest x-rays show elevation of the left mainstem bronchus and a double density along the right border of the cardiac silhouette, indicating enlargement of the LA. Greater prominence of the pulmonary vasculature in the upper than in the lower portions of the lung fields (cephalization) is a manifestation of high LA pressure. **F,** In the lateral view, the cardiac silhouette is enlarged, both anteriorly and posteriorly, indicating right and possibly left cardiac enlargement. A thin anterior pericardial stripe[*] indicated by an arrow suggests the absence of a pericardial effusion.

[*] An anterior pericardial stripe is seen near the sternodiaphragmatic angle as a thin linear opacity bordered on each side by 2 radiolucent layers. The anterior radiolucent layer is the pericardial fat and the posterior, subepicardial fat. When a pericardial effusion occurs, the anterior pericardial stripe increases to 5 mm or more in thickness.

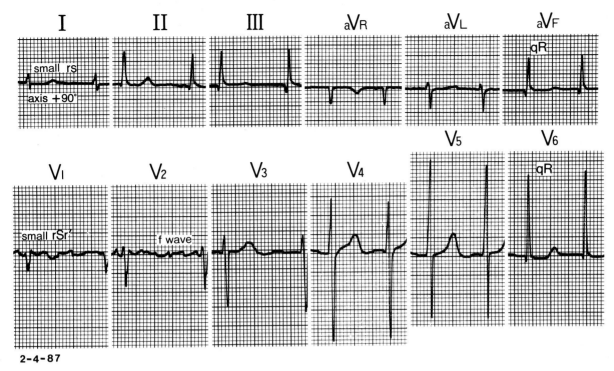

I   II   III   aVR   aVL   aVF

small rs
axis +90°

qR

V₁   V₂   V₃   V₄   V₅   V₆

small rSr′   f wave   qR

G   2-4-87

Fig. 21-2. *(Continued)* **G**, His ECG shows AF with a rate of 80 to 90. The QRS voltage in both I and V₁ is low. Small f waves are observed in V₁ and V₂. The QRS axis is about +90°. The small rs in I and the rSr′ in V₁, accompanied by AF, raises a suspicion of MS. A tall qR pattern in V₆ and an upright T wave suggest diastolic LV overloading and favor MR. These findings correlate with those of the echo and indicate dominant MR plus inconspicuous MS.

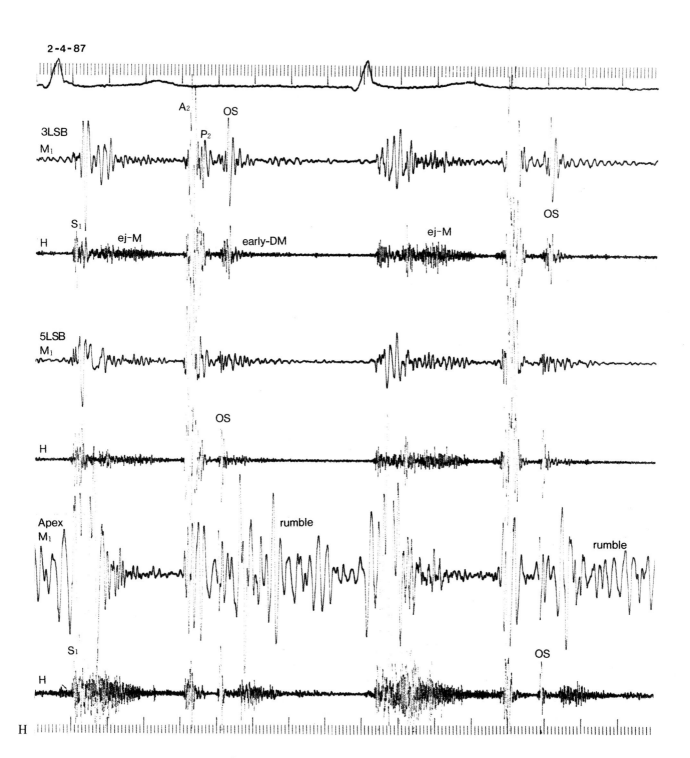

Fig. 21-2. (*Continued*) **H**, PCG shows a narrow S_2 split, late opening snap (OS), and an accentuated S_1 recorded at the base. A soft ejection murmur (ej-M) and an early diastolic murmur (early-DM) are in the same region. The early diastolic murmur is more characteristic of AR on auscultation: however, on the PCG it appears to begin with the OS, and may represent transmission of the high-frequency components of the MS murmur. A decrescendo-shaped murmur and a delayed early diastolic murmur are at the apex. This systolic murmur is not the usual plateau or spindle-shaped MR murmur. However, it is a pansystolic murmur of MR and the unusual shape may be caused by an overlapping ejection murmur from the base. At the apex, a medium frequency recording shows a diastolic rumble.

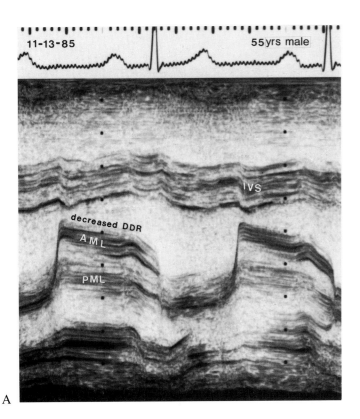

A

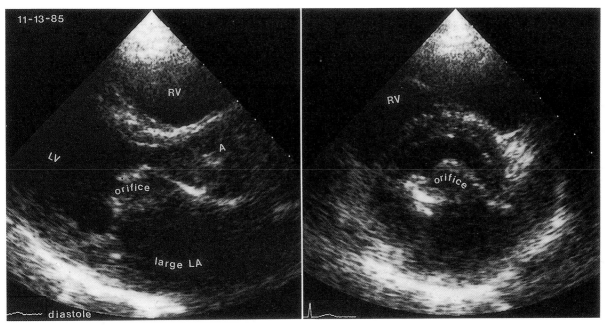

B ... diastole

C

Fig. 21-3. A, During the early days of echo when only M-mode was available, a diagnosis of MS was made by noting a decreased diastolic descent rate (known as DDR or EF slope) of the anterior mitral leaflet (AML). In cases of MS, The EF slope becomes shallow, resembling a trapezoid. Furthermore, both the AML and the posterior mitral leaflet (PML) are composed of multiple-layers of strong echoes due to calcium and they become parallel with each other. This 55-year-old man with MS and AS shows a typical trapezoid configuration in his M-mode recording.

Fig. 21-3. *(Continued)* **B,** On the left, a long-axis echo of the same patient shows a small mitral orifice with some doming. **C,** On the right, his short-axis view shows a reduced mitral opening with some calcification of the posterior mitral leaflet (PML) indicating the presence of MS.

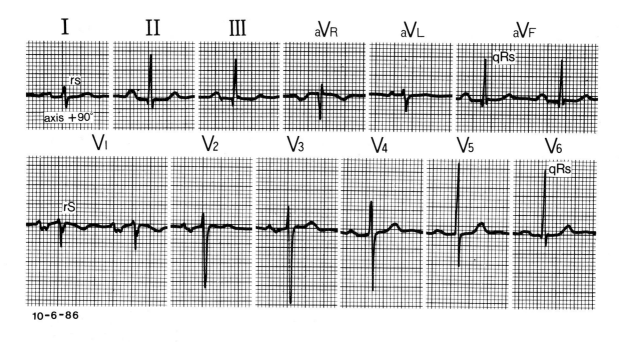

| I | II | III | aVR | aVL | aVF |

rs
axis +90°

qRs

| V₁ | V₂ | V₃ | V₄ | V₅ | V₆ |

rŠ

qRs

D   10-6-86

Fig. 21-3. *(Continued)* **D**, An ECG of the same patient shows a widely notched P in lead I. The P wave in V₁ is typical of LA overloading, as manifested by a large area of terminal P negativity. The QRS axis is about +90°. Leads I and V₁ are of low voltage. The overall findings in this case correlate with MS.

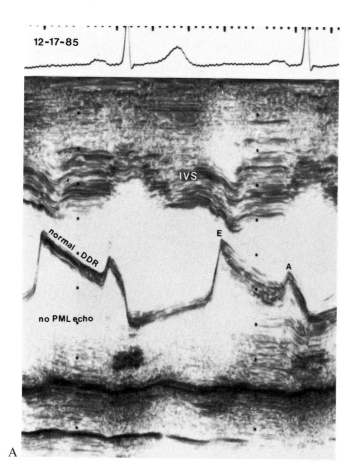

12-17-85

IVS

normal · DDR

E

A

no PML echo

A

Fig. 21-4. A, The M-mode echo of this 50-year-old man is an example of how an erroneous diagnosis can be made based on M-mode echo alone. The diastolic descent rate (DDR or EF slope) is nearly normal and there are no multiple layered echoes, so that this may be considered only slightly abnormal.

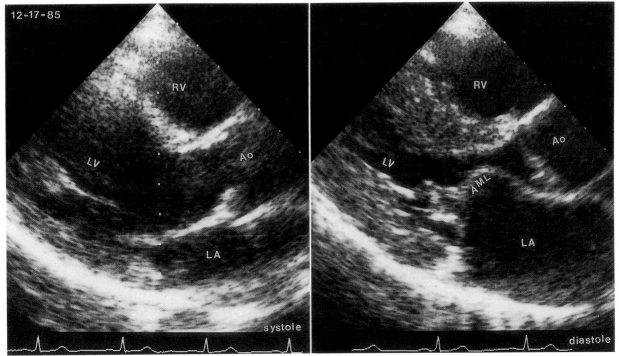

Fig. 21-4. *(Continued)* **B**, His long-axis echo on the right shows poor mitral valvular opening during diastole with doming of the anterior mitral leaflet (AML) indicating that the belly of the leaflet remains soft. When an echo beam is directed at this dome, the M-mode recording may show a normal M-shaped mitral valve which causes us to overlook MS. Both the AML and the posterior mitral leaflet (PML) are thickened and their movements are limited.

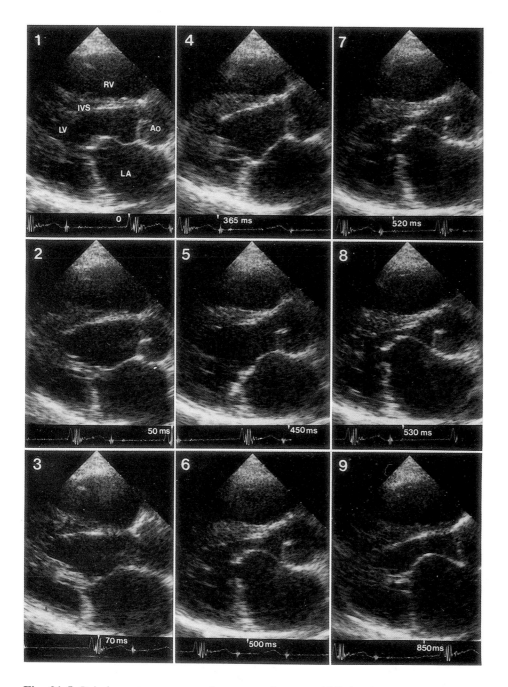

Fig. 21-5. It is important to recognize an opening snap (OS) in diagnosing MS. The OS occurs early in diastole, and it may disappear with a severely stiffened mitral valve. Pliability of the anterior mitral leaflet is necessary to produce the OS. Serial long-axis echoes of a 39-year-old woman with MS and AR clearly demonstrate the cause of the OS. The numbers indicate the delay from the peak of the R wave in milliseconds (ms). Figure 1 shows 0 ms and indicates an end-diastolic phase. The aortic valve is closed but mitral valve is still open. Figure 2 show aortic valve opening and mitral closure. Figure 5 at 450 ms shows the beginning of mitral opening. Figure 6 at 500 ms shows doming of the AML toward the IVS, at 530 ms maximum doming occurs and this coincides with the OS in a simultaneously-recorded PCG. According to this, the OS is assumed to be due to doming of a pliable AML during maximum opening of a stenotic mitral valve.

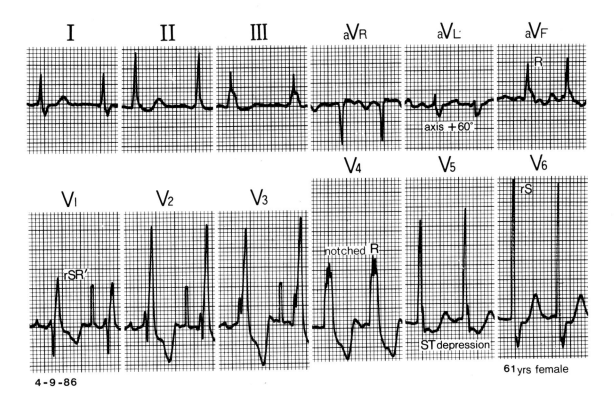

Fig. 21-6. A, This 61-year-old woman has MS and AR. Her ECG reveals AF, and there is an rSR′ in V₁ and V₂ with broad QRS complexes of RBBB. The QRS axis is about +60°. The configuration is not that of MS and is probably from concomitant ischemic heart disease. The slightly sagging ST depressions in leads II and III are probably a digitalis effect. The tall QRS in V₅ and V₆ may indicate associated AR and/or MR.

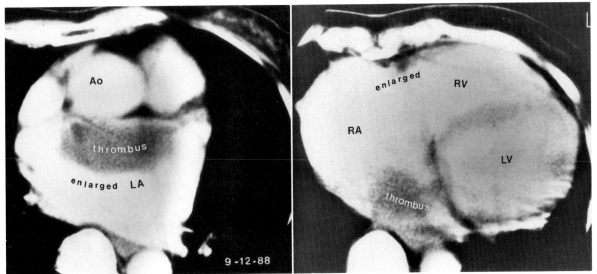

Fig. 21-6. *(Continued)* **B,** A cardiac CT section at the level of the LA on the left shows a large thrombus attached to the anterior wall of an enlarged LA. **C,** On the right, an enlarged RA is seen and the IVS is oriented nearly 90° in the coronal plane, indicating right-sided cardiac enlargement. The LV is also large and there is a negative defect in the LA suggesting the thrombus.

21. Mitral Stenosis and Regurgitation   *357*

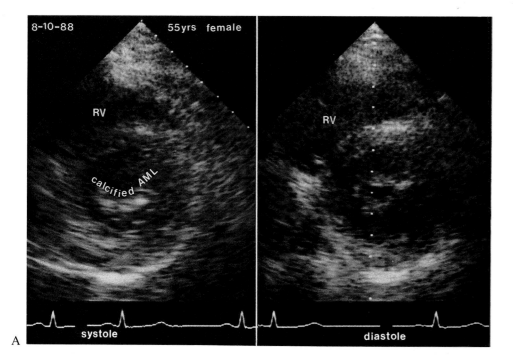

Fig. 21-7. A, These short-axis echoes are from a 55-year-old housewife who gradually developed exertional dyspnea. They show a calcified mitral valve in systole. In diastole on the right, limited opening of the mitral valve is seen. However, there is no enlargement of either the RV or LV.

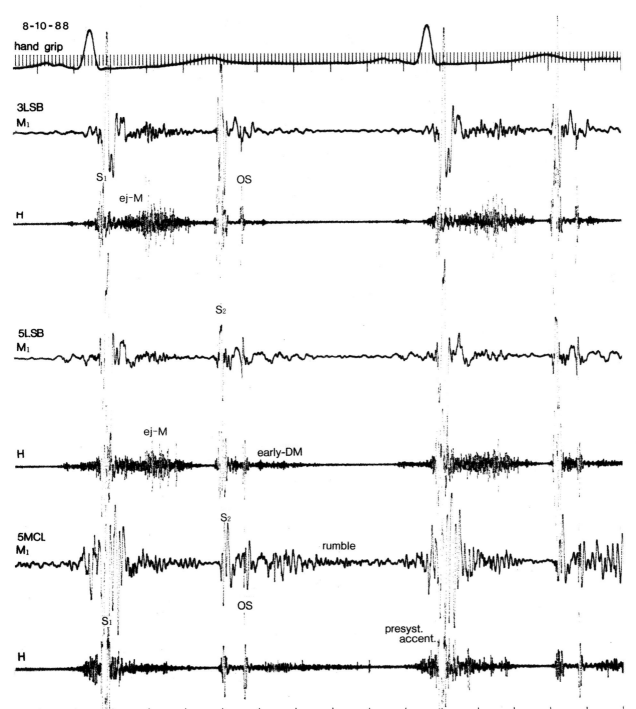

Fig. 21-7. *(Continued)* **B**, Her PCG shows an ejection murmur (ej-M) at the 3LSB and 5LSB. An opening snap (OS) is present from the base to the apex. A soft early diastolic murmur (early-DM) of probable AR is best seen at the 5LSB. At the apex, a medium frequency tracing shows a diastolic rumble with presystolic accentuation (presyst. accent.). The S_1 is also accentuated. This is a typical case of combined aortic and mitral valvular disease with dominant MS.

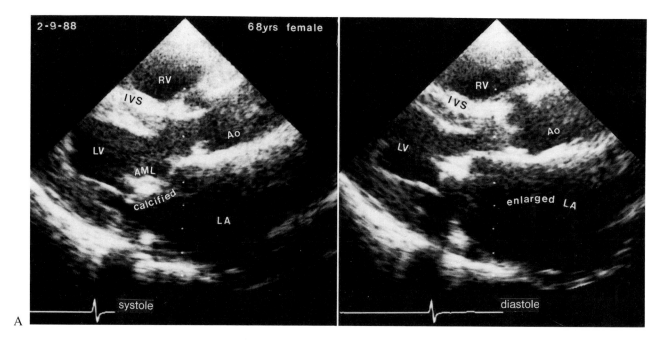

Fig. 21-8. A, This 68-year-old woman has AS and MS as well as AR and MR. Long-axis echoes show a calcified anterior mitral leaflet (AML) with limited opening. There is an enlarged LA but no LV or RV dilatation. Both the anterior and posterior walls of the Ao are calcified, with limited movement of the aortic valve especially in systole. The IVS has strong echoes and its thickness is indeterminate. The patient has diabetes mellitus which may be the cause of the strong echoes which represent either deposits of metabolic products or degeneration.

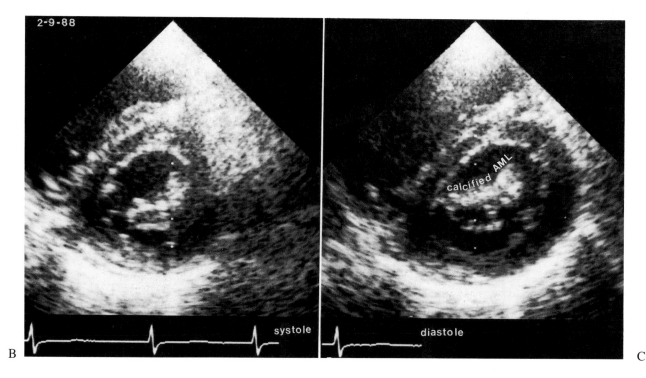

Fig. 21-8. *(Continued)* **B**, Short-axis echoes of the same patient show a calcified AML and valve which appear to close incompletely. **C**, During diastole, the mitral opening is severely limited. There is no apparent RV enlargement.

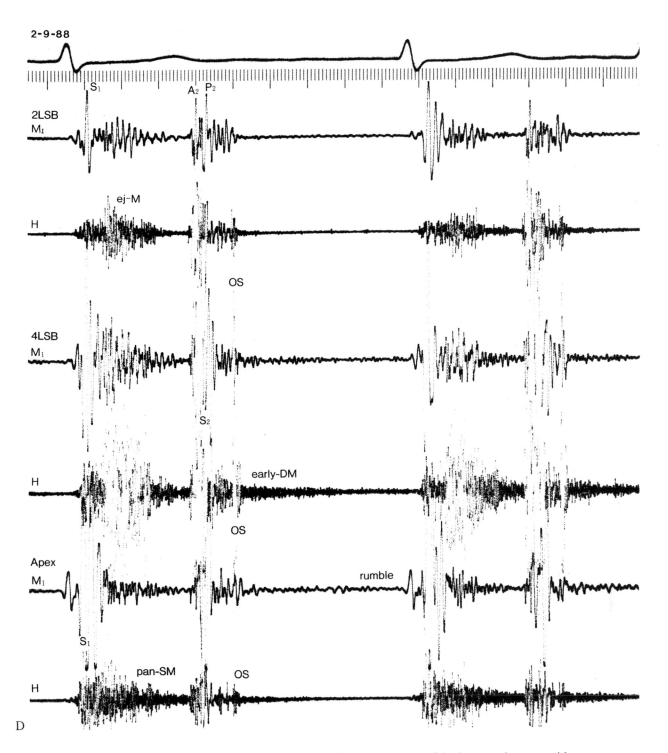

Fig. 21-8. *(Continued)* **D**, Her PCG shows an accentuated S$_1$ from the base of the heart to the apex with an opening snap (OS). A coarse rejection murmur (ej-M) is seen at the 2LSB. There is a pansystolic decrescendo murmur from the 4LSB to the apex. Its configuration, though, is different from an ordinary MR murmur at the 4LSB, and may be caused by an overlapping ejection murmur from the cardiac base. At the apex a decrescendo systolic murmur is commonly seen with mild or moderate MR associated with dominant MS. An early diastolic murmur (early DM) seems to begin with A$_2$ and last until the next S$_1$, probably from AR. There is also a faint diastolic rumble at the apex.

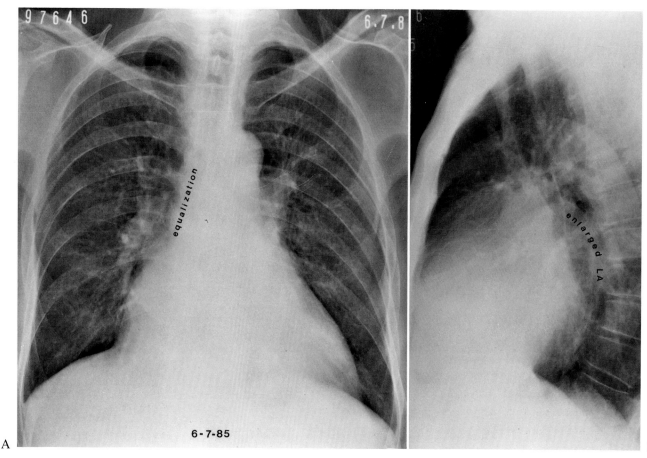

A

B

Fig. 21-9. These chest x-rays are from a 59-year-old man with combined valvular heart disease. The patient has dominant MS with moderate MR and mild AR. His frontal chest x-ray shows generalized cardiomegaly with an enlarged LA. The peripheral pulmonary vascularity is about the same in both upper and lower lung fields on the right (equalization indicating passive congestion). **B**, On the lateral view, an enlarged LA is clearly visible.

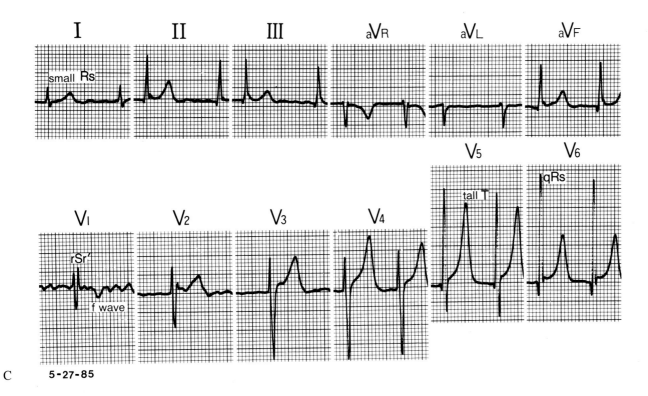

Fig. 21-9. *(Continued)* **C,** An ECG of the same patient demonstrates AF with a rate of about 85. There is an rSr′ pattern in V₁ and V₂ with a relatively small QRS in leads I and V₁, a common feature in MS. As can be judged from the rate of his AF, the patient is probably receiving digitalis. However, the tall T waves in V₄ to V₆ suggest diastolic LV overloading possibly caused by the combination of both the MR and AR.

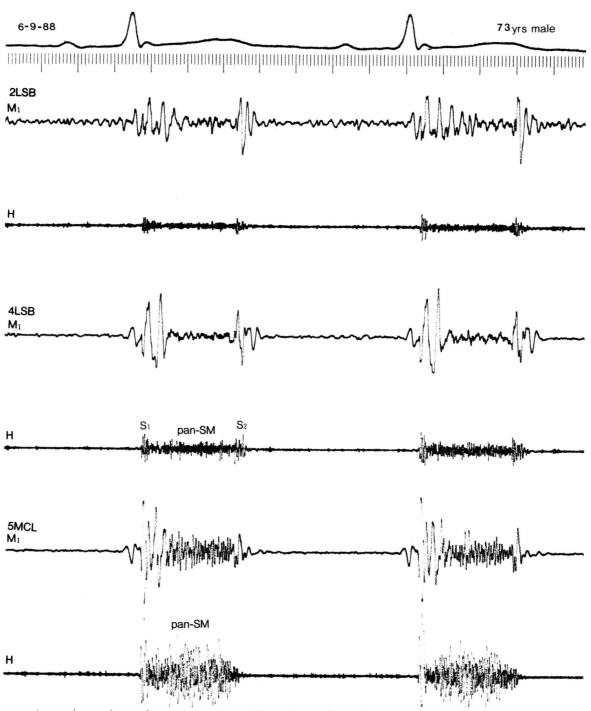

Fig. 21-10. A, PCG from a 73-year-old man with a pansystolic murmur (pan-SM) that is loudest at the apex but also audible at the cardiac base. Other than an accentuated S_1 at the apex, there is no S_3 to suggest severe MR.

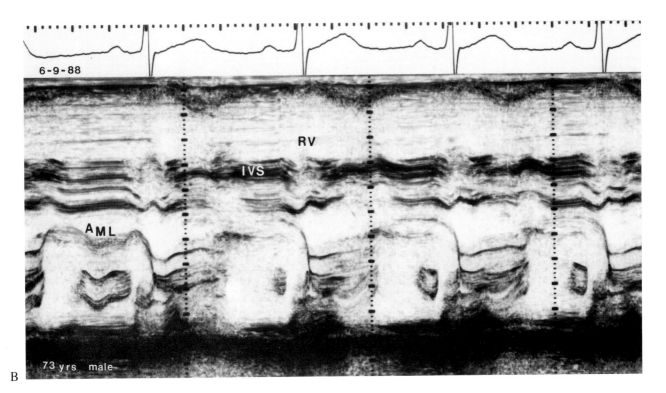

B

Fig. 21-10. *(Continued)* **B,** His M-mode recording shows a most unusual finding — a diastolic box-like echo in the center of the mitral valve. Although the posterior mitral leaflet (PML) is not clear, mitral valve closure seems to occur at the normal site, and this box-like echo is not the PML. During systole, a multiple-layered echo is present most likely caused by the anterior mitral leaflet (AML) and PML.

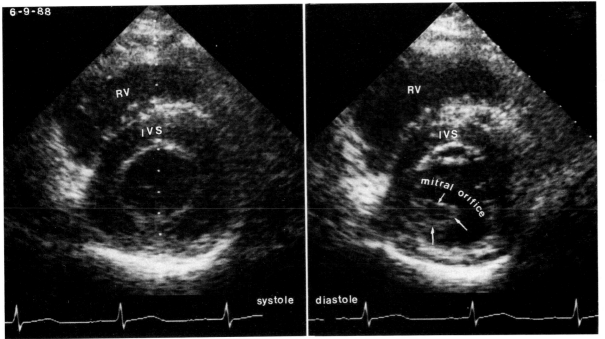

C

D

Fig. 21-10. *(Continued)* **C,** Short-axis echoes show no apparent mitral valvular closure during systole. **D,** During diastole, there is a protruding echo in the mitral orifice (arrows). This echo appears to be the same one observed in the M-mode recording.

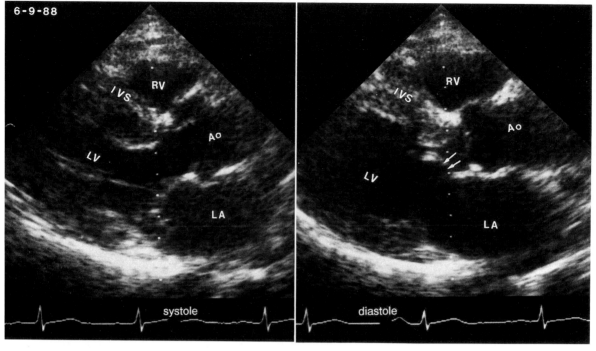

Fig. 21-10. *(Continued)* **E,** The long-axis echoes show no specific chamber enlargement. There may be a slight protrusion of the PML into the LA during systole. **F,** In diastole, the mitral valve opens completely, but there seems to be a diverticulm-like defect on the AML (arrows) which is better seen in video. The defect is probably the cause of an inexplicable echo found in the M-mode recording. The patient is asymptomatic and his ECG and chest x-rays are unremarkable.

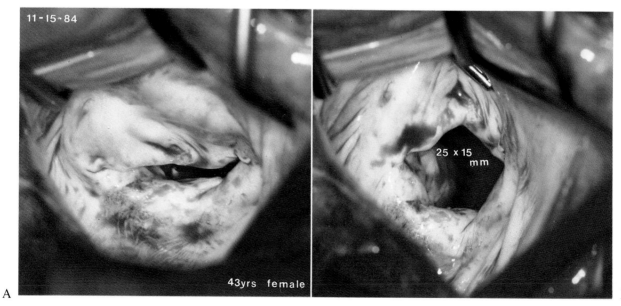

Fig. 21-11. A, This 43-year-old woman has MR and MS. At surgery, both the AML and PML were thickened and the commissures were fused. **B,** The mitral orifice was estimated to be 25 × 15 mm.

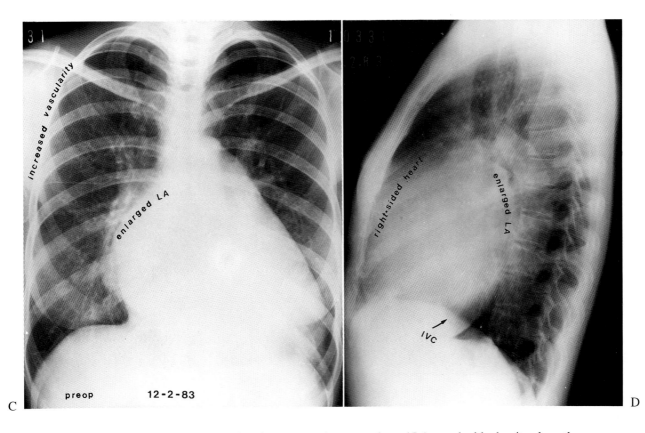

C

D

Fig. 21-11. *(Continued)* **C,** Her preoperative chest x-rays show an enlarged LA as a double density along the right cardiac border. The main PA is dilated and there is increased peripheral pulmonary vascularity in the upper portions of the lung fields, indicating equalization or cephalization. This is a common x-ray feature of MS. **D,** On the lateral view, an enlarged LA is visualized and right-sided cardiac enlargement is seen. The inferior vena cava (IVC) crosses the posterior cardiac border below the level of the diaphragm: this usually indicates LV enlargement. A dilated right-sided heart may be the cause of the displaced cardiac border posteriorly.

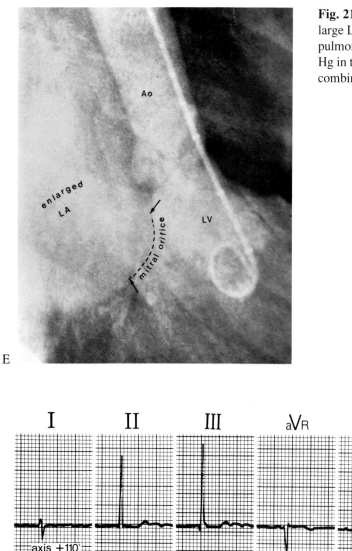

Fig. 21-11. *(Continued)* **E,** Her preoperative angiogram shows a large LV to LA regurgitation. The pressure was 26 mm Hg in the pulmonary capillaries, 106/81 mm Hg in the Ao, and 120/20 mm Hg in the LV. The cardiac index was 3.7. This is a typical case of combined MS and MR.

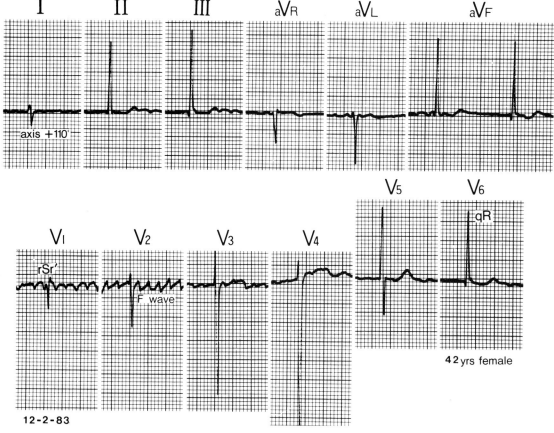

Fig. 21-11. *(Continued)* **F,** Her preoperative ECG shows AF with a rate of about 75. The QRS axis is nearly +110°. There is an rSr′ pattern in V_1 and qR in V_6. The relatively small QRS in leads I and V_1 suggests MS; however, absence of the s wave in V_6 indicates a concomitant MR or AR.

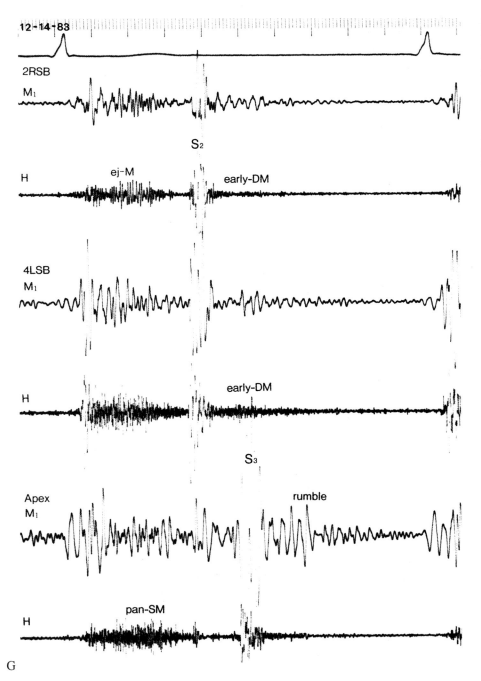

12-14-83

2RSB
M₁

S₂

H   ej-M   early-DM

4LSB
M₁

H   early-DM

S₃

Apex
M₁   rumble

H   pan-SM

G

Fig. 21-11. *(Continued)* **G,** Her PCG shows an ejection murmur (ej-M) and an early diastolic murmur (early DM) of AR at the base of her heart which is transmitted to the 4LSB. There is a spindle-shaped pansystolic murmur at the apex with a large S₃ followed by a diastolic rumble. The S₁ is not accentuated. These findings indicated combined valvular disease consisting of MS and MR and AR.

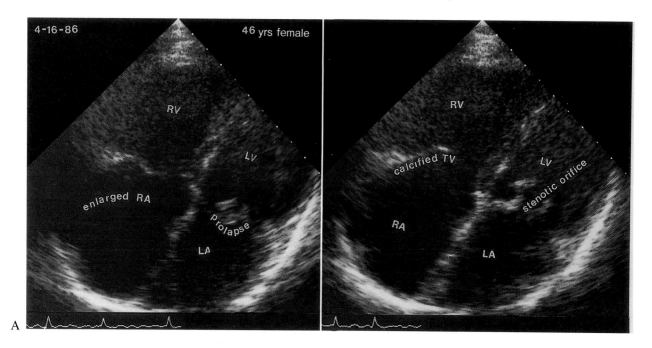

Fig. 21-12. A, This 46-year-old woman has MS. The echoes in the apical four-chamber view show some strong echoes from the tricuspid valve suggesting tricuspid stenosis (TS), an infrequent finding. The mitral valve is thickened and its opening is limited, indicating MS. Both the RA and RV are dilated, suggesting the presence of both TS and tricuspid regurgitation (TR).

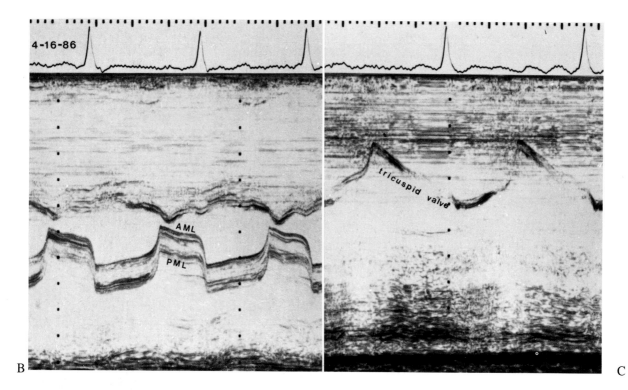

Fig. 21-2. *(Continued)* **B,** Her M-mode echoes show multiple-layered strong echoes from the anterior mitral leaflet (AML). The movement of the posterior mitral leaflet (PML) is parallel to the AML. The diastolic descent rate or EF slope is greatly diminished, indicating significant MS. **C,** On the right, the tricuspid valvular movement also shows a decrease in the EF slope, indicating TS. Occasionally, a relative TS and/or TR occurs as a result of MS, but tricuspid calcification is rarely observed.

Chapter 22 Mitral Valve Prolapse

Pathophysiology and Clinical Clues

In the "click murmur syndrome," mitral valve prolapse (MVP) is characterized by auscultatory findings and is now well established by echo. An abnormality of the mitral complex, including the mitral valve, mitral annulus and chordae tendineae results in a systolic click and/or mitral regurgitation. One cause is an imbalance in the area of the mitral leaflets and the LV cavity, which causes the mitral leaflets to protrude into the LA during systole. This often occurs in the Marfan syndrome, the narrow chest syndrome, and occasionally in hyperthyroidism. In these conditions it is usually caused by myxomatous transformation of the mitral leaflets together with elongated chordae. An early click is difficult to differentiate from an ejection sound, but unlike the ejection sound it changes with posture and/or respiration. There may be no symptoms from the prolapse itself unless the mitral regurgitation is severe. Chest pains and/or sudden death can occur but are rare. The vague chest discomfort felt by some patients with MVP is often caused by extrasystoles.

Approaches to the diagnosis of MVP are as follows:

★★★ The cardiac echo shows mitral leaflets, either anterior or posterior, protruding into the LA during systole. The LA and LV are enlarged if the MR is severe. The Doppler echo identifies the MR.

★★★★ Auscultatory findings typically show mid- to late-systolic clicks and a late-systolic murmur. However, a pansystolic murmur without transmission to the left axillary area is frequent.

★★ Chest x-rays may show an enlarged LA and/or LV.

★★ The ECG may show diastolic LV overloading if the MR is severe. Various types of arrhythmias including atrial and ventricular tachycardia have been reported. The T waves may be negative or notched in the aVF and LV leads.

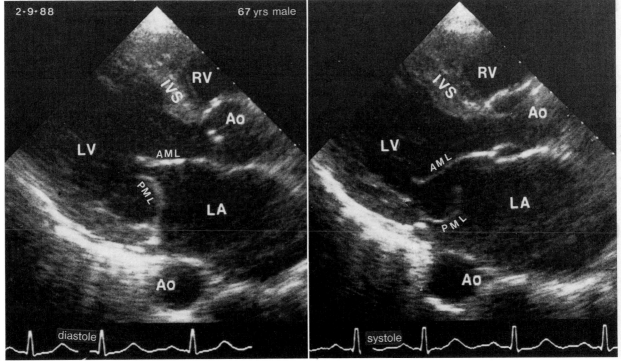

Fig. 22-1. These long-axis echoes of a 67-year-old asymptomatic man demonstrate typical MVP. **A,** During diastole, the mitral valve opens; both anterior mitral leaflet (AML) and posterior mitral leaflet (PML) appear to be elongated. **B,** During systole, the PML protrudes into the LA as doming. The coaptation of the leaflets is apparently incomplete. (Courtesy of S. Ogata, MD).

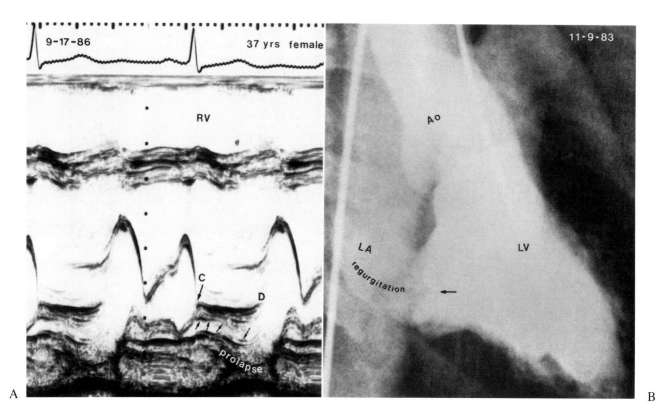

Fig. 22-2. An M-mode echo and a left ventriculogram are from a 37-year-old woman with hyperthyroidism accompanied by MVP. **A**, Her M-mode recording on the left shows normal E and A waves. Mitral valvular closure is indicated by C and a large arrow. Normally, there is a slight linear upward echo from points C to D, the point of onset of mitral valve opening. In this case, between the C and D a sagging extra echo approaches point D, indicating posterior mitral leaflet (PML) prolapse (small arrows). **B**, On the right, her left ventriculogram shows a volcano-like mitral valve allowing regurgitation into the LA.

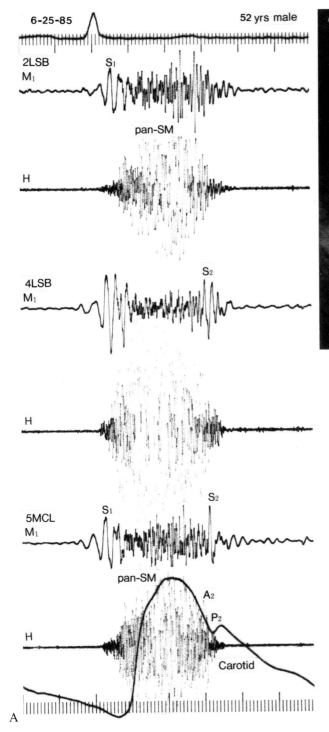

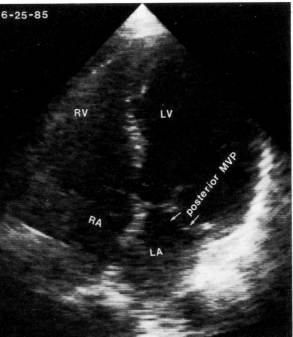

B

Fig. 22-3. This is another case of hyperthyroidism associated with MVP in a 52-year-old man. **A**, His PCG reveals a loud pansystolic regurgitant murmur from the 2LBS to the apex, resembling a VSD. **B**, His echo in the apical four-chamber view on the right shows the PML to be prolapsed into the LA during systole.

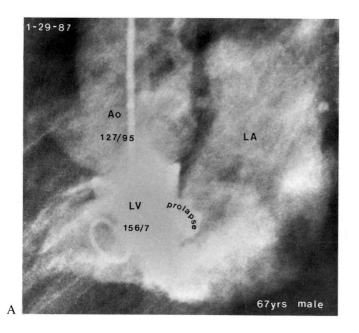

Fig. 22-4. A, This is a left ventriculogram from a 67-year-old man with a heart murmur showing the MVP with contrast medium leaking from the LV to the LA. The pressures in the LV and the Ao were 156/7 mm Hg and 127/95 mm Hg respectively. Thus there was about a 30 mm Hg pressure gradient between the LV and the Ao. The pulmonary capillary pressure was normal.

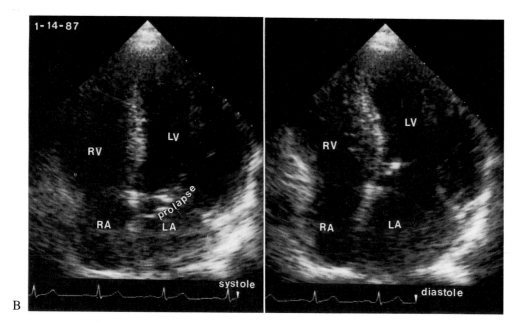

Fig. 22-4. *(Continued)* **B,** The apical four-chamber views show a strong echo on the AML and appears to indicate incomplete closure and protrusion into the LA in systole. There is no specific chamber enlargement.

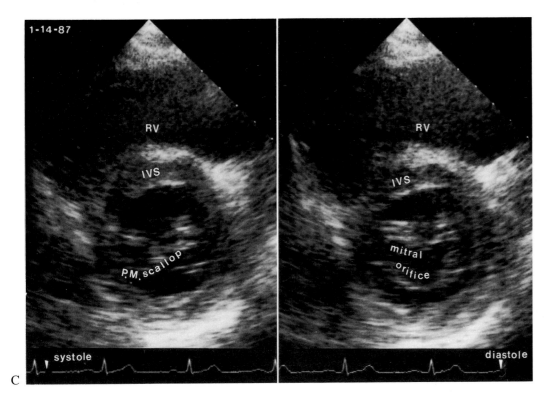

Fig. 22-4. *(Continued)* **C**, The short-axis echoes of the same patient show a prolapse of a posteromedial scallop (P.M. scallop) of the PML during systole.

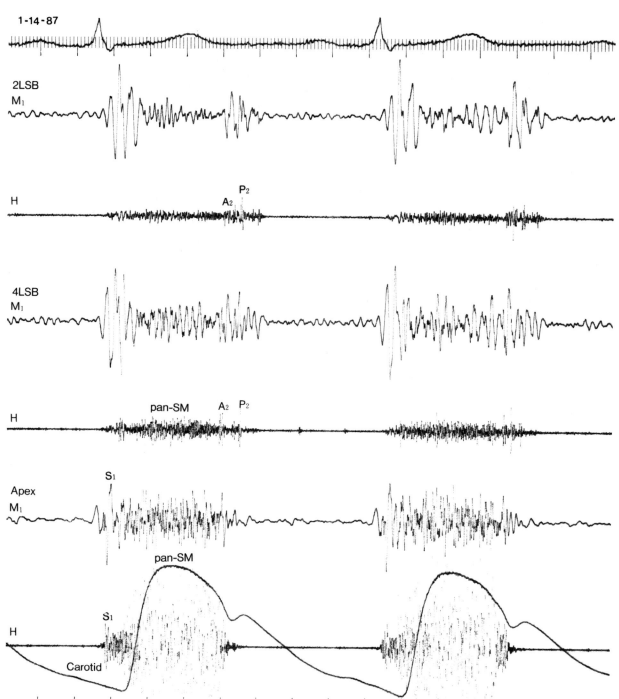

Fig. 22-4. *(Continued)* **D**, A PCG of the same patient shows splitting of S_2 with a crescendo regurgitant murmur maximal at the apex. There is a small vibration after P_2 which may be a short pulmonary regurgitant (PR) murmur. The apical murmur did not radiate well into the axillary region, an important characteristic of some MVP murmurs.

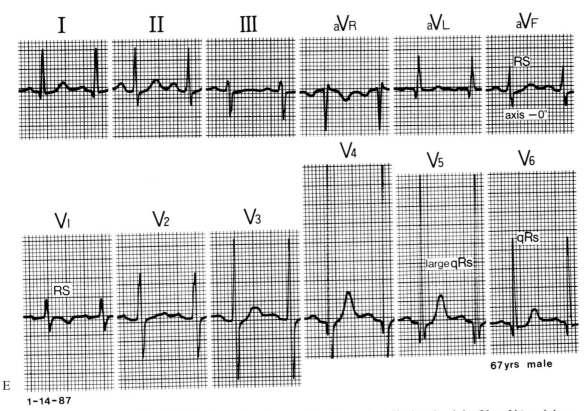

1-14-87

Fig. 22-4. *(Continued)* **E,** His ECG shows that the transitional zone is shifted to the right (V$_1$ to V$_3$) and there is a large QRS complex in V$_4$ and V$_5$ correlating with counterclockwise rotation of the heart. The large QRS complexes in V$_3$ to V$_5$ are frequently observed in counterclockwise rotation, since a tortuous ascending Ao twists the heart anteriorly causing the heart to abut against the sternum. Therefore, tall QRS complexes in the LV leads in this case do not necessarily indicate LV overloading.

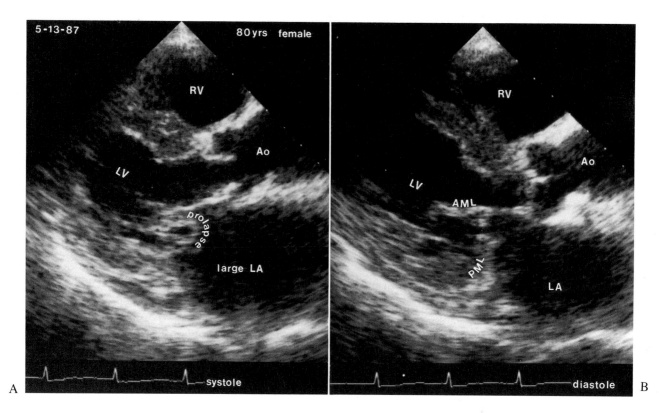

Fig. 22-5. A, UCG from an 80-year-old woman with hypertension. Long-axis echoes show marked MVP during systole. Her video showed the AML to be elongated and prolapsed into the LA.

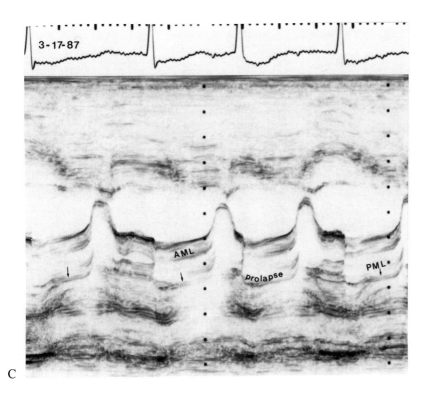

C

Fig. 22-5. *(Continued)* C, An M-mode echo of the same patient shows that the PML sags toward the LA, and there are multiple echoes of the mitral valve suggesting MVP. Multiple layering of echoes may also represent the redundancy of mitral leaflet tissue.

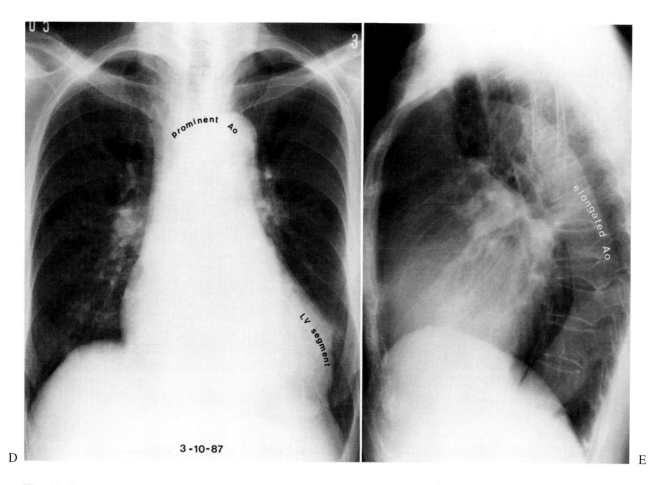

Fig. 22-5. *(Continued)* **D,** Chest x-rays show generalized cardiac enlargement and a prominent aortic arch. **E,** A tortuous Ao and LA enlargement are observed in the lateral view.

5-13-87

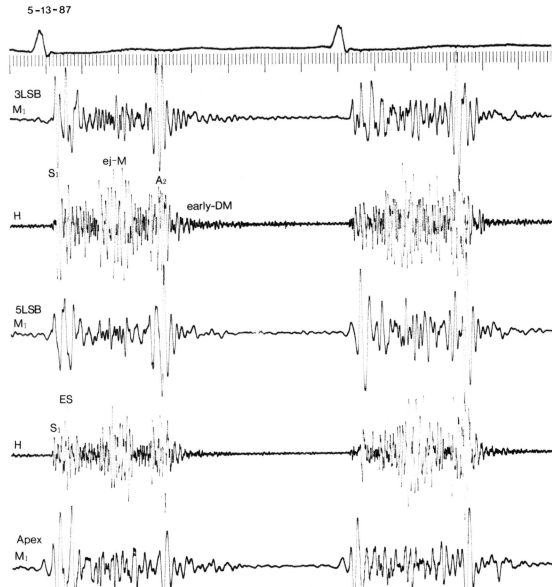

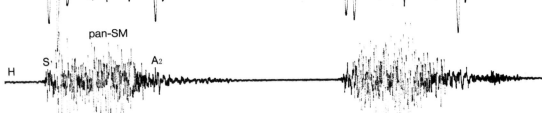

F

Fig. 22-5. *(Continued)* **F,** Her PCG shows a coarse ejection murmur (ej-SM) with slight mid-systolic accentuation and a soft early diastolic murmur (early DM) at the 3LSB. At the apex, there is a pansystolic murmur (pan-SM) extending beyond the A$_2$. The duration of the ejection murmur at the base is rather long and may overlap a regurgitant murmur.

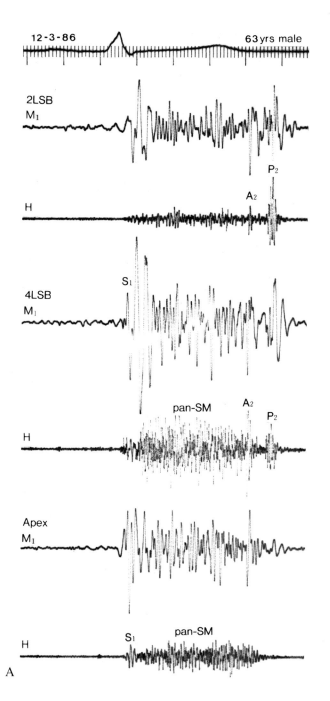

Fig. 22-6. A, PCG from a 63-year-old asymptomatic man with a heart murmur showing wide splitting of the S$_2$ at the 2LSB to 4LSB. A spindle-shaped pansystolic murmur (pan-SM) is seen in all regions. Because it is maximum at 4LSB, it is most unlikely that this murmur is of rheumatic origin, but could indicate MVP.

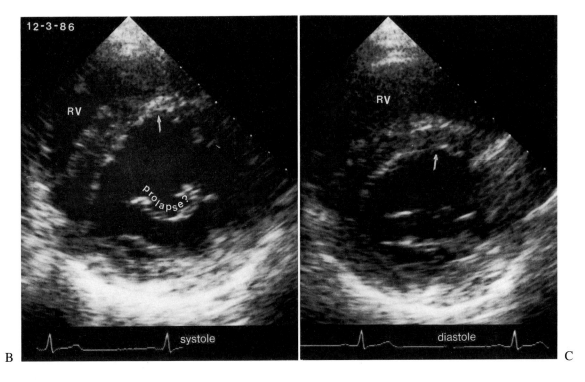

Fig. 22-6. *(Continued)* **B and C**, Short-axis echoes show probable MVP of the medial portion in systole. There is reduced thickness of the anterior portion of the IVS during both systole and diastole with some strong echoes (arrows). This suggests a fibrotic change in the IVS.

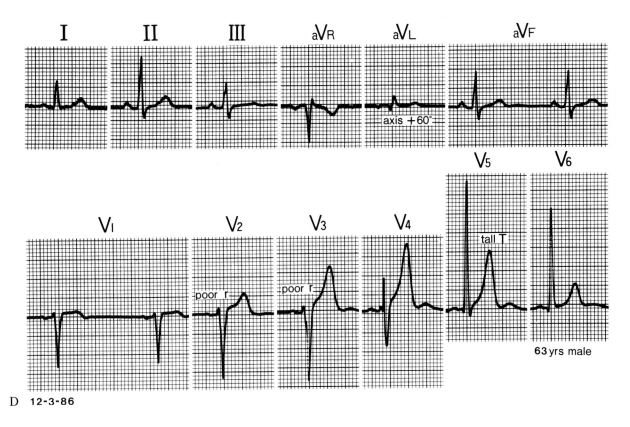

Fig. 22-6. *(Continued)* **D**. His ECG shows poor r/S ratio progression in V_2 and V_3 which correlates with echo changes in the septum. A tall T wave in V_3 to V_5 appears to show diastolic LV overloading.

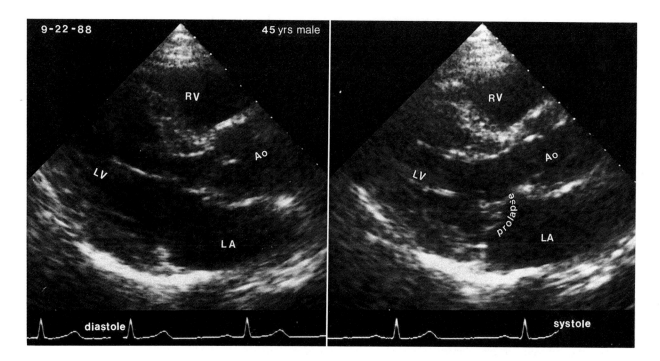

Fig. 22-7. This 45-year-old asymptomatic man has a pansystolic murmur at his apex. Long-axis echoes show no chamber enlargements but the AML protrudes into the LA during systole indicating MVP. The definition of the MVP by long-axis view may be difficult in some cases since there are many borderline cases.*

* When drawing a straight line from the distal end of the posterior aortic wall (which merges into the AML) to the hinging point of the PML as the base line, many true MVPs will not bulge beyond this line in systole. Thus false negative findings may result. Where the distal edge of the posterior wall of the Ao continues into AML, there is a short relatively immovable portion (observed by video) which is recommended as the point from which to draw the base line.

Chapter 23 Arteriosclerosis of the Aorta and Associated Sigmoid Septum

Pathophysiology and Clinical Clues

Elongation and/or tortuosity of the Ao may result from arteriosclerosis. The heart is suspended by the great vessels, and may be twisted either by elongation and/or tortuosity of the Ao resulting in counterclockwise rotation of the heart. Dilatation and calcification of the aortic arch are concomitant findings in counterclockwise rotation of the heart, but left ventricular hypertrophy and/or dilatation are not necessarily associated with counterclockwise rotation of the heart. Counterclockwise rotation of the heart may be the cause of the sigmoid septum commonly seen on echo in the elderly, i.e. the upper portion of the IVS protrudes below the aortic valve during diastole. In some cases, it may even obstruct the left ventricular outflow tract (LVOT) during systole, simulating hypertrophic subaortic stenosis.

Approaches to diagnosing arteriosclerosis of the aorta and sigmoid septum are as follows:

★★★★ Chest x-ray shows a dilated Ao including the ascending portion and the aortic arch. Concavity of the main PA segment is a feature if counterclockwise rotation is present. In the lateral view the descending Ao is imaged below the mid-portion of the cardiac silhouette. Calcification in the aortic wall is also a common finding.

★★★★ The ECG may show the septal q wave shifted to the right as far as V_3 (termed qV3 pattern) indicating counterclockwise rotation of the heart.

★★★★ Long-axis echoes show the sigmoid septum with a sharp aortoseptal angulation which may cause obstruction of the LVOT.

★★ On auscultation there is often a nonspecific aortic ejection murmur which is usually enhanced by amyl nitrite inhalation.

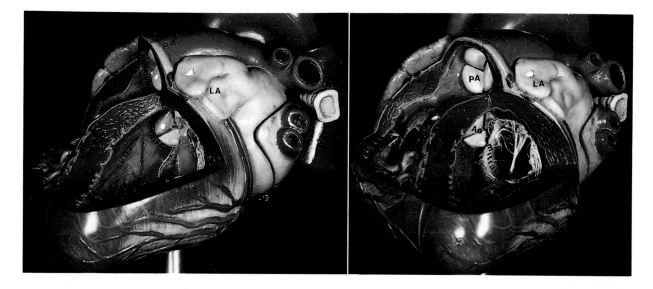

Fig. 23-1. This cardiac model illustrates the relationship between the IVS and the ventricles. The IVS protrudes into the RV below the pulmonary valve to comprise the right ventricular outflow tract (RVOT). The IVS forms a concavity at the left ventricular outflow tract (LVOT). This physiologic curvature of the IVS may be altered by counterclockwise rotation of the Ao from elongation and/or tortuosity caused by arteriosclerosis. Posteroinferior to the pulmonary valve, the right cusp and noncoronary cusp of the aortic valve are observed. The LVOT is behind the curvature of the IVS.

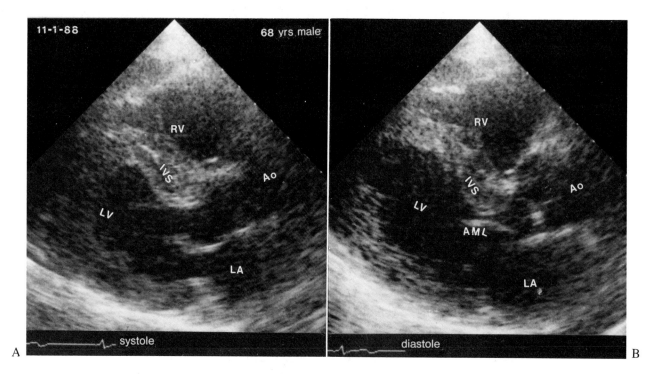

Fig. 23-2. A, This is from a 68-year-old asymptomatic man with a sigmoid septum. Long-axis echoes show the sigmoid septum protruding below the Ao during both diastole and systole. **B,** The anterior mitral leaflet (AML) touches the septum in diastole. The distal portion of the Ao seems enlarged. The aortoseptal angulation is very sharp.

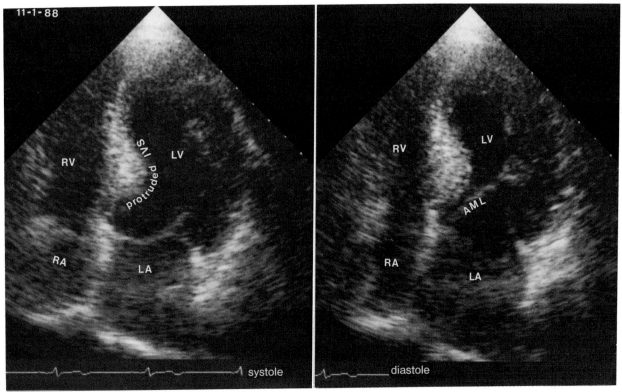

Fig. 23-2. *(Continued)* **C,** The apical four-chamber views show marked protrusion of the septum into the LVOT. The apical portion of his heart seems to be twisted toward the RV side. Since the degree of the systolic septal protrusion is different in the long-axis and the four-chamber view, the sigmoid septum is probably not causing obstruction of the LVOT during systole at rest.

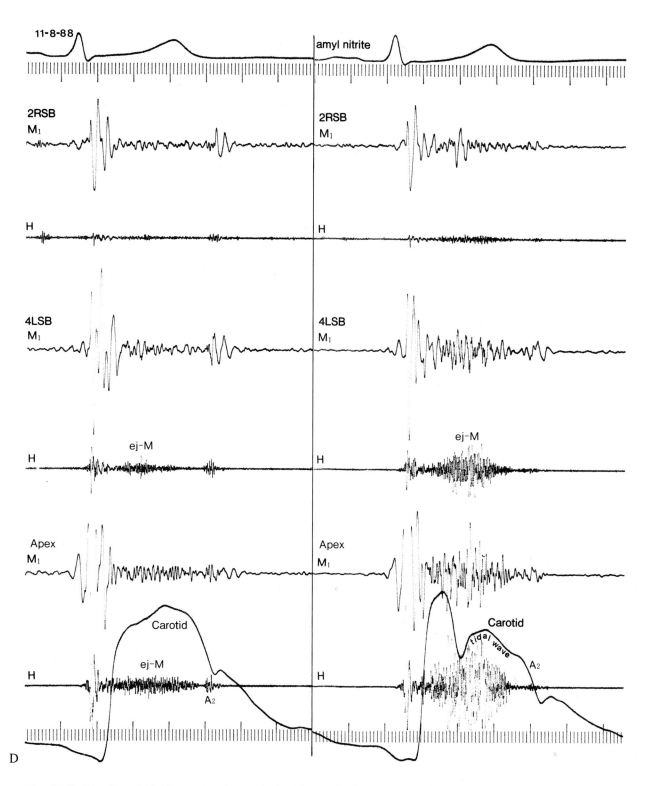

Fig. 23-2. *(Continued)* **D,** The patient has an insignificant ejection murmur (ej-M) at his apex. After amyl nitrite inhalation, however, his PCG shows a coarse ejection murmur. Simultaneous with the change of the murmur, the carotid tracing developed an abrupt descent of the percussion wave followed by a large tidal wave, often seen in cases of hypertrophic cardiomyopathy. Therefore, it is assumed that, with provocation, protrusion of the sigmoid septum can cause LVOT obstruction.

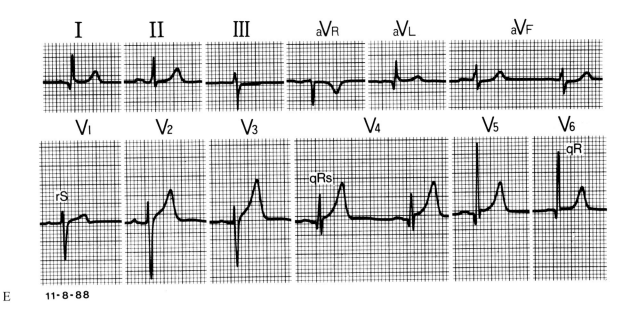

E   11·8·88

Fig. 23-2. *(Continued)* E, An ECG of the same patient shows a possible small q wave in V_3 which is inconclusive. When the normal septal q wave extends to V_3, it suggests counterclockwise rotation of the heart which is frequently concomitant with the sigmoid septum. Counterclockwise rotation of the heart may be caused by elongation and tortuosity of the Ao.

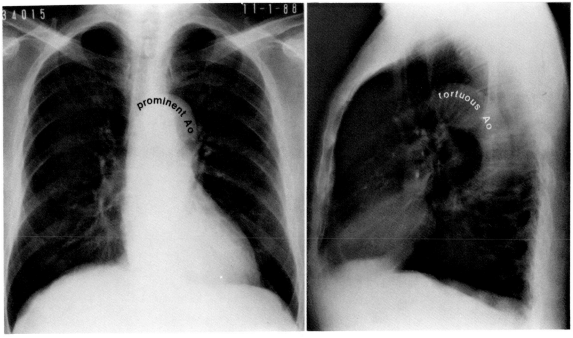

F   G

Fig. 23-2. *(Continued)* F, His chest x-rays show a prominent aortic arch. The main PA is not imaged because of the counterclockwise rotation. G, On the lateral view, a tortuous elongated descending Ao is visible, which appears to twist the upper portion of the heart posteriorly while the apex remains unchanged.

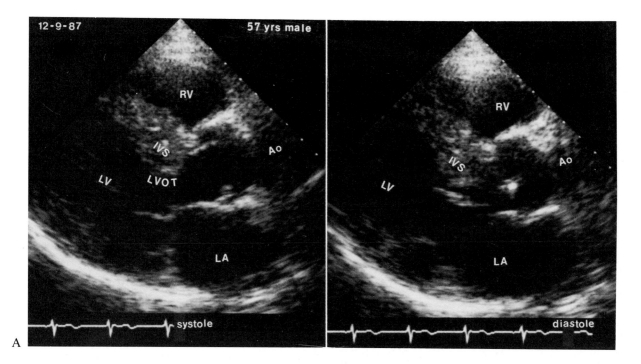

Fig. 23-3. A, This is a 57-year-old asymptomatic man with hypertension (160/90). Long-axis echoes show a sigmoid septum protruding into the LVOT during both systole and diastole. The degree of protrusion is about the same in both. Otherwise there are no remarkable findings.

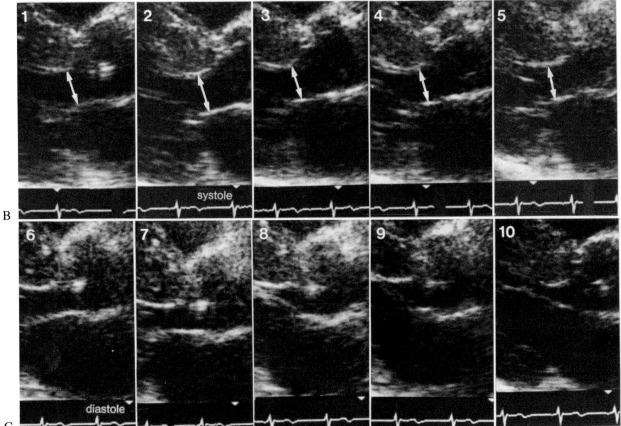

Fig. 23-3. *(Continued)* **B,** Serial long-axis echoes of the same patient focused on the IVS and the Ao show interesting findings. Figure 1 is during end-diastole and the aortic valve is closed. Figures 2 to 5 are during systole, and the IVS protrudes beneath the aortic ring. The maximum protrusion occurs in late-systole (Figures 4 to 5). The approximate width of the left ventricular outflow (LVOT) is indicated by arrows. **C,** During diastole, the LVOT again becomes narrower when the AML approaches the IVS.

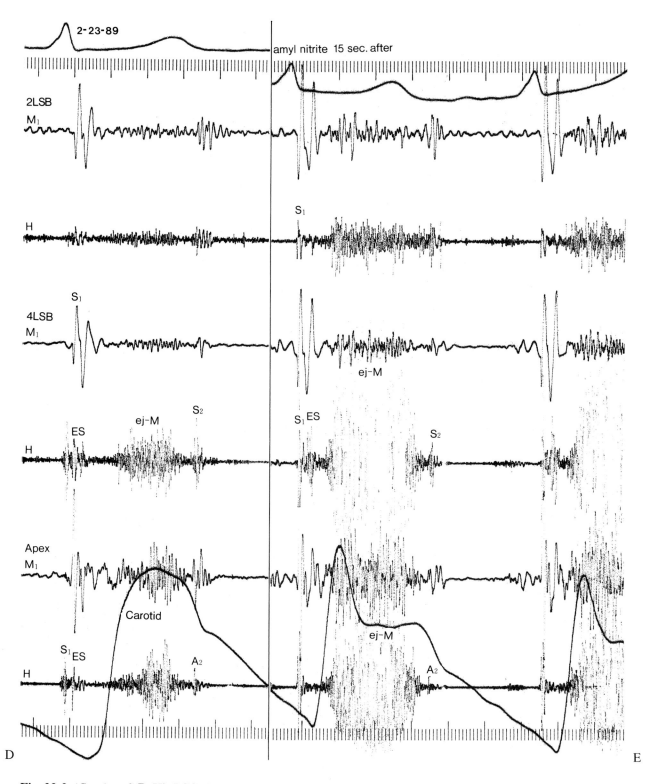

Fig. 23-3. *(Continued)* **D**, His PCG shows a soft ejection sound (ES) and ejection murmur (ej-M) accentuated toward late-systole at the 4LSB and transmitted to the apex. **E**, However, amyl nitrite inhalation (right) produced a coarse ejection murmur, and the carotid tracing showed an abrupt descent of the percussion wave followed by a prominent tidal wave. The ejection murmur has its peak toward late systole, which may indicate that this murmur is a result of the LVOT obstruction caused by the sigmoid septum.

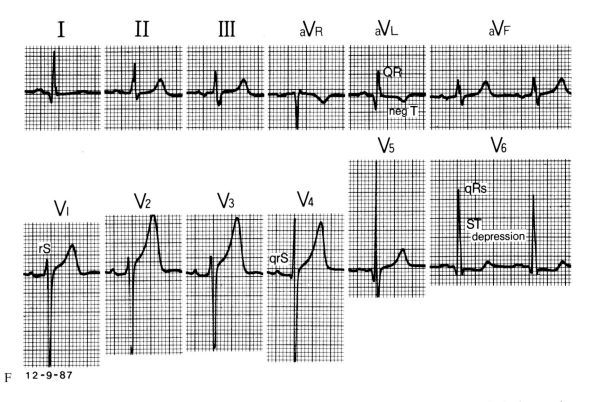

Fig. 23-3. *(Continued)* **F**, His ECG shows a qRS pattern in V$_4$ which may suggest counterclockwise rotation of the heart. There is a horizontal ST depression in V$_6$ indicating myocardial ischemia.

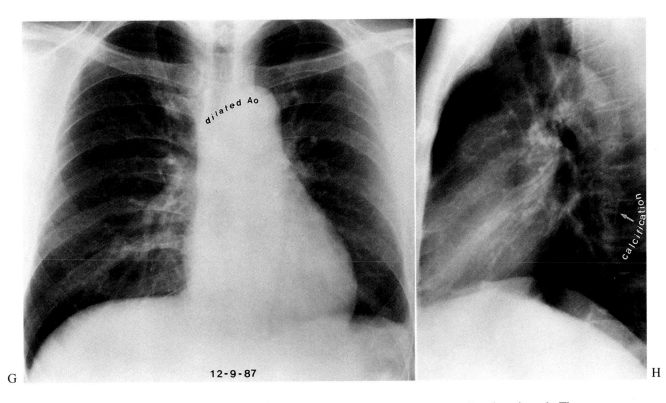

Fig. 23-3. *(Continued)* **G**, The frontal chest x-ray of the same patient demonstrates a dilated aortic arch. The main PA segment is not clearly visible. **H**, In the lateral view, a dilated aortic arch is seen and there is a linear calcification in the posterior wall of the descending Ao (arrow).

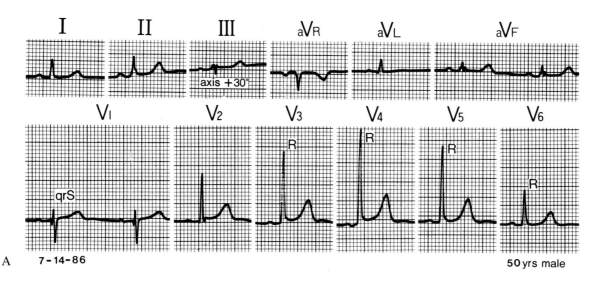

Fig. 23-4. A, ECG from a 50-year-old asymptomatic man who had an abnormal ECG at his annual physical. The QRS axis is normal (+30°) and there is a qrS pattern in V_1 and an R wave in V_2 to V_6 with upright T waves. The absence of an initial septal q wave in the LV leads together with a q wave in V_1 suggests an incomplete LBBB pattern or a corrected transposition of the great arteries (C/T). But there is no left-axis deviation as is commonly seen in C/T. However, with the transition zone shifted to between V_1 and V_2, marked counterclockwise rotation of the heart was suspected.

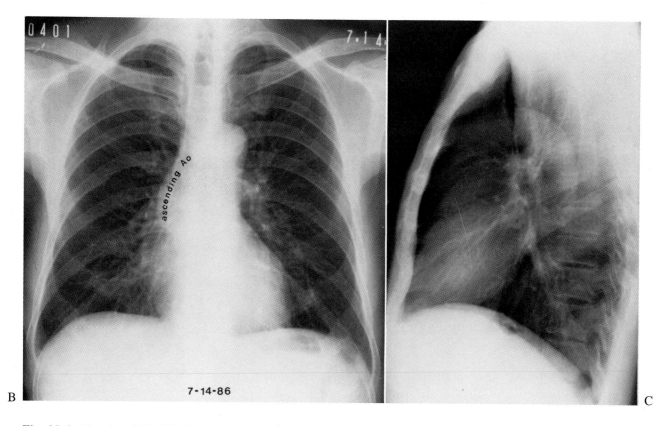

Fig. 23-4. *(Continued)* B, His chest x-rays reveal a prominent ascending Ao with a relatively large aortic arch. The main PA segment is concave. These findings are typical of counterclockwise rotation of the heart. C, The lateral view shows some increase in posteroanterior thoracic diameter which may be the cause of our inability to record his echo.

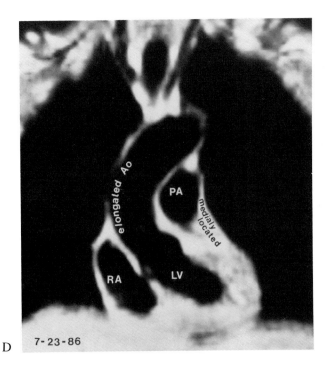

Fig. 23-4. *(Continued)* **D**, To verify the presence of counterclockwise rotation of the heart, MRI was performed. The coronal section of the MRI shows marked elongation of the ascending Ao with a medially-located main PA that correlated with the chest x-ray findings.

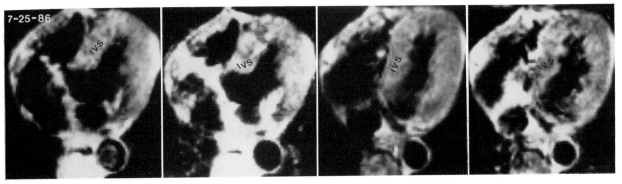

Fig. 23-4. *(Continued)* **E**, Serial MRI sections show a protruding upper portion of the septum in the LVOT region. Both the septum and the LV free wall seem to show symmetric hypertrophy. The septum is not oriented at the usual 45° angle due to counterclockwise rotation.

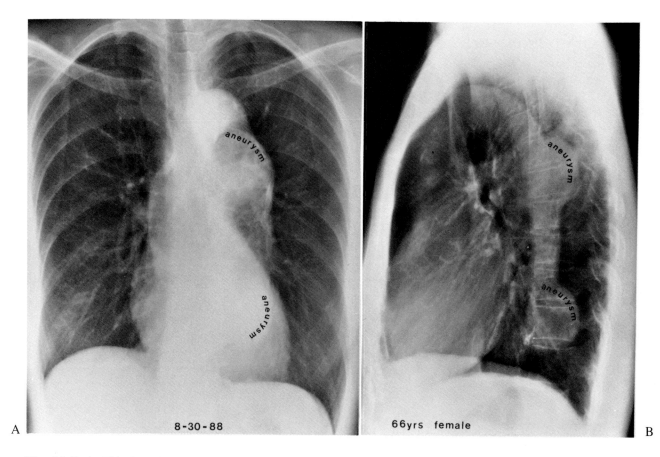

A

8-30-88

66yrs female

B

Fig. 23-5. A, This is a 66-year-old noncardiac patient who has aneurysms in her Ao. Her chest x-rays demonstrate a tortuous and elongated Ao with a large aneurysm which overlaps the left pulmonary artery. There is another aneurysm in the distal descending Ao just above the level of the diaphragm. B, On the lateral view, 2 aneurysms are clearly visible.

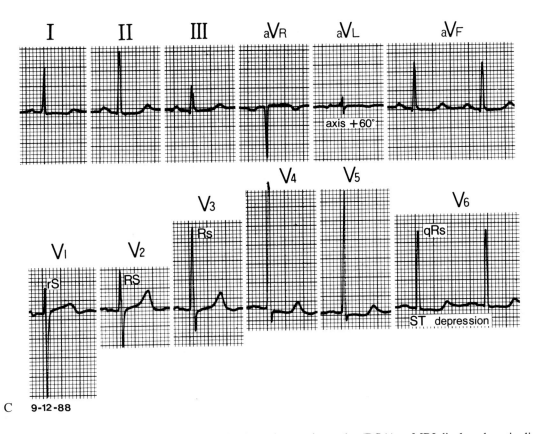

I   II   III   aVR   aVL   aVF

axis +60°

V1   V2   V3   V4   V5   V6

rS   RS   Rs   qRs

ST depression

C   9-12-88

Fig. 23-5. *(Continued)* **C,** Neither digital subtraction angiography (DSA) or MRI disclosed aortic dissection. Her ECG shows a transitional zone at V₂ suggesting counterclockwise rotation of her heart. There are horizontal ST depressions in the LV leads which indicate myocardial ischemia. The elongation and tortuosity of her Ao could be the cause of this counterclockwise rotation.

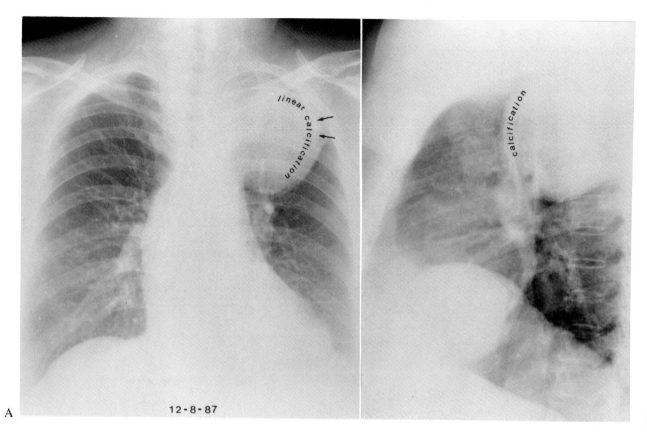

A

B

Fig. 23-6. A, These chest x-rays are from a 78-year-old woman with vague back pain. There is a huge mass next to the aortic arch and it cannot be separated from the Ao. The mass contains a linear calcification a few mm medial to the outer margin (arrows). **B,** On the lateral view, the mass appears to be attached to the aortic arch.

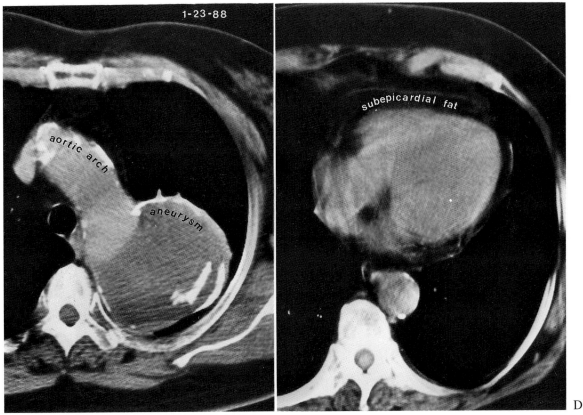

C   D

Fig. 23-6. *(Continued)* **C,** An enhanced cardiac CT section at the level of the aortic arch demonstrates a huge aneurysm with thrombus formation. There are 2 layers of calcifications. **D,** A CT section below the mitral valve shows no cardiac enlargement; there is abundant subepicardial fat surrounding the entire cardiac surface. This would show an extra echo space in the echo.

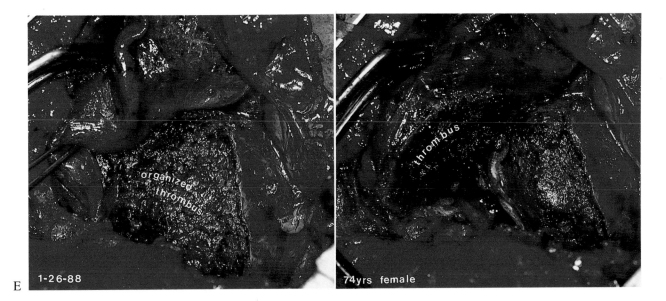

E

Fig. 23-6. *(Continued)* **E,** Because of her vague back pain, possibly caused by this aneurysm, a 5 × 5 cm thrombosed aneurysm was resected at surgery. The patient's recovery was uneventful.

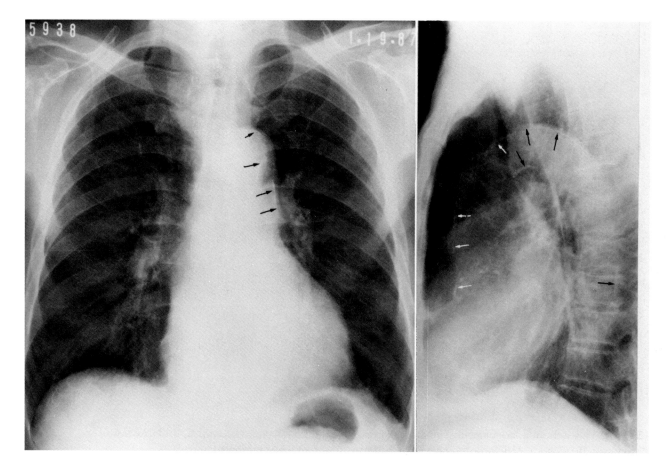

Fig. 23-7. These chest x-rays are from a 72-year-old man with arteriosclerosis of the Ao. They show fine linear calcifications from the ascending Ao to the descending Ao, simulating the aortitis syndrome. Calcification due to arteriosclerosis is usually thick, scattered along the Ao, and different from the aortitis syndrome in which the calcification is usually fine. In this case, however, in spite of calcification resembling aortitis, there is neither dilatation of the Ao nor any variation in its diameter. Therefore, this probably represents arteriosclerosis.

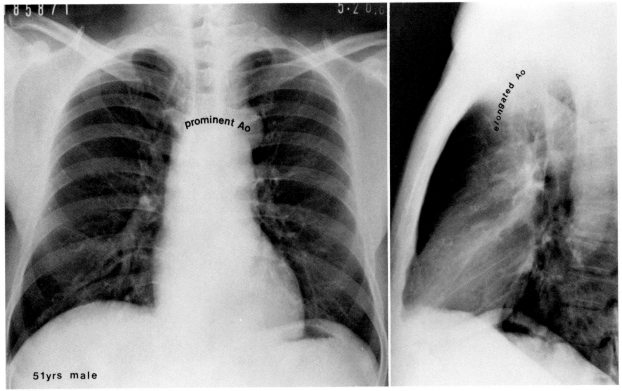

A | 51yrs male

B

Fig. 23-8. A, This is from a 51-year-old asymptomatic man with a prominent aortic arch. **B,** In the lateral view, however, there is no obvious aortic aneurysm, and the ascending Ao is elongated.

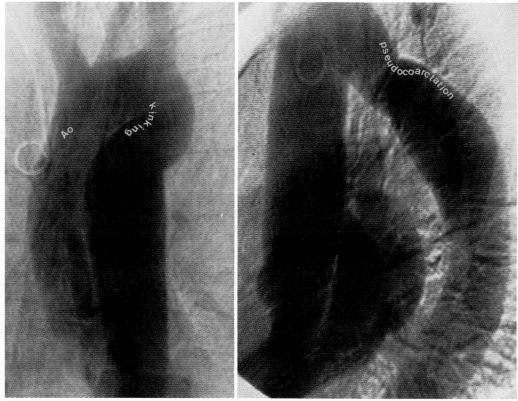

C

Fig. 23-8. *(Continued)* **C,** His DSA study shows marked kinking of the descending Ao below the aortic arch, producing a pseudocoarctation. This is an example of the difficulty in differentiating the causes of dilatation of the Ao by conventional radiography.

Chapter 24 Congestive Heart Failure

Pathophysiology and Clinical Clues

Congestive heart failure (CHF) consists of an imbalance between tissue oxygen requirements and supply, causing dyspnea, high venous pressure, and accumulation of fluid. In LV failure, the effect of volume and pressure proximal to the aortic valve is termed preload; that distal to the aortic valve is termed afterload. An example of the former is MS; the latter, hypertension or AS. In cases of mild CHF, the symptoms and signs include nocturia, nocturnal dyspnea, and weight gain. These symptoms are often overlooked. With severe CHF, orthopnea and peripheral edema with symptoms of dyspnea on exertion and fatigue are familiar symptoms.

The clinical approaches to diagnosing CHF are

★★★★ The chest x-ray reveals an abnormal distribution of pulmonary vasculature. Normally, the peripheral pulmonary vasculature is more prominent in the lower than in the upper lung fields, and this is termed "caudalization." When vasculature is equal in both lung fields, it is termed "equalization," and suggests a slight increase in the LA pressure. If the peripheral vasculature is more prominent in the upper than in the lower lung fields, it is termed "cephalization" and is caused by moderate to severe increase in LA pressure. Furthermore, interstitial edema causes hazy margins of the PA at the hilum, peripheral perivascular, peribronchial cuffing,[*] and septal lines. In acute CHF, butterfly or "bat-wing" appearances occur with pleural effusions on the right, or bilaterally.

★★★★ The ECG often shows LA overloading manifested by a biphasic P wave with increased area of terminal negativity in V_1 providing there is normal sinus rhythm. A negative U wave and prolongation of the QT interval may be present.

★★★★ On auscultation there may be an S_3. Mitral regurgitation may be present due to papillary muscle dysfunction secondary to LV dilatation or fibrosis.

★★★★ The echo reveals an enlarged LV and/or RV with decreased amplitude of motion of the anterior mitral leaflet (AML) and of the LV posterior wall (LVPW). There may occasionally be pericardial effusions.

---

[*] Peribronchial cuffing is seen as a cross-sectional view (ring) of a bronchus near the upper part of the hilum. The normal thin, sharply outlined ring becomes thicker and indistinct due to edema of the walls and connective tissue around the walls.

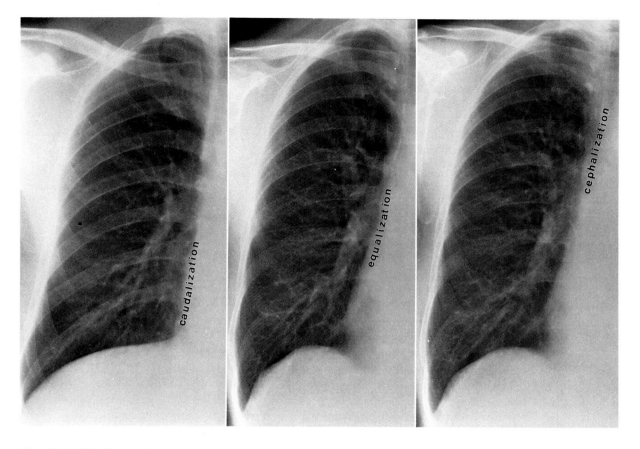

Fig. 24-1. This illustration demonstrates various types of peripheral pulmonary vascularities. On the left, normal peripheral pulmonary vascularity is greater in the lower lung field than that in the upper lung field, termed caudalization. In the middle, mild congestion is shown as equalization of the peripheral pulmonary vascularity in both the upper and lower lung fields. On the right, there is greater vascularity in the upper lung fields than in the lower, indicating cephalization. These abnormal distributions are caused by various degrees of elevation of LA pressure and differ from those of increased whole pulmonary blood flow, i.e., left to right shunts.

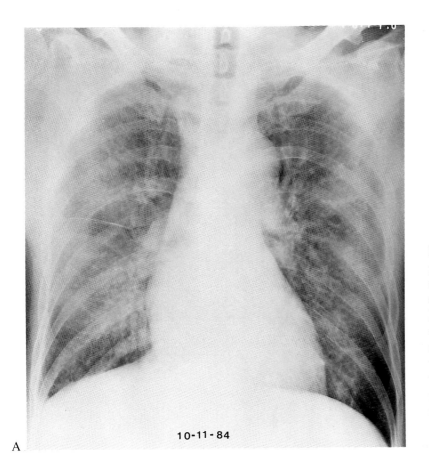

Fig. 24-2. A, This chest x-ray is from a 62-year-old man with persistent tachycardia of several hours duration. He had experienced similar tachycardias which had resolved upon lying down. The present attack occurred suddenly when he abruptly arose from his chair, suggesting paroxysmal supraventricular tachycardia (PSVT). On admission, his frontal chest x-ray showed diffuse, predominantly interstitial, pulmonary infiltration. The minor fissure was also thickened indicating the subpleural edema and/or the presence of a small amount of pleural fluid.

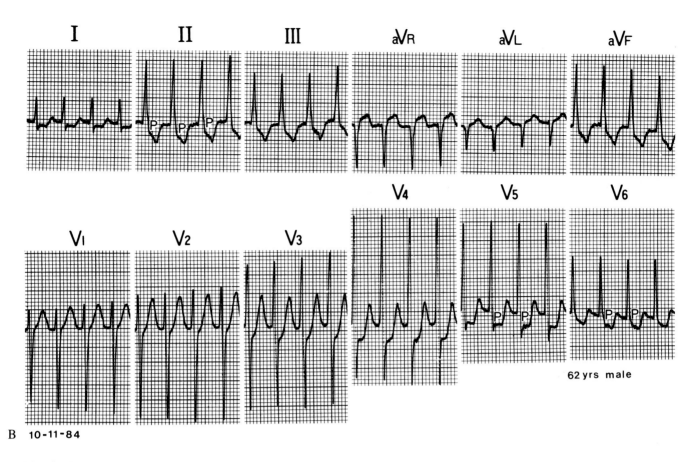

| I | II | III | aVR | aVL | aVF |

| V1 | V2 | V3 | V4 | V5 | V6 |

62 yrs male

B 10-11-84

Fig. 24-2. *(Continued)* **B,** His ECG made at nearly the same time showed tachycardia with a regular rate of 200. The QRS complex is narrow, and negative P waves following the QRS complexes indicate PSVT with retrograde P waves due to re-entry. The ST depression, especially in V$_3$ to V$_6$, suggests ischemic heart disease (IHD).

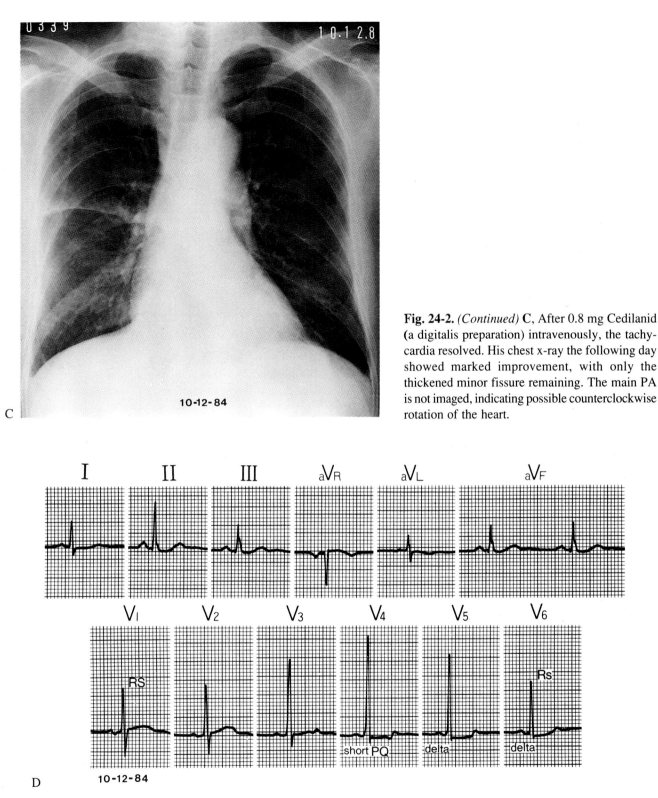

Fig. 24-2. *(Continued)* **C**, After 0.8 mg Cedilanid (a digitalis preparation) intravenously, the tachycardia resolved. His chest x-ray the following day showed marked improvement, with only the thickened minor fissure remaining. The main PA is not imaged, indicating possible counterclockwise rotation of the heart.

Fig. 24-2. *(Continued)* **D**, His ECG recorded the same day, shows sinus rhythm at a rate of 60. The P-R interval is nearly 0.14 seconds; however, V_4 to V_6 reveals a small delta wave. Rs patterns in V_1 to V_3 are suspicious of the A-V pre-excitation type A and the tachycardia was due to a W-P-W syndrome. The delta wave is upright in all precordial leads and the tall R waves in the RV leads suggest that activation progresses in a posteroanterior direction. In general, unless the atrial tachycardia lasts more than 48 hours, or is very rapid, CHF is uncommon.

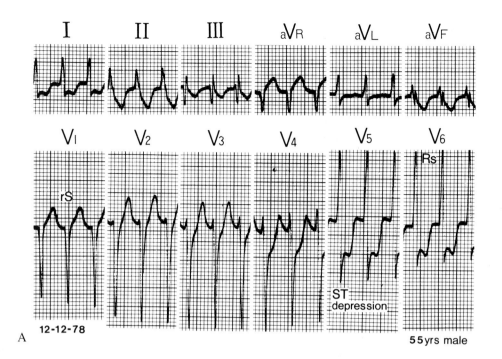

A   12-12-78

55 yrs male

Fig. 24-3. A, This is another case of PSVT with CHF. The patient is a 55-year-old man who had a typical history of PSVT. On admission his heart rate was 200. The QRS complex is narrow and the P waves are not identified. Marked ST depressions are observed in leads I, and V_4 to V_6 suggesting concomitant IHD.

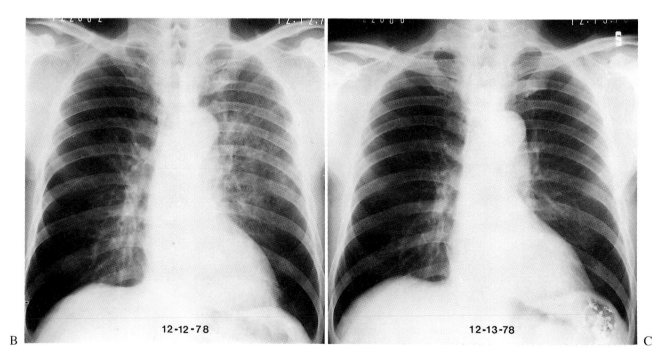

B   12-12-78   12-13-78   C

Fig. 24-3. *(Continued)* **B,** Chest x-rays on admission shows diffuse peripheral vascular congestion in his upper left lung field, indicating acute pulmonary edema. However, his right lung field is fairly clear. This congestion, limited to the left lung, may be due to the fact that the patient remained in the left lateral decubitus position until he was admitted. **C,** His frontal chest x-ray made the following day shows complete resolution of the congestion.

V6

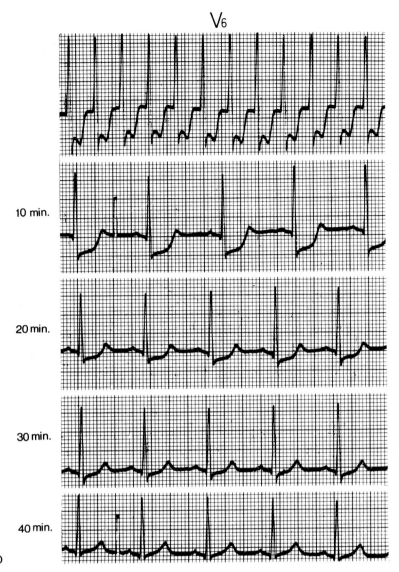

10 min.

20 min.

30 min.

40 min.

D

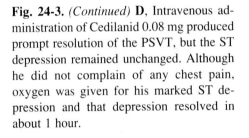

Fig. 24-3. *(Continued)* **D,** Intravenous administration of Cedilanid 0.08 mg produced prompt resolution of the PSVT, but the ST depression remained unchanged. Although he did not complain of any chest pain, oxygen was given for his marked ST depression and that depression resolved in about 1 hour.

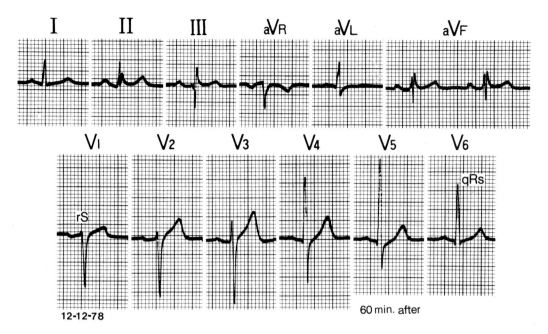

Fig. 24-3. *(Continued)* **E**, After resolution of the ST depression, there is a biphasic P wave with abnormal negativity in V_1 suggesting LA overloading.

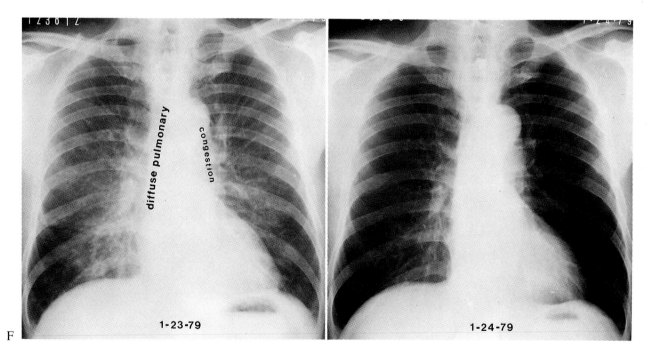

Fig. 24-3. *(Continued)* **F**, Interestingly, this patient had a similar episode of PSVT a month later that ceased on admission. His frontal chest x-ray showed identical congestion mainly in his right lung field with some on the left. **G**, This congestion also resolved the following day. Although PSVT usually does not cause CHF, CHF may result if there is concomitant heart disease, or if there is an extremely rapid heart rate of prolonged duration.

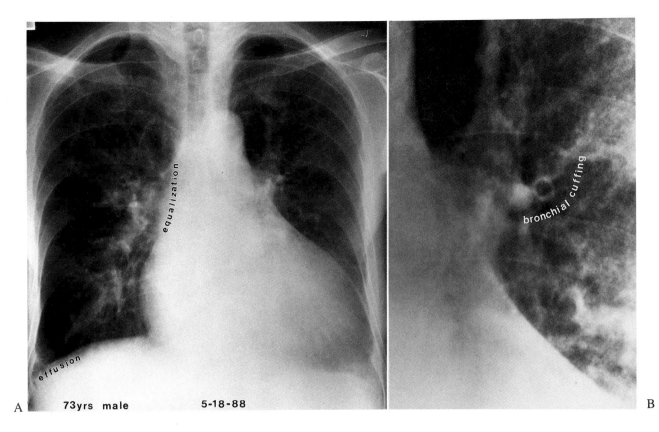

A   73yrs male   5-18-88   B

Fig. 24-4. A, These chest x-rays are from a 73-year-old man with combined valvular heart disease. On his first visit he complained of exertional dyspnea, and his heart is enlarged bilaterally with pleural effusion on both sides. The margin of his right central artery is hazy and the peripheral pulmonary vascularity shows "equalization." **B,** A magnified view of the left hilum shows the haziness of the left PA and bronchial cuffing.

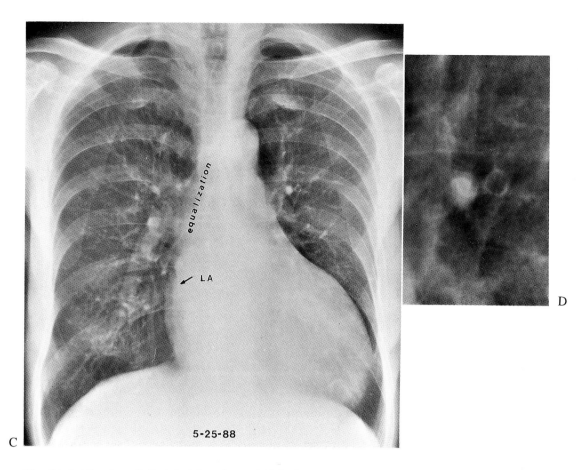

C

D

Fig. 24-4. *(Continued)* **C**, Administrations of digitalis and a diuretic for 1 week resolved his symptoms as well as his chest x-ray findings. The cardiac silhouette shows a prominent LV segment, but there is resolution of the bilateral pleural effusions. The peripheral pulmonary vascularity remains that of "equalization"; however, the previous haziness of his central artery on the right is now absent. **D**, A magnified view of the left hilum shows a hazy peripheral pulmonary artery as a white circle, but the peripheral bronchus appears relatively clear.

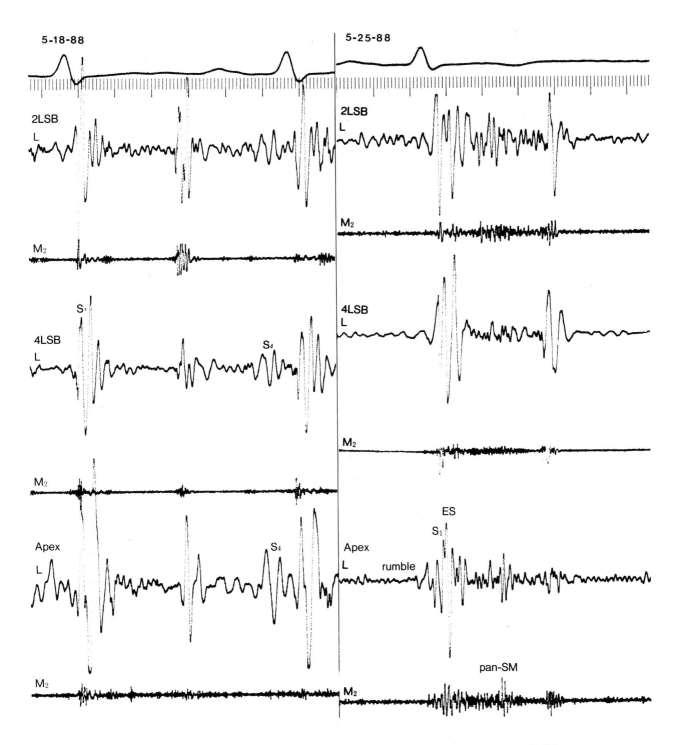

Fig. 24-4. *(Continued)* **E,** His PCGs made the same day as his chest x-ray show a loud S_4 from the 4LSB to the apex. One week later, this S_4 resolved and there was an ejection sound (ES), and a possible regurgitant murmur of MR at the apex. Auscultation suggested MR plus MS and AR.

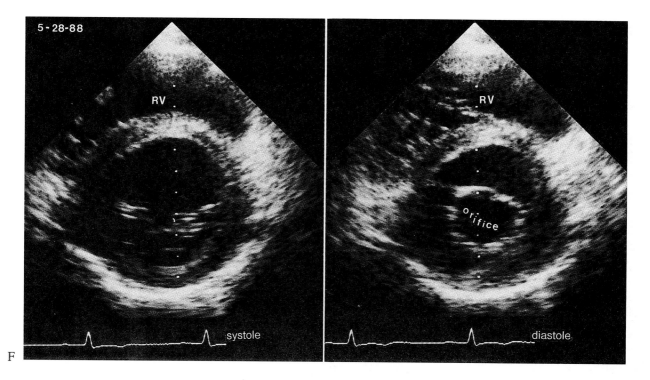

Fig. 24-4. *(Continued)* **F,** Ten days after his initial visit, he became asymptomatic. Short-axis echoes demonstrate a slightly limited opening of the mitral valve but there is no obvious calcification. Both the size of LV and the RV are not remarkable.

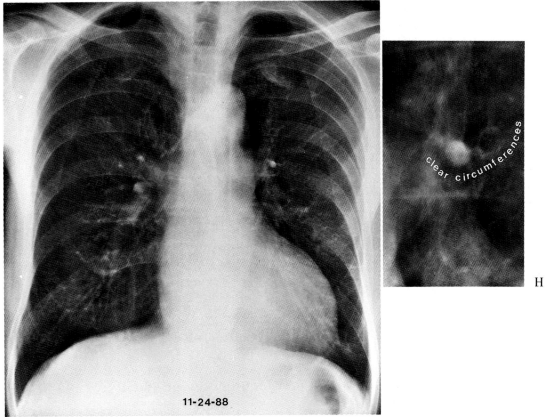

G

H

Fig. 24-4. *(Continued)* **G,** Frontal chest x-ray of the same patient nearly 6 months later shows marked reduction in cardiac size. The margin of the central artery on the right is clear and there is less peripheral pulmonary vascularity in his upper lung fields. **H,** A magnified view of his left hilum now shows clear circumferences of both the peripheral PA and the bronchus which indicates a resolution of the interstitial edema. This finding should be emphasized in determination of the presence of CHF when the cardiac silhouette shows no appreciable change in its size.

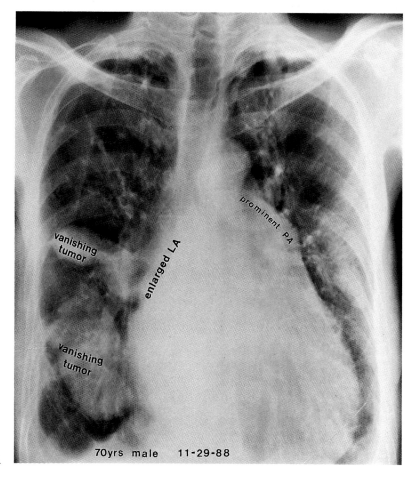

vanishing
tumor

enlarged LA

prominent PA

vanishing
tumor

70yrs male   11-29-88

A

Fig. 24-5. A, This 70-year-old retired school principal was admitted for exertional dyspnea. Although he had many annual physical examinations, he was not told of any heart murmur. Over the past few years, he began to notice exertional dyspnea which had increased for several days before admission. On admission, his frontal chest x-ray showed cardiomegaly with bilateral pleural effusions. In the mid- and lower-lung fields on his right, there were 2 tumor-like densities. Despite a relatively small aortic arch, his main PA was prominent. An enlarged LA was seen as a double density along the right cardiac margin. Peripheral pulmonary vascularities were increased. At first impression, it looked like the last stages of atrial septal defect.

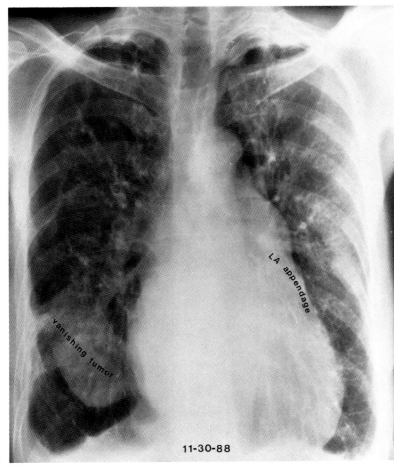

vanishing tumor

LA appendage

11-30-88

B

Fig. 24-5. *(Continued)* **B,** Intravenous administration of digitalis and a diuretic acted promptly; there is a residual tumor-like density only in the lower lung fields. A previously unidentified LA appendage was apparent. The pulmonary vascularity showed cephalization. Because of an enlarged LA, a Lutembacher syndrome* was suspected.

* Lutembacher is one of the congenital heart diseases with ASD associated with MS.

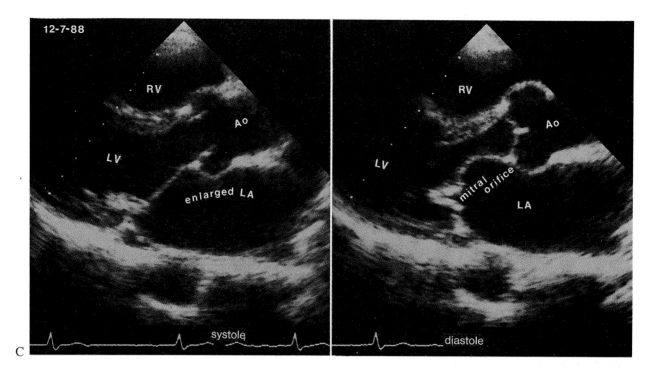

Fig. 24-5. *(Continued)* **C,** Long-axis echoes made 7 days later show a dilated LA with moderately severe MS. Auscultation revealed a high pitched AR-like murmur that was probably due to pulmonary regurgitation, i.e., a Graham-Steell murmur.

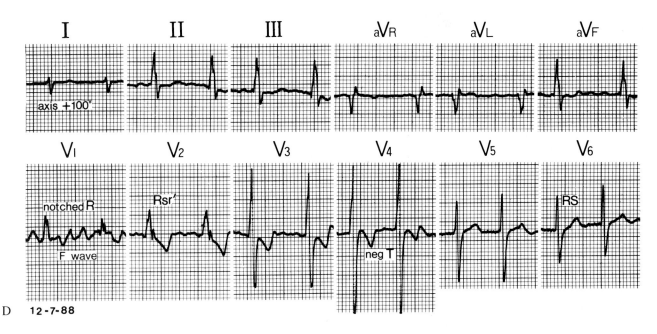

I II III aVR aVL aVF

axis +100°

V₁ V₂ V₃ V₄ V₅ V₆

notched R Rsr' RS

F wave neg T

D 12-7-88

Fig. 24-5. *(Continued)* **D,** ECG made the same day as the echo shows AF with a rate of about 90 to 120. Despite adequate digitalis, he showed a rapid heart rate, and hyperthyroidism was suspected for which Inderal 20 mg was effective. His ECG shows a QRS axis of about +100° with small QRS complexes in both leads I and V₁. V₁ shows a relatively tall and notched R wave. These findings are compatible with MS and, with negative T waves in V₂ to V₄, suggest severe RV overloading. If, in spite of digitalis, there is an upright T wave in V₅ and V₆, concomitant AR and/or MR should be suspected.

Fig. 24-5. *(Continued)* **E,** His frontal chest x-ray 3 weeks later shows a prominent main PA and LA enlargement. The peripheral pulmonary vascularity is that of cephalization with a minimal residual pleural effusion on the right.

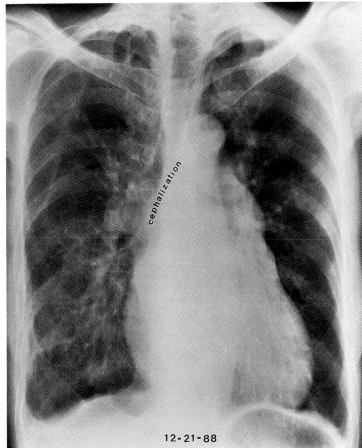

cephalization

12-21-88

E

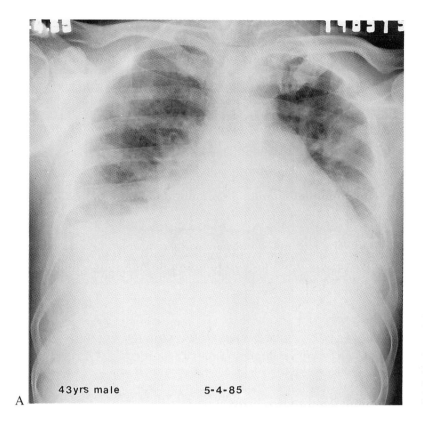

A

Fig. 24-6. A, This is from a 43-year-old man with an upper respiratory infection of 3 days duration. On admission, his portable chest x-ray showed marked cardiac enlargement with pulmonary congestion and bilateral pleural effusions.

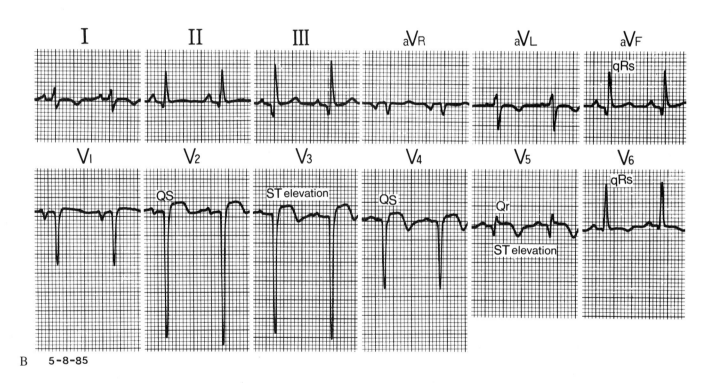

B   5-8-85

Fig. 24-6. *(Continued)* B, An ECG 4 days later showed wide Q waves in leads III and aVF and V_1 to V_5, indicating extensive myocardial involvement. ST elevations are also seen in V_1 to V_5 suggesting that there is either an acute infarct or an old aneurysm.

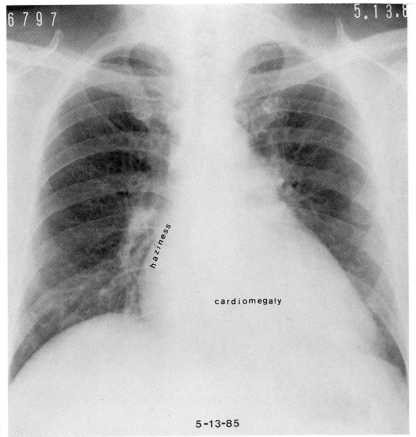

Fig. 24-6. *(Continued)* **C,** With treatment for CHF, his frontal chest x-ray 9 days after admission revealed cardiac enlargement with a decrease in the degree of CHF. The CHF is indicated by the haziness of the central pulmonary arteries. If there is marked cardiac enlargement with negligible CHF, one must suspect pericardial effusion.

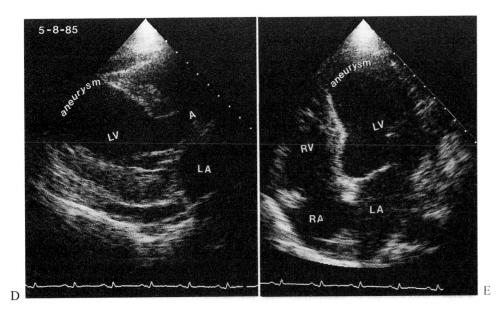

Fig. 24-6. *(Continued)* **D,** His echoes 3 days after admission showed an extra-echo space (EES) due to pericardial effusion behind the left ventricular posterior wall (LVPW) in the long-axis view. **E,** Aneurysmal dilatation of the LV at the apex in the apical four-chamber view on the right is evident.

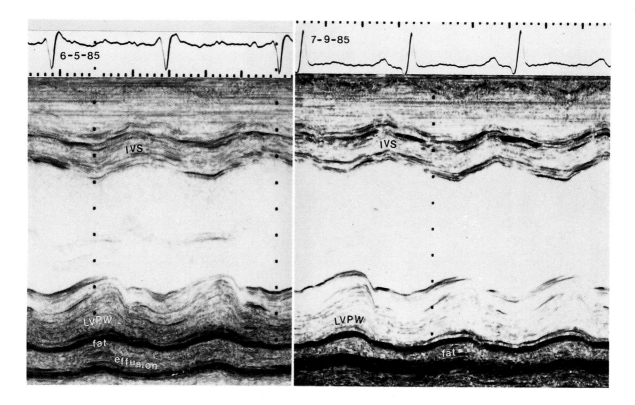

Fig. 24-6. *(Continued)* **F**, His M-mode echo (left) made about a month later shows a double-layered EES behind the LVPW, indicating subepicardial fat proximally and pericardial effusion distally. On the right, nearly 2 months after admission, his M-mode echo shows resolution of the pericardial effusion. The subepicardial fat remains.

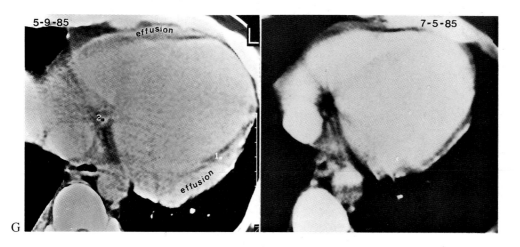

Fig. 24-6. *(Continued)* **G**, Cardiac CT sections made the same day of the M-mode echoes show pericardial effusions both anteriorly and posteriorly which resolved 2 months later.

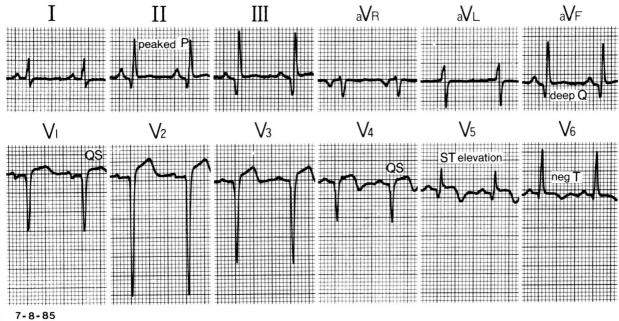

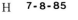
H   7-8-85

Fig. 24-6. *(Continued)* **H,** An ECG made about 2 months after admission shows that the QS pattern remained unchanged in V₁ to V₄ with very little regression of the ST elevations. Interpretation of the peaked P in lead II in this case is difficult. MI involvement of the RA usually causes AF, which is not the case here. Myocarditis and/or pulmonary embolism seems to be a better explanation, but this is not conclusive.

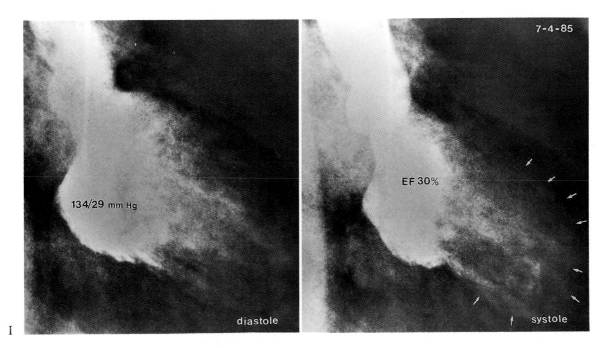

I

Fig. 24-6. *(Continued)* **I,** Finally, left ventriculography and coronary angiography were performed. The ejection fraction (EF) was 30% and hypokinesis of the apical portion of his LV was observed, which correlated well with the echo findings. Pressure in the LV was 134/29 mm Hg, indicating LV failure.

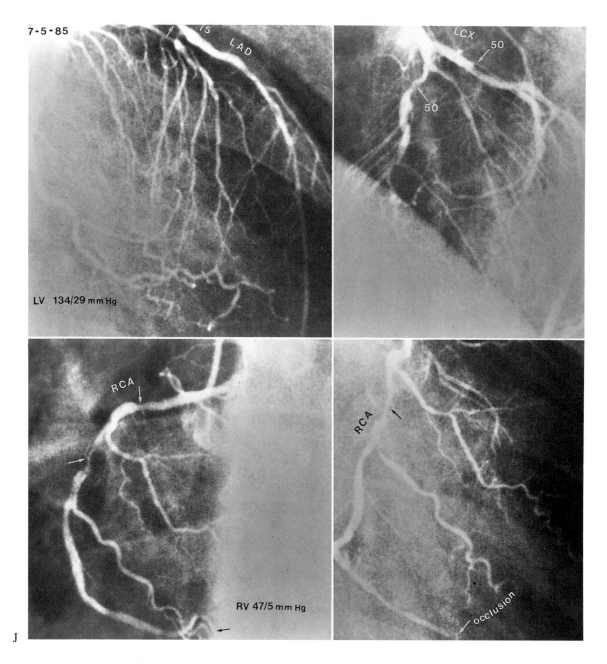

7-5-85

75
LAD

LV 134/29 mm Hg

LCX
50

50

RCA

RV 47/5 mm Hg

RCA

occlusion

J

Fig. 24-6. *(Continued)* **J,** His coronary angiogram revealed three-vessel disease. On the top left, the left anterior descending artery (LAD) showed 75% obstruction near the diagonal branch, and 50% occlusion in the left circumflex artery (LCX) on the right. In the bottom row, the right coronary artery (RCA) was also severely occluded and its peripheral circulation was made via collaterals from the LCX on the left lower row. To review, this case involves a 43-year-old patient with an old silent MI. His upper respiratory infection prior to admission, without abnormal blood chemistries does not suggest acute MI. A pericardial effusion is also unusual for acute MI and leads us to suspect myocarditis. Since his chest x-rays showed marked cardiac enlargement on admission, myocarditis superimposed on an old silent MI was considered. The patient did not return for further treatment.

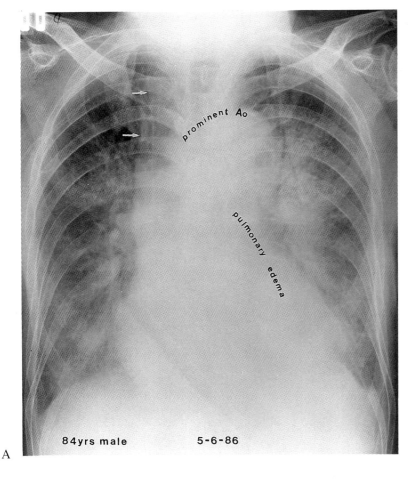

Fig. 24-7. A, Chest x-ray of an 84-year-old man with acute dyspnea shows acute pulmonary edema and a dilated superior vena cava (SVC) (arrows). His aortic arch (Ao) is also prominent. Since this x-ray is portable and therefore in the anteroposterior projection, accurate measurements are impossible; however, the cardiac base seems enlarged, suggesting the presence of a pericardial effusion.

84yrs male   5-6-86

A

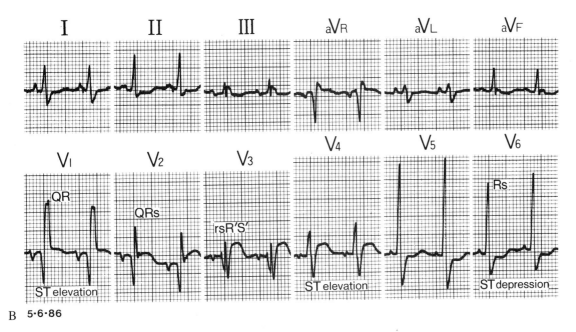

B 5·6·86

Fig. 24-7. *(Continued)* **B,** The ECG on admission shows a RBBB. A Q in V_1 and V_2 with upward convex ST elevations in V_1 to V_4 suggests an acute anteroseptal MI. The ST depressions seen in V_5 to V_6 are probably not the reciprocal changes of an anteroseptal MI, but represent previously existing subendocardial ischemia or fibrosis.

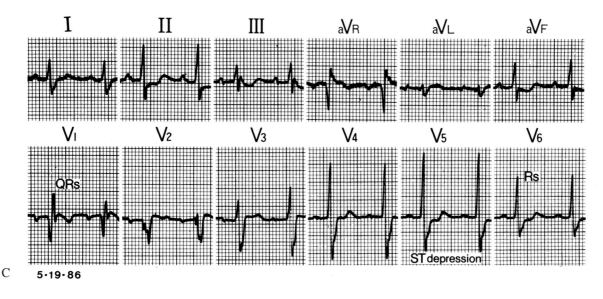

C 5·19·86

Fig. 24-7. *(Continued)* **C,** About 2 weeks later, his ECG shows a QRs pattern in V$_1$ and the previously noted ST elevations in V$_1$ to V$_3$ have resolved.

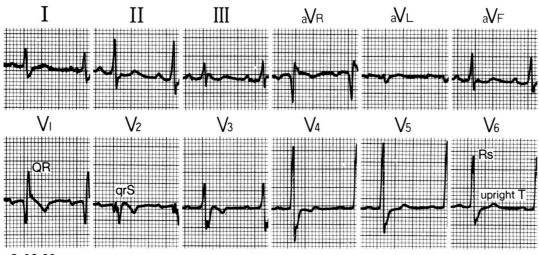

D 5-26-86

Fig. 24-7. *(Continued)* **D,** Three weeks later his ECG shows a QR in V$_1$ and a qrS pattern in V$_2$. There are no previously described ST elevations or depressions, and the T waves in the LV leads are upright, indicating resolution of the myocardial damage in the LV region.

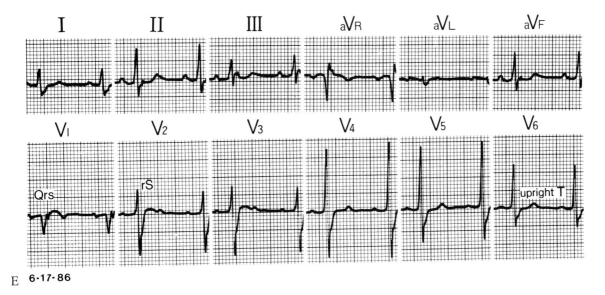

I   II   III   aVR   aVL   aVF

V1   V2   V3   V4   V5   V6

Qrs   rS   upright T

E   6·17·86

Fig. 24-7. *(Continued)* **E,** His ECG 5 weeks after admission, shows resolution of the ST elevation. The RBBB pattern has resolved and a Qrs pattern is seen in V₁. There are notched T waves in V₁ and V₂, indicating residual abnormal repolarization in these regions.

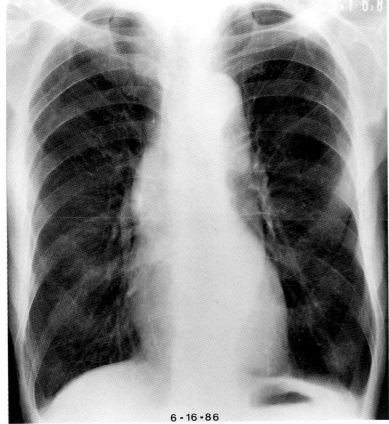

F   6 · 16 · 86

Fig. 24-7. *(Continued)* **F,** Frontal chest x-ray of the same patient 5 weeks after admission shows his heart is in the center of his thorax and his diaphragm is low. The ascending Ao is elongated and the main PA is not imaged, indicating counterclockwise rotation of the heart. However, there is no evidence of CHF. This case demonstrates that chest x-rays and ECG showing severe abnormalities do not always mean a poor prognosis. He recovered uneventfully.

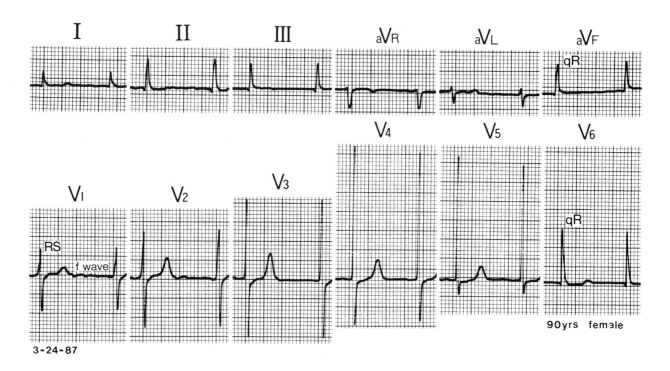

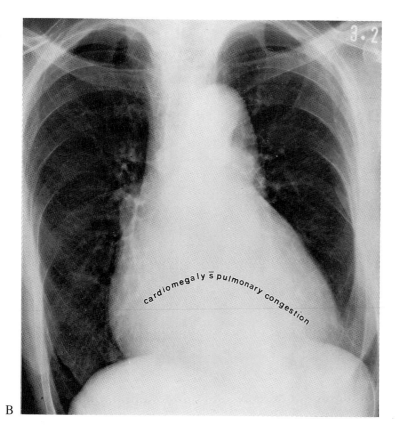

Fig. 24-8. A, This 90-year-old woman experienced gradually increasing shortness of breath over the past several years. She had not sought medical assistance. Her ECG on admission showed AF at the rate of about 100. Despite the low voltage in the extremity leads, V₃ and V₄ show large QRS complexes with upright T waves.

Fig. 24-8. *(Continued)* **B,** Her frontal chest x-ray shows marked cardiomegaly without pulmonary congestion, suggesting pericardial effusion.

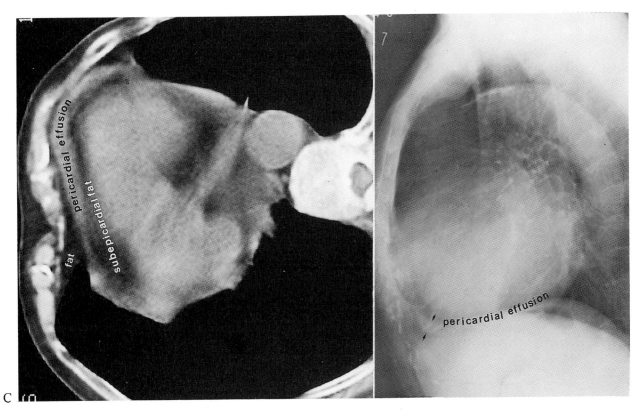

C

D

Fig. 24-8. *(Continued)* **C,** On the left, a cardiac CT scan reveals increased anteroposterior diameter of her thorax. The cardiac CT scan is illustrated in the right lateral decubitus position in order to facilitate a clear comparison with her lateral x-ray. Abundant subepicardial fat is seen both anteriorly and posteriorly with a widened anterior pericardial space, indicating a small pericardial effusion. A triangular radiolucent region between the sternum and the heart indicates the pericardial fat. **D,** In the lateral x-ray, the anterior pericardial stripe is increased in width correlating with the CT finding.* In the present case, a radiolucent zone which encases the cardiac silhouette represents subepicardial fat. There is another radiolucent zone beneath the sternum representing pericardial fat. Between these 2 radiolucent layers is a band-like opacity, which represents the anteriorly-located pericardial effusion.

* Normally, the anterior pericardial stripe is less than 2 to 3 mm in width, and it may become greater than 5 mm in cases of pericardial effusion.

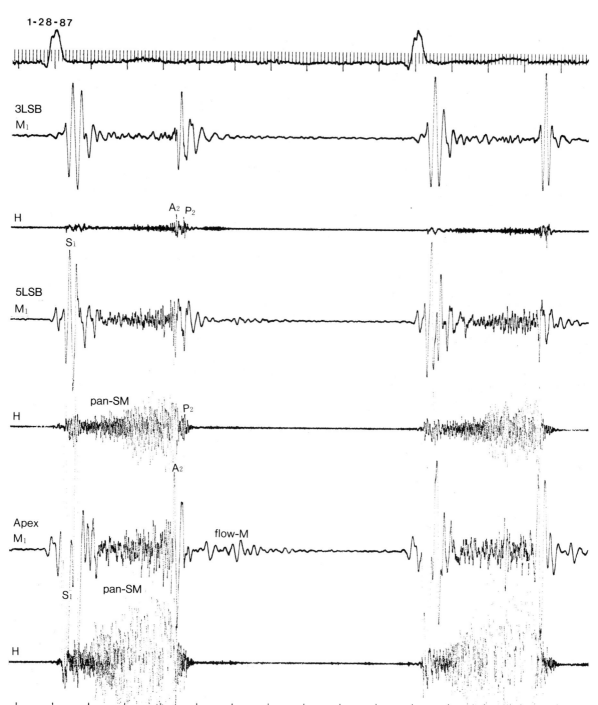

Fig. 24-8. *(Continued)* **E,** A PCG of the same patient shows narrow splitting of S_2 at the base of the heart. A harsh crescendo regurgitant murmur is present at the 4LSB to 5LSB and loudest at the apex.

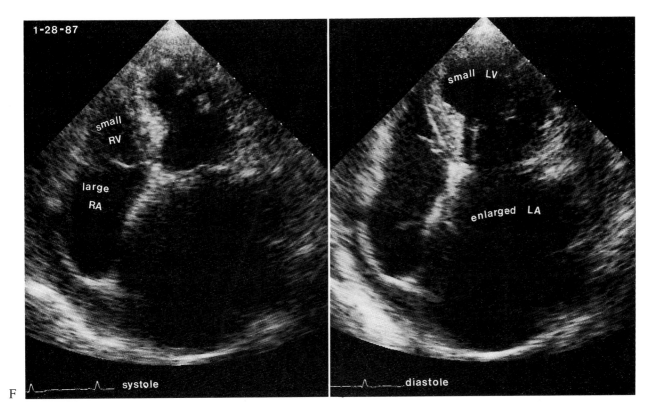

Fig. 24-8. *(Continued)* **F,** Her echoes in the apical four-chamber view show marked dilatation of the LA with a small LV. The RA is also larger than the RV, indicating that this is not a usual MR or tricuspid regurgitation (TR) in spite of the regurgitant murmur. During systole, there is neither mitral nor tricuspid valvular prolapse. Enlarged atria without dilated ventricles suggest reduced compliance of the ventricles, as in restrictive cardiomyopathy. The causes of this condition may be ischemic heart disease (IHD) with ventricular fibrosis, amyloidosis, or other unusual conditions.

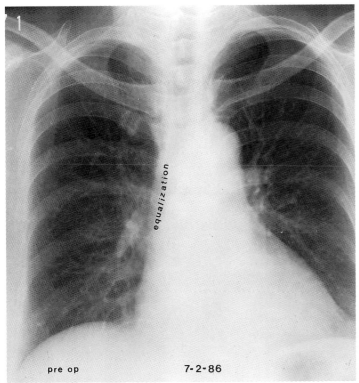

Fig. 24-9. A, This 62-year-old nurse with orthopnea had no history of rheumatic valvular disease or hypertension. On admission, her frontal chest x-ray showed an enlarged cardiac silhouette, especially of the LV. The peripheral pulmonary vasculature showed equalization of the upper and lower lung fields and there was a regurgitant murmur from the cardiac base to the apex. Ruptured chordae tendineae causing MR was suspected from her echo and mitral valve replacement was performed 3 weeks later.

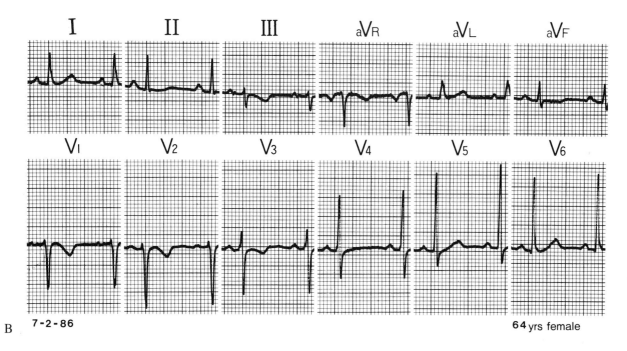

B   7-2-86   64 yrs female

Fig. 24-9. *(Continued)* **B,** Her ECG shows negative T waves in V_1 to V_3 suggesting right-sided cardiac overloading. There are no other remarkable findings.

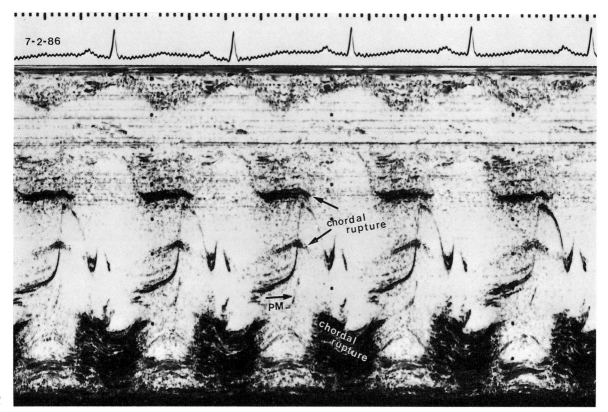

Fig. 24-9. *(Continued)* **C,** Her echo in the video demonstrates ruptured chordae tendineae that swing freely in the LV cavity. This was difficult to reproduce. Her M-mode echo shows shaggy echoes around the mitral leaflets representing chordal rupture.

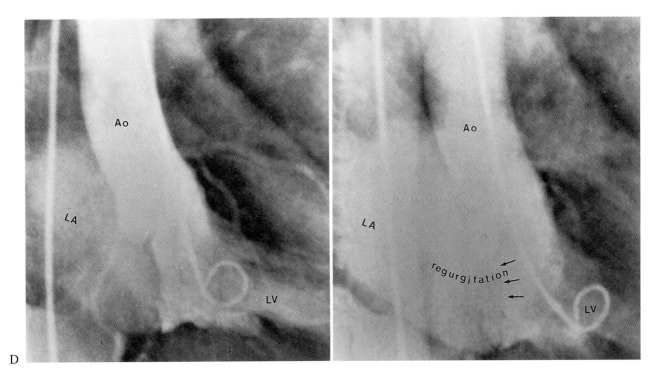

D

Fig. 24-9. *(Continued)* **D**, Her preoperative left ventriculogram shows a marked mitral regurgitation.

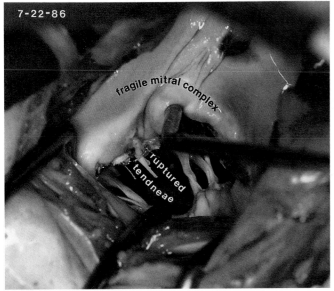

E

Fig. 24-9. *(Continued)* **E**, At surgery, her mitral valve and its surrounding tissues were very fragile, as in the Marfan syndrome. Several myxomatous chordae tendineae were ruptured, causing severe MR.

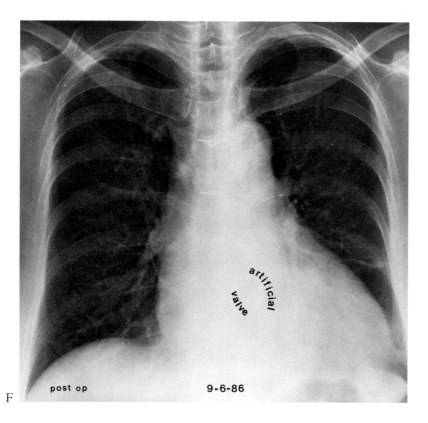

F

post op   9-6-86

Fig. 24-9. *(Continued)* **F,** A frontal chest x-ray made nearly 50 days postoperatively shows resolution of her pulmonary congestion. Her heart is still enlarged and the artificial mitral valve is seen.

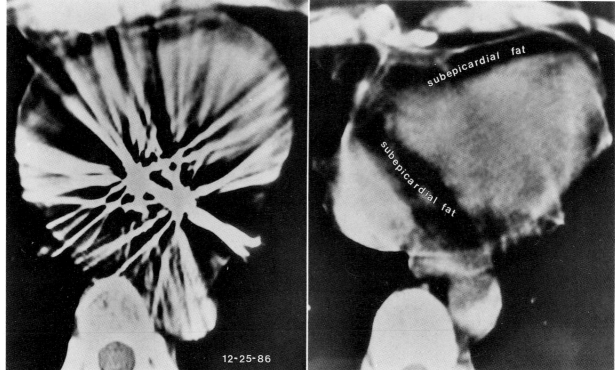

G   12-25-86   H

Fig. 24-9. *(Continued)* **G,** A cardiac CT scan made at the level of the mitral valve about 6 months postoperatively shows strong streak artifacts from the artificial mitral valve on the left. **H,** A CT slice below the level of the mitral valve on the right shows a rather small cardiac silhouette with abundant subepicardial fat deposits. There was no evidence of pericardial effusion.

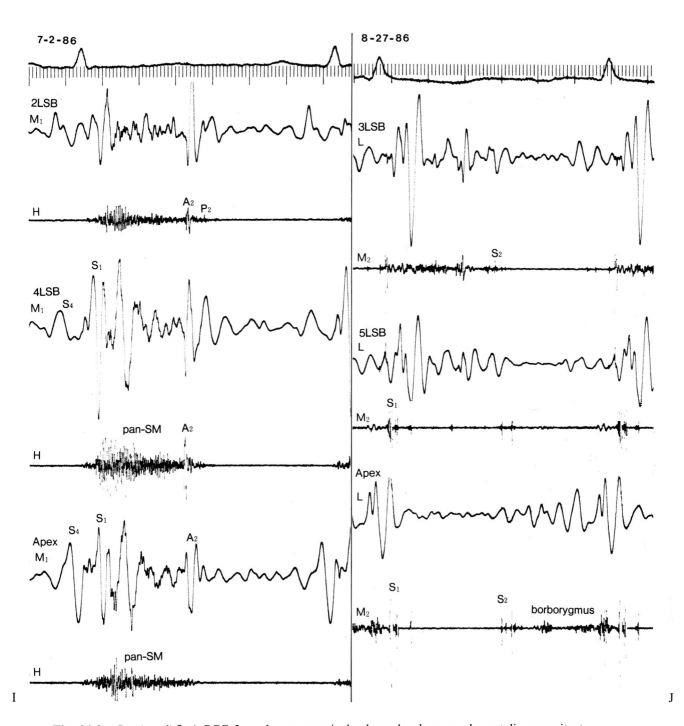

Fig. 24-9. *(Continued)* **I,** A PCG 3 weeks preoperatively showed a decrescendo systolic regurgitant murmur from the 2LSB to the apex. There was narrow splitting of S_2, a loud S_4 at the apex and no S_3, OS, or rumble to suggest rheumatic valvular disease. **J,** PCG 5 weeks postoperatively shows resolution of the regurgitant murmur. Multiple clicks are observed in both systole and diastole, due to the artificial mitral valve.

Chapter 25 Ischemic Heart Disease

Pathophysiology and Clinical Clues

The old term "arteriosclerotic heart disease" has been replaced by either "coronary artery disease" or "atherosclerotic artery disease" which implies the presence of coronary artery obstructions with or without symptoms. The term "ischemic heart disease" (IHD) refers to clinical manifestation of coronary artery disease and is now popularly used to pay respect to William Heberden of Birmingham, England, for his first clear description of effort angina. Its important risk factors include heredity, hypertension, diabetes, obesity, hyperlipidemia, and smoking. These risk factors are irregularly combined, and result in a mosaic theory. Many classifications of IHD have been proposed, but, the author clinically categorizes IHD as:

1. Angina of effort
2. Angina at rest
3. Variant angina, or vasospastic angina
4. Intermediate form; unstable angina, impending infarction
5. Myocardial infarction (MI)

The duration of chest discomfort in angina is less than 10 minutes; when effort angina begins to last longer than usual, comes on more easily, or begins to occur at rest, it is the intermediate form. In such cases, the chest discomfort lasts up to 30 minutes. If the chest oppression lasts longer than 30 minutes, it is myocardial infarction (MI). If it occurs with ST elevation at rest or with effort, it is vasospastic.

The left coronary artery bifurcates about 1 cm distal to its orifice to become the left anterior descending (LAD) and left circumflex (LCX) coronary arteries supplying the interventricular septum (IVS), as well as the lateral and posterior regions of the heart. The inferior or diaphragmatic surface of the cardiac apex may be nourished by the terminal portion of the LAD or right coronary artery (RCA). Involvement of the LAD usually results in anteroseptal infarction and changes in V_1 to V_4, while LCX obstruction causes lateral wall involvement manifested by changes in aV_L and/or V_5 and V_6. Involvement of either the peripheral portion of the LAD or RCA may produce an inferior MI and this is reflected by changes in aV_F. Since the atrioventricular nodal artery is a branch of the RCA, involvement of the RCA often produces an A-V block in addition to changes in aV_F.

Approaches to the diagnosis of IHD are as follows:

★★★★ The ECG shows an abnormal Q wave and/or either ST elevation or depression. T waves in the involved regions often become negative. An exercise ECG is necessary for the symptomatic cases with relatively normal resting ECG.

★★★★ The echo may show reduced thickness of the involved portion and/or aneurysmal dilatation of the left ventricle (LV). Reduced contractility is often seen. In M-mode echo, a relatively tall A wave may be observed if there is decreased compliance of the LV.

★★ The chest x-ray may show aneurysmal dilatation of the LV. There may be a calcified coronary artery.

★★ Auscultation often shows an S_4 with or without the S_3. A mitral regurgitation murmur of papillary muscle dysfunction may occur.

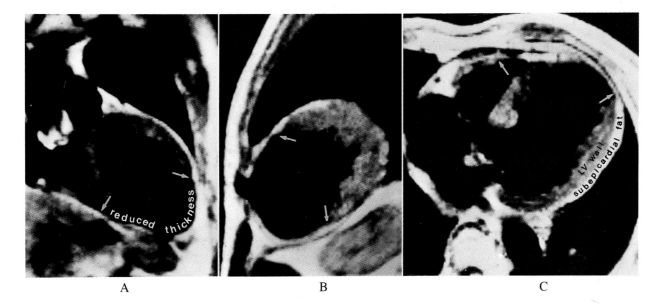

A   B   C

Fig. 25-1. Coronal, sagittal, and transaxial MRI sections of a 60-year-old man with anteroseptal and inferior myocardial infarctions show reduced wall thickness between the 2 white arrows. **A,** The apical portion of the heart is so thin that the myocardium is nearly unrecognizable. **B,** The sagittal section shows that the anteroseptal region and its inferior portions are markedly reduced in thickness, indicating MI. **C,** A transaxial section reveals reduced wall thickness in the same region with aneurysmal dilatation.* These changes may be caused by obstructions of the LAD, but distal right or LCX obstruction might account for the inferior involvement.

* On the transaxial section, there is a broad, bright, band-like structure (high signal intensity) surrounding the myocardium, indicative of subepicardial fat that will not be recognizable on the CT scan. This indicates that the nongated cardiac CT scan may not disclose the subepicardial fat layer, especially at the left ventricular posterior wall (LVPW), because of its motion and superimposed lung tissue (partial volume effect). Thus, the absence of subepicardial fat on cardiac CT does not exclude its presence.

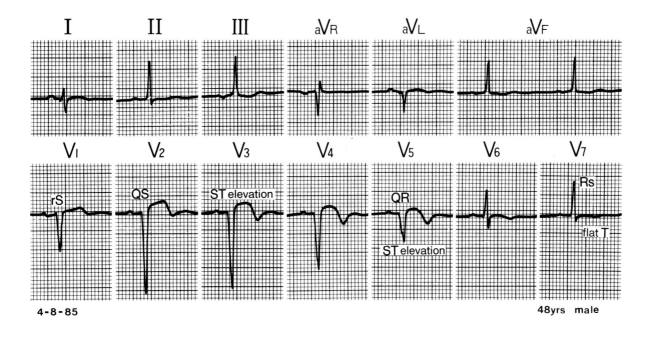

A

Fig. 25-2. **A,** This 48-year-old man had an anteroseptal MI. He continued to show ST elevations in V_2 to V_5 3 weeks after the onset of the attack, suggesting an aneurysm.

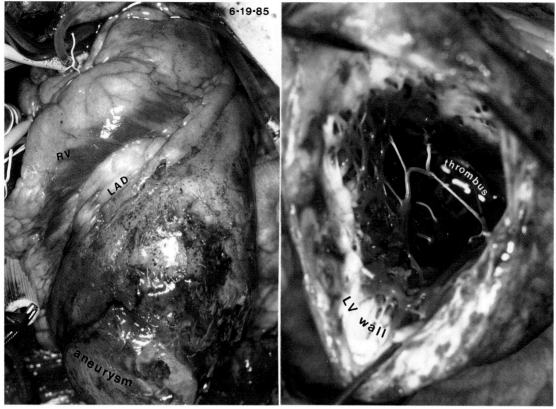

B   C

Fig. 25-2. *(Continued)* **B,** Because of recurrent attacks of CHF, resection of the aneurysm was performed. Surgery revealed adhesive pericarditis and a 3 × 5 cm aneurysm at the cardiac apex. **C,** There were multiple new and old thrombi in the LV cavity.

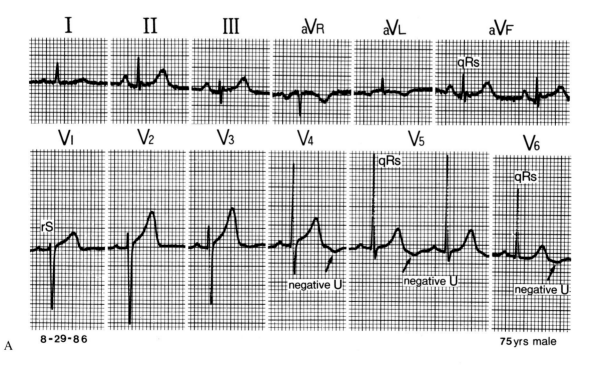

A

Fig. 25-3. A, This ECG from a 75-year-old man with exertional dyspnea shows markedly negative U waves in leads V₄ to V₆; otherwise, there are no abnormal ST·T changes. The negative U waves may be secondary to myocardial ischemia and are indicative of suppressed LV function which often precedes a MI and/or congestive heart failure.

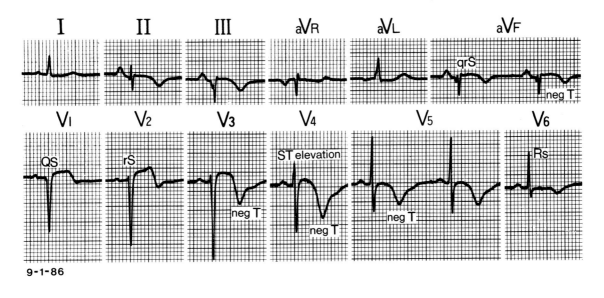

B   9-1-86

Fig. 25-3. *(Continued)* **B,** Three days later, the patient visited the out-patient clinic because of no improvement in his exertional dyspnea. His ECG now reveals a q in III and aVF, a QS pattern in V$_1$ with ST elevations, and inverted T waves in the left precordial and inferior limb leads. These, with qrS patterns in aVF, indicate an acute anteroseptal and inferior MI. Since there is no initial q wave in V$_6$, the QS pattern in V$_1$ may not indicate myocardial necrosis, but it does suggest abnormal septal activation, probably from a MI involving the interventricular septum.

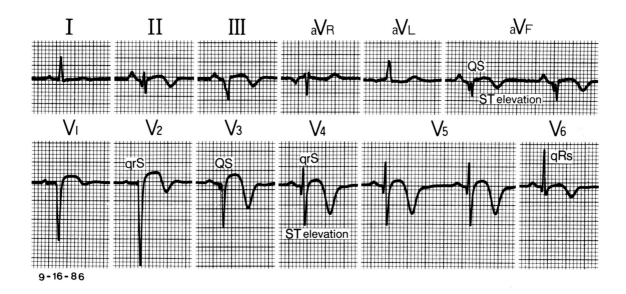

C   9-16-86

Fig. 25-3. *(Continued)* **C,** An ECG 3 weeks later shows QS and qrS patterns with ST elevations in the precordial leads and in aVF, which indicate evolution of an anterior and inferior MI with an apical aneurysm. The septal q waves in V$_6$ indicate normal septal conduction. Therefore QS in V$_1$ is due to myocardial necrosis.

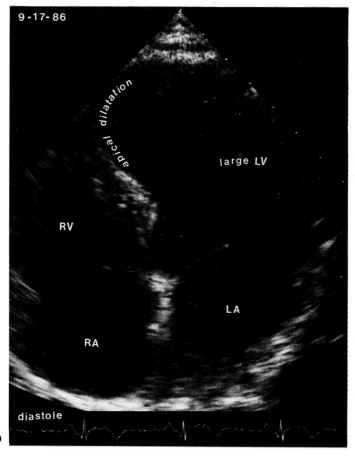

9-17-86

apical dilatation

large *LV*

RV

LA

RA

diastole

D

Fig. 25-3. *(Continued)* **D**, The echo in the apical four-chamber view of the same patient reveals a large apical aneurysmal dilatation. The aneurysm protrudes into the RV, which may be the cause of the dilated RA.

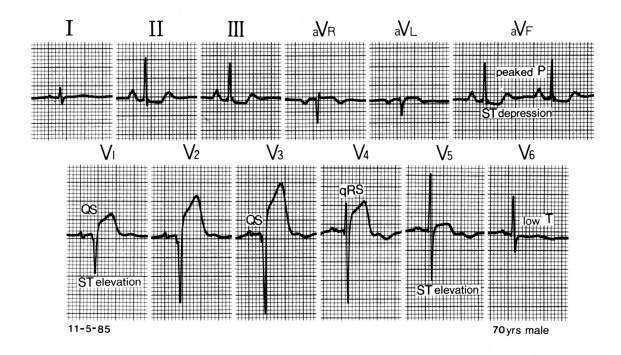

I   II   III   aVR   aVL   aVF

V1   V2   V3   V4   V5   V6

peaked P

ST depression

QS

qRS

QS

low T

ST elevation

ST elevation

11-5-85

70 yrs male

A

Fig. 25-4. A, This 70-year-old man experienced acute chest oppression and had ST elevations in leads V$_1$ to V$_5$ and aVL with reciprocal ST depressions in II, III and aVF, pointing to an anterolateral infarction, hyperacute stage.[*]

[*] With myocardial injury, the electrodes facing the injured region show ST elevations. If the injured region is large, there will be ST depressions on the opposite side of the heart. In this case, a large region of myocardium is severely injured, as indicated by marked ST elevations in V$_1$ to V$_5$. If the T waves are upright in leads with an elevated ST segment, the infarct is usually only a few hours old and is in the hyperacute stage.

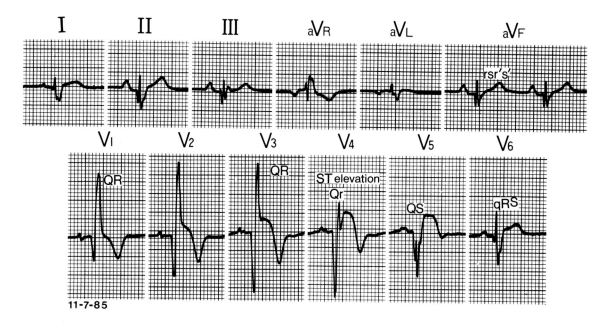

B

Fig. 25-4. *(Continued)* **B,** The ECG tracing of the same patient 2 days later showed a QR pattern in V_1 to V_4 with wide QRS complexes, indicating RBBB. Retrospectively, the presence of the septal q wave in the initial tracing was seen only in V_6, and it was very small for the QRS complex. This could raise the suspicion of abnormal septal activity and forecast a RBBB or LBBB.

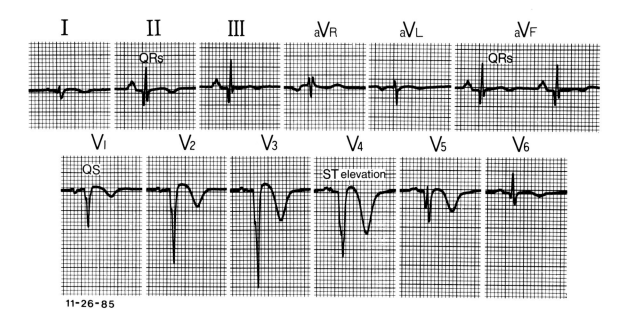

C

Fig. 25-4. *(Continued)* **C,** The RBBB was transient and resolved in 1 week. The ST segments usually return to the base line in about 2 weeks, but they remained elevated 5 weeks after the attack, suggesting an aneurysm.

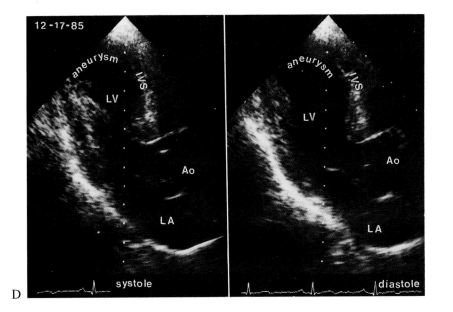

D

Fig. 25-4. *(Continued)* **D,** His echoes in the apical two-chamber view reveal an enlarged LV cavity with aneurysmal dilatation at the apical region.

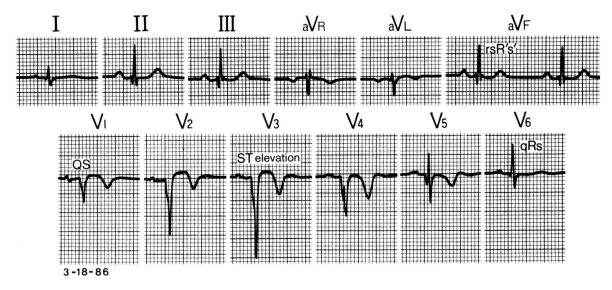

E

Fig. 25-4. *(Continued)* **E,** His ECG made 5 months later shows a QS pattern in V_1 and rS in V_2 to V_4. There is an initial septal q wave in V_6 indicating a normal septal activation. Therefore, the QS in V_1 represents myocardial necrosis. The previously noted ST elevations are still present in V_1 to V_4, but the degree has been markedly reduced.

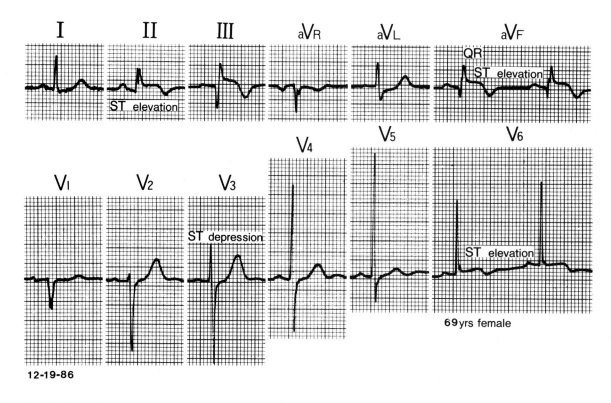

A   **12-19-86**

Fig. 25-5. A, This 69-year-old woman experienced chest pain during sleep. Marked ST elevations are seen in II, III, aVF and V₆ with a relatively deep Q wave in aVF indicating an acute inferolateral MI. In addition, depressed ST segments in V₁ to V₄ are reciprocal changes and suggest posterior involvement.

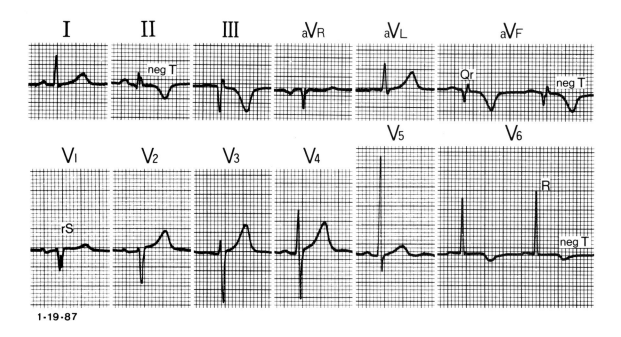

B   **1-19-87**

Fig. 25-5. *(Continued)* **B,** An ECG 4 weeks later shows resolving ST elevations. However, the negativity of the T waves is increased in the same leads. Increased amplitude of the R wave frequently occurs in V₁ to V₃ in cases of posterior MI. This is not the case here, suggesting that an old anteroseptal infarction is counterbalancing it. Poor r/S progression in V₂ and V₃ is indicative of anteroseptal myocardial necrosis.

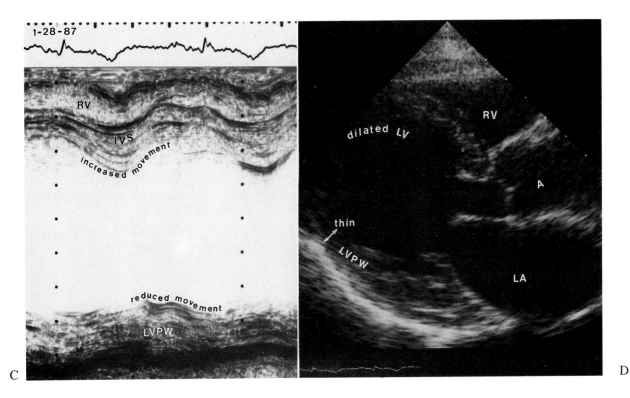

C

D

Fig. 25-5. *(Continued)* **C,** Her echoes show a posterior MI. An M-mode recording shows reduced movement of the left ventricular posterior wall (LVPW). The interventricular septum's (IVS) movement is increased to compensate for the LVPW. **D,** A long-axis echo shows a dilated apical portion of the LV cavity suggesting an anteroseptal MI. The LVPW is reduced in thickness below the mitral valve which correlates with posteroinferior involvement.

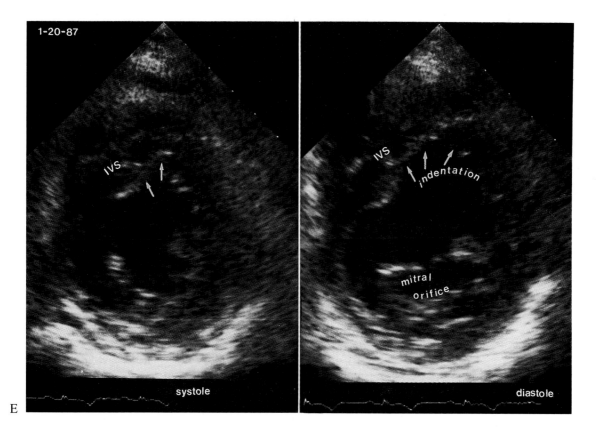

E

Fig. 25-5. *(Continued)* **E,** Short-axis echoes reveal a deformed IVS during both systole and diastole that was caused by the protrusion into the RV cavity which made an indent on the LV side.

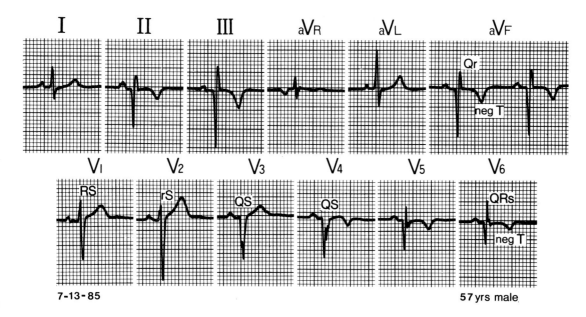

A

Fig. 25-6. A, This 57-year-old man had an old inferoposterior infarction and developed anteroseptal infarction. His initial ECG shows deep Q waves in leads II, III, aVF and V_3 to V_6. Inferior MI is indicated by the Qr pattern in aVF and posterior infarction is shown by the tall R wave in V_1. This is because of a reciprocal change caused by a loss of posteriorly-directed potential which is counterbalanced by anteriorly-directed potentials. However, there is no ST depression in V_1 to V_3 to indicate that the posterior infarction is not recent. In addition, the QS pattern in V_3 and V_4 indicates anteroseptal infarction and Qr waves in V_5 and V_6 indicate lateral involvement.

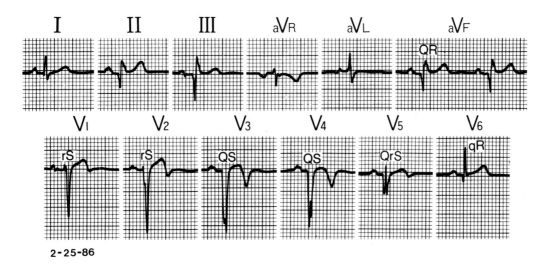

Fig. 25-6. *(Continued)* **B,** His ECG 1 year later shows reduced depths of Q waves in II, III, aVF and V$_6$ together with a reduction of the R waves in V$_1$ to V$_3$ with slight ST elevations in these precordial leads. These findings indicate that he had an old inferoposterior MI, then developed a new anteroseptal MI. Surprisingly, he had been asymptomatic.

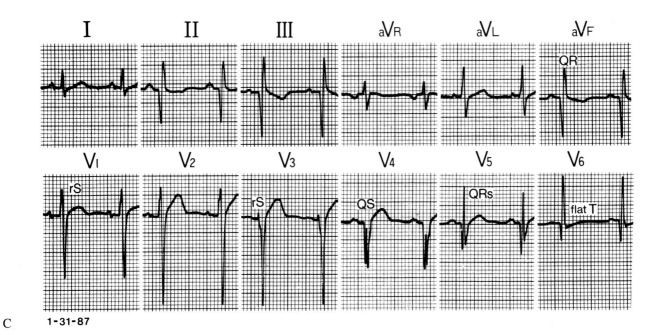

C   1-31-87

Fig. 25-6. *(Continued)* **C,** The patient's uneventful recovery from repeated MIs is clear in the upright T waves in V$_3$ to V$_5$ which were previously inverted. The R waves in V$_1$ and V$_2$ show increases in their amplitude.

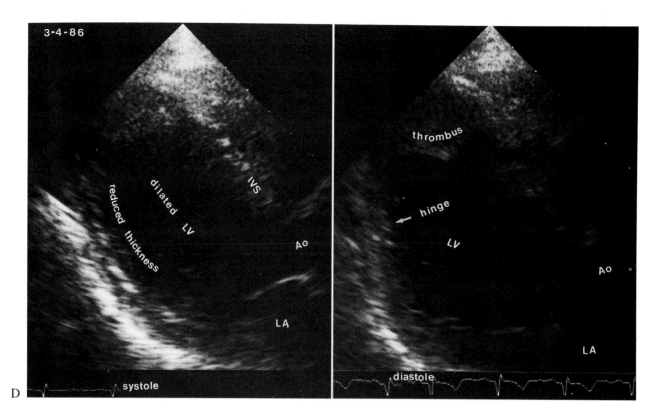

Fig. 25-6. *(Continued)* **D**, His echoes in the apical four-chamber view reveal a dilated LV cavity with reduced thickness of the LVPW. The apical portion of the LV has a hinge which suggests the presence of an aneurysm distal to the hinge. There is a smoke-like echo suggesting stasis in the aneurysm.

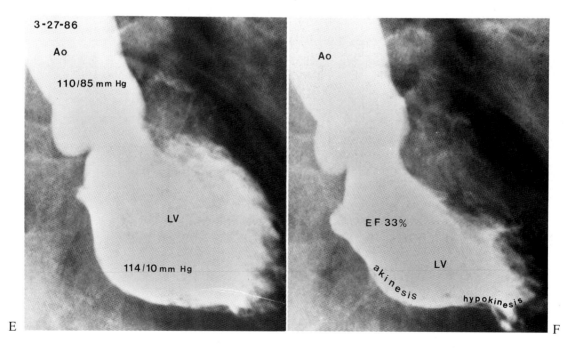

Fig. 25-6. *(Continued)* **E**, The patient finally agreed to have a ventriculogram which showed akinesis of the inferior wall and hypokinesis of the apical portion of the LV. **F**, His ejection fraction (EF) was 33%.

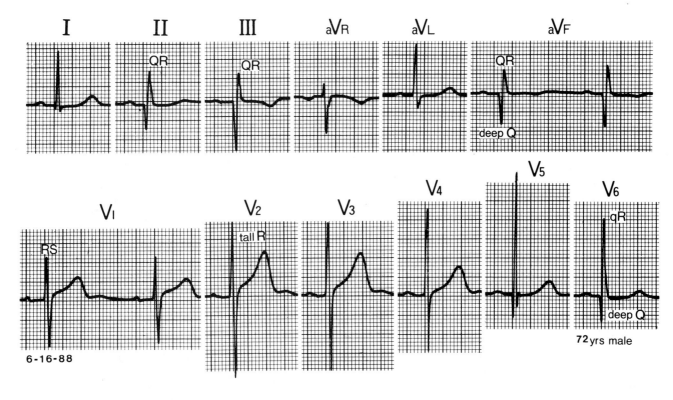

A

Fig. 25-7. A, This ECG is from a 72-year-old man who had a posteroinferior MI 2 years ago. A deep Q wave is seen in II, III, aVF, and V5 and V6. There is a relatively tall R wave in leads V1 to V3 which is a reciprocal change of a posterior MI. However, the posterior MI is not recent since there is no ST depression in V1 to V3.

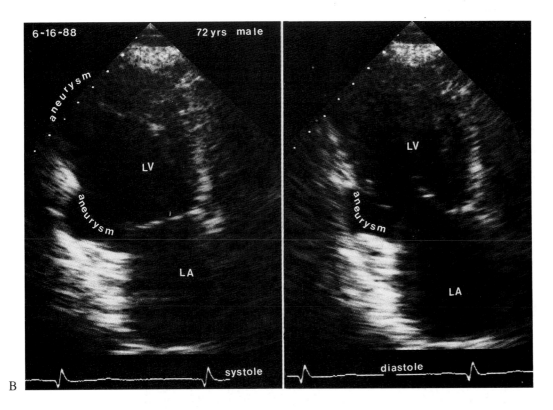

B

Fig. 25-7. *(Continued)* **B**, His echoes in the apical two-chamber view made on the same day as the ECG show a dilated LV cavity with reduced thickness of the LVPW below the mitral valve. The cardiac apex appears to show aneurysmal dilatation with some smoke-like echoes indicating possible stasis.

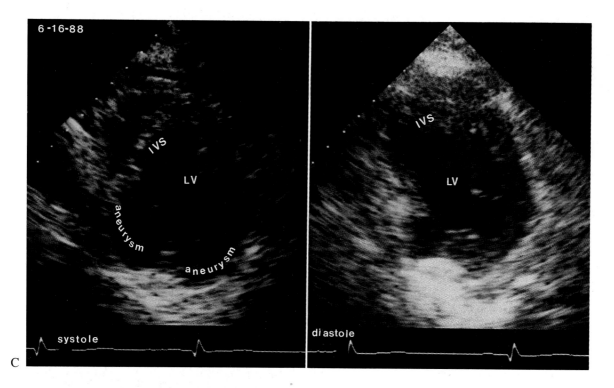

Fig. 25-7. *(Continued)* **C**, Short-axis echoes show a deformed LV cavity due to aneurysmal dilatation of the LVPW.

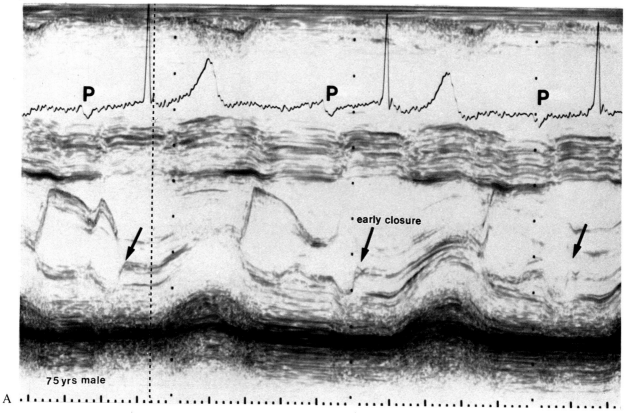

Fig. 25-8. A, This is an M-mode echo of a 75-year-old man with hypertension. He had a first degree A-V block, and the early P wave and atrial contraction are causing early closure of the mitral valve preceding the QRS complex. Mitral closure normally coincides with the terminal portion of the QRS complex of the ECG believed to be a result of LV contraction. Contrary to this conventional hypothesis, mitral closure may be accomplished entirely by atrial contraction and relaxation.

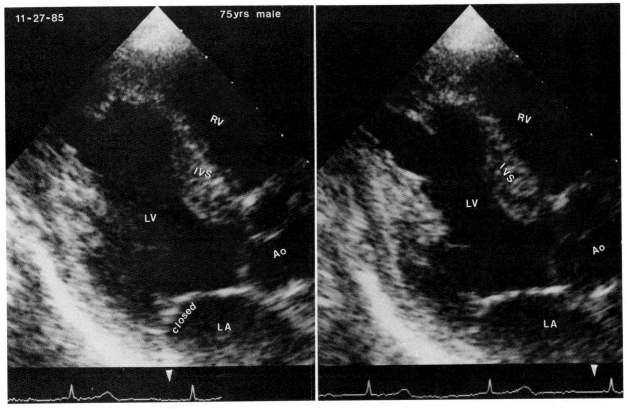

Fig. 25-8. *(Continued)* **B,** Echoes in the apical two-chamber view of the same patient show early mitral closure preceding the QRS complex of the ECG, indicated by an arrowhead immediately after the P wave. This confirms that mitral closure may begin before the onset of isovolumic contraction of the LV. The same mechanism probably contributes to mitral closure even with normal P-R intervals. Note that a sigmoid septum is also present.

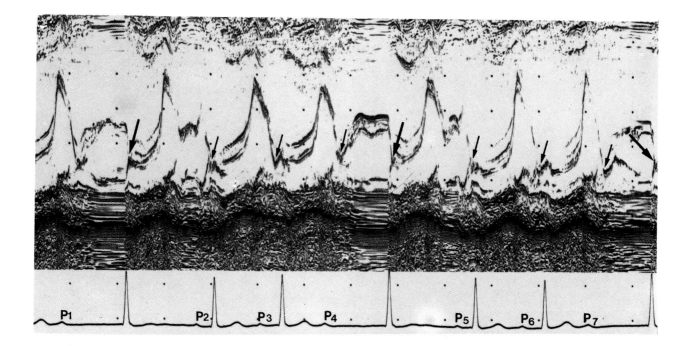

Fig. 25-9. This is an example of early mitral closure occurring in a 19-year-old healthy male student who has a transient first degree A-V block. The P-R interval is prolonged as indicated by P_1. The mitral valve closes nearly completely immediately after the P_1 reopens, then abruptly closes simultaneously with the R wave in the ECG. P_2 has a normal P-R interval but the mitral valve closes slightly earlier than the R wave as in the P_5. P_3 has a slightly prolonged P-R interval and the mitral valve closure occurs immediately after the P_3 which is not abrupt. It is not clear, but the valve may reopen and close simultaneously with or slightly earlier than the R wave. Immediately after P_4, the mitral valve closes and reopens, then it abruptly closes simultaneously with the R wave. P_7 shows a similar pattern. This demonstrates that with a normal P-R interval, the mitral valve does not close abruptly, suggesting that it occurs without benefit of ventricular contraction. When the ventricular contraction influences the mitral valve, it causes an abrupt closure and results in an intensified S_1.

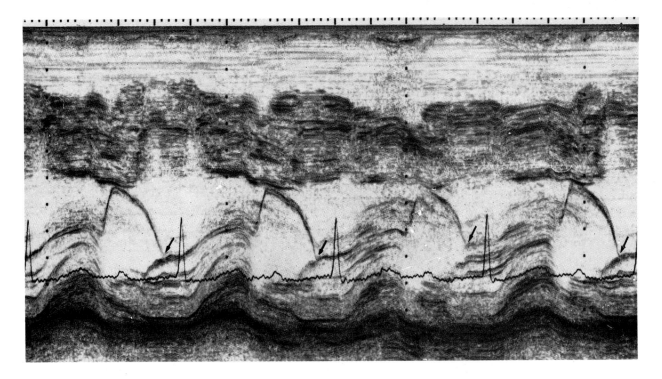

A

Fig. 25-10. A, This 77-year-old woman also has first degree A-V block and early mitral closure. Her M-mode echo shows early closure as indicated by the arrows which precede the QRS complex. There is no re-opening of the mitral valve following the early closure. Assuming a reduction of left atrial (LA) pressure as a result of its active relaxation, the resulting suction may draw the mitral valve toward the LA.

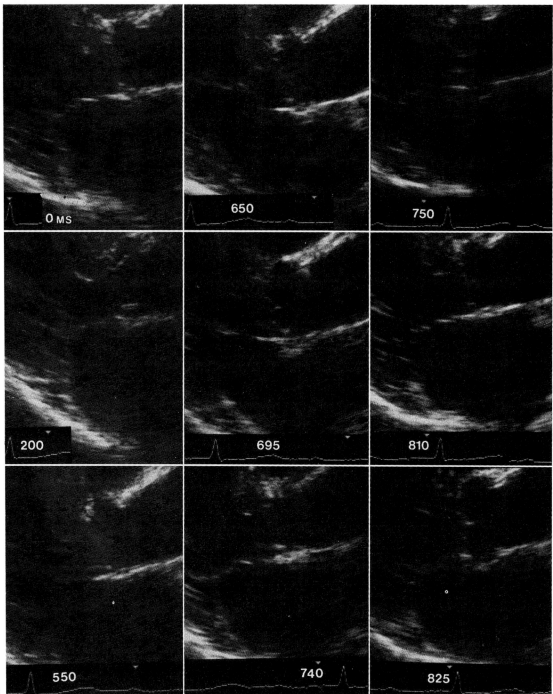

B

Fig. 25-10. *(Continued)* **B,** Serial tracings of the long-axis echo seem to clarify the cause of the early mitral closure. The number in each frame indicates the delay in milliseconds (ms) from the peak of the R wave of the ECG. At 0 ms, at the beginning of isovolumic contraction, the aortic and mitral valves are closed. At 200 ms, the aortic valve is open and the mitral valve remains closed. At 550 ms, the beginning of diastole, the mitral valve is open and remains open until 695 ms. At 740 ms, the mitral valve is closed; this occurred before the QRS complex of the ECG. At 750 ms, the mitral valve reopens, and its final closure occurs from 810 ms to 825 ms. This serial tracing confirms that early closure of the mitral valve precedes the QRS complex of the ECG. Presystolic closure is assumed to be due to the contraction and relaxation of the LA initiated by the early appearance of P wave.

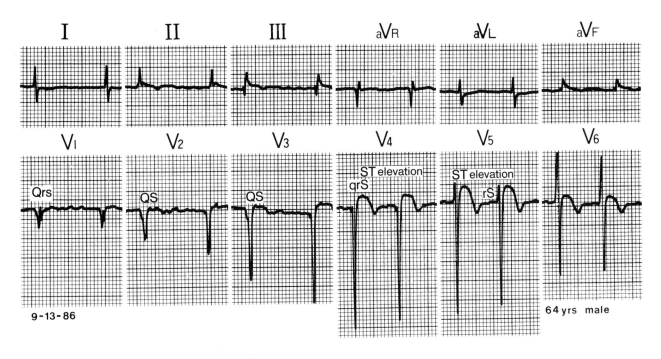

Fig. 25-11. A, This ECG from a 64-year-old man was made 3 days after the onset of acute chest pain. The rhythm is AF with a rate of about 100. ST elevation is seen in V_4 to V_6 with a Q in V_1 and V_4. The transitional zone is beyond V_6 indicating a markedly clockwise rotation of his heart. This is probably from loss of anterior force by an extensive MI.

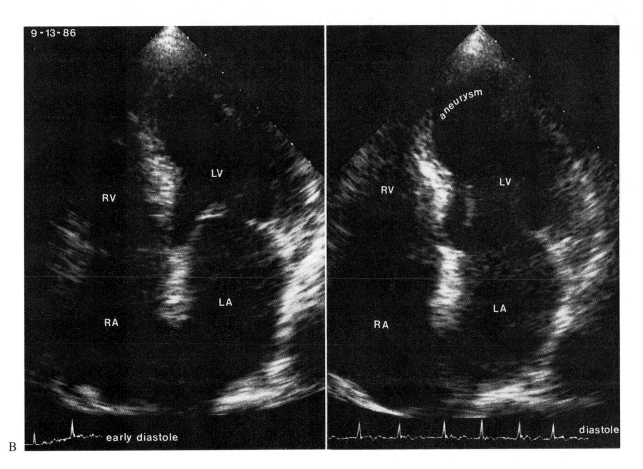

Fig. 25-11. *(Continued)* **B,** His echoes in the apical four-chamber view show reduced thickness of the IVS and anterior portion of the LV causing aneurysmal dilatation which is more readily seen during diastole.

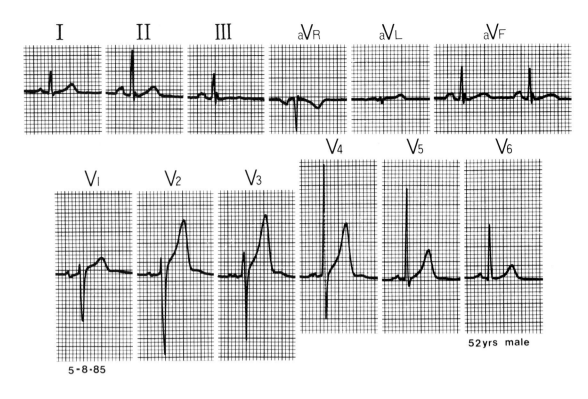

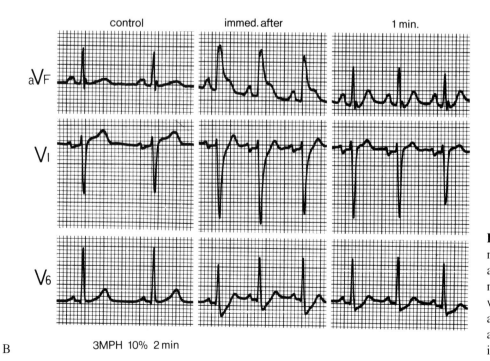

Fig. 25-12. A, This is the ECG of a 52-year-old man with effort angina. A widely notched P is seen in the precordial leads suggesting an intra-atrial conduction defect. There are neither ST nor T wave changes that suggest myocardial ischemia.

Fig. 25-12. *(Continued)* **B,** Treadmill exercise at 3 miles per hour on a 10% slope for 2 minutes produced marked ST elevation in lead aV$_F$ with ST depressions in leads V$_1$ and V$_6$, indicating severe inferior, and possible posterior, myocardial injury.

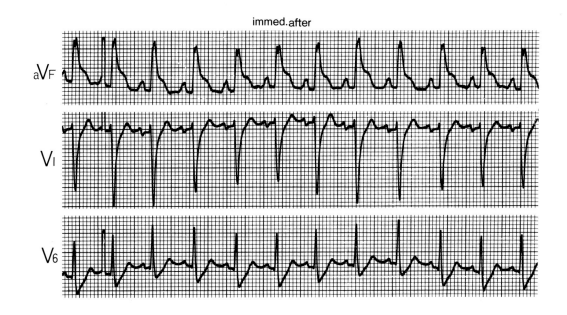

Fig. 25-12. *(Continued)* C, Recordings immediately following this exercise show persistent ST elevations in aVF, with ST depressions in leads V₁ and V₆. The P wave increased in amplitude in aVF, and the P wave in V₁ showed greater terminal negativity. One minute later, the ST elevation was resolved but the ST depressions persisted in V₆ for 3 minutes. After 15 minutes, the T waves in aVF and V₆ did not completely revert to the control state and the P wave remained the major sign of an abnormal pattern. An elevation of the LV end-diastolic pressure from LV dysfunction can cause LA overloading, and manifest P wave changes; this same LV dysfunction reduces coronary circulation and causes the ST·T changes. In this case, the ST elevations after exercise suggest coronary spasm.

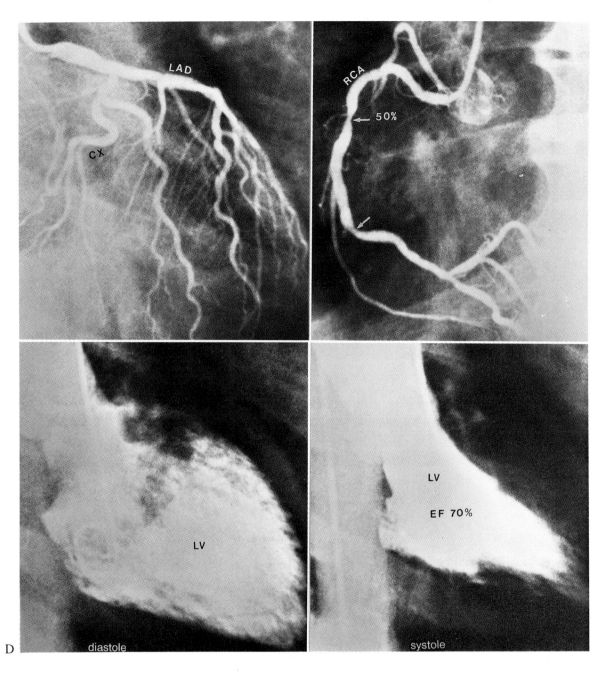

Fig. 25-12. *(Continued)* **D,** Coronary angiography of the same patient revealed only 50% stenotic lesions in the right coronary artery (RCA) with an ejection fraction (EF) of 70%. The patient is under medical management with symptomatic improvement.

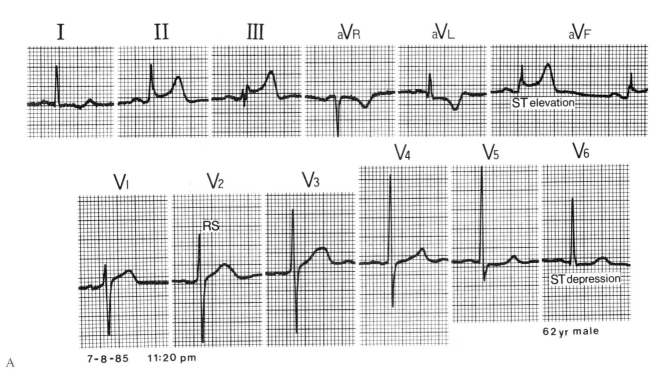

Fig. 25-13. A, This ECG of a 62-year-old man with acute nocturnal chest pain shows ST elevations in leads II, III, and aVF with reciprocal ST depressions in aVL suggesting an acute inferior MI. There is slightly increased amplitude of the T wave in the RV leads as shown by the T in V_1 being taller than the T in V_6. Also the slightly tall R wave in V_1 to V_3 suggests the presence of a concomitant posterior MI.

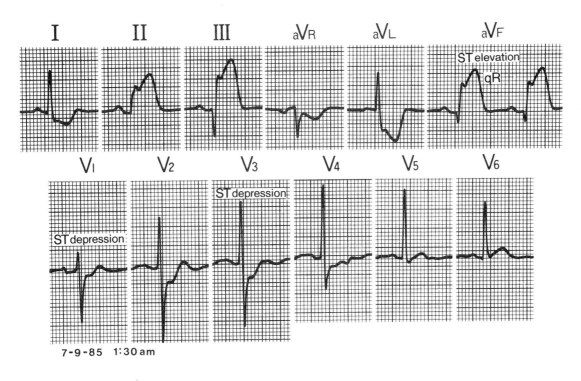

Fig. 25-13. *(Continued)* **B,** An ECG of the same patient made 2 hours later shows increased ST elevations in leads II, III and aVF with the addition of ST depressions in V_2 to V_5 indicating acute posterior involvement.

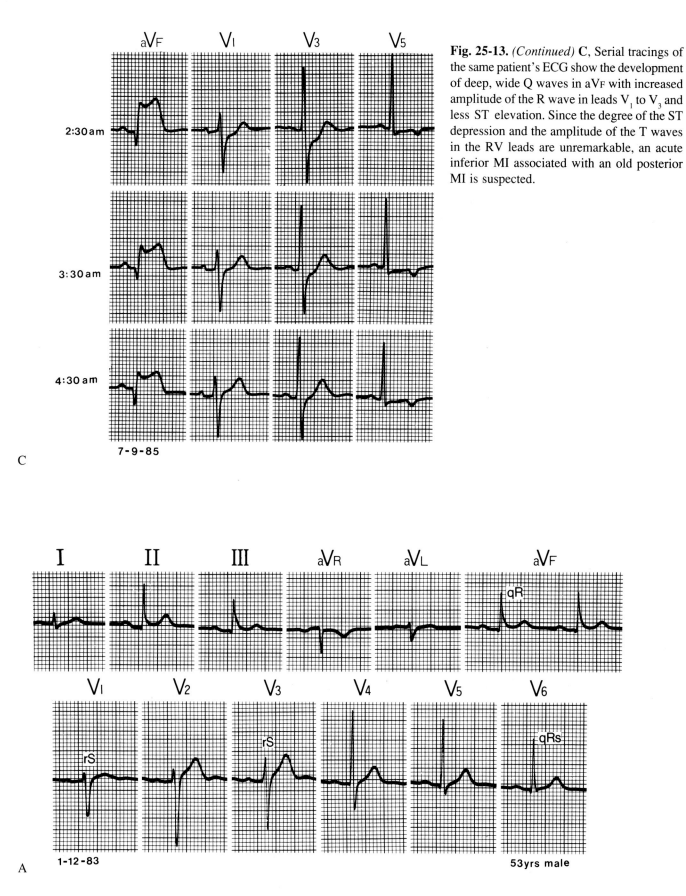

Fig. 25-13. *(Continued)* **C**, Serial tracings of the same patient's ECG show the development of deep, wide Q waves in aVF with increased amplitude of the R wave in leads V_1 to V_3 and less ST elevation. Since the degree of the ST depression and the amplitude of the T waves in the RV leads are unremarkable, an acute inferior MI associated with an old posterior MI is suspected.

Fig. 25-14. A, This is a 53-year-old man with hypertension. His initial ECG shows slight ST elevation in leads V_1 to V_5 which could be normal.

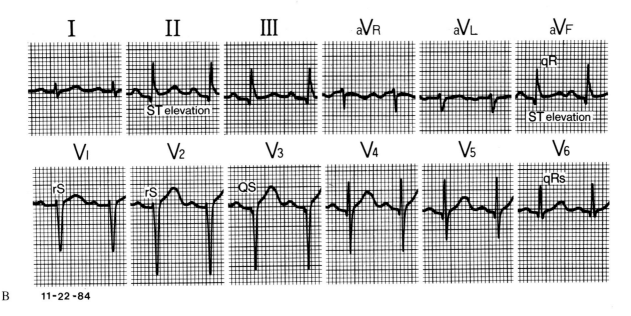

B   11-22-84

Fig. 25-14. *(Continued)* **B,** An ECG 20 months later during palpitations shows an increase in the depth of the q wave and the ST elevation in II, III, and aVF, with poor r/S progression from V_1 to V_3. ECG also shows a QS pattern in V_3 and an increased depth of the q wave in V_4 to V_6. These changes imply an anteroinferior MI.

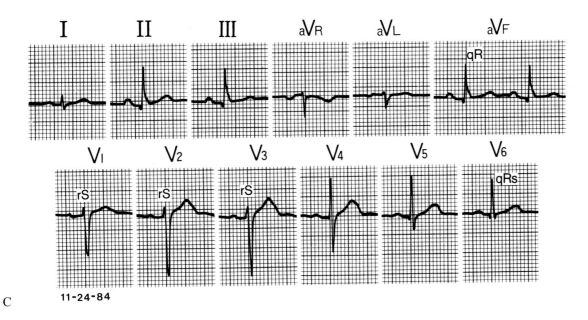

C   11-24-84

Fig. 25-14. *(Continued)* **C,** An ECG of the same patient 2 days later shows resolution of the tachycardia and the ST elevations. The previously shown QS in V_3 assumed an rS pattern with a poor r/S ratio compared to the initial tracing, which suggests a small non-Q wave MI, but this seems most unlikely since the change was very rapid.

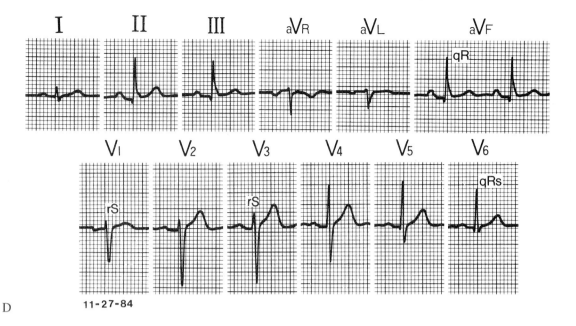

D   11-27-84

Fig. 25-14. *(Continued)* **D,** An ECG made about 2 weeks later reveals no significant change since the previous ECG. The patient's main symptom was palpitation lasting only a few hours, and there was no evidence of abnormal blood chemistry to suggest myocardial ischemia. Transient QS patterns have been observed during asthmatic attacks from depression of the diaphragm, but there was no episode and no emphysema. Either a tachycardia caused a hidden necrosis to be unmasked, or a silent infarct occurred with complete recovery by spontaneous reperfusion. Hidden necrosis can be uncovered by myocardial ischemia from shock, anemia, and angina.

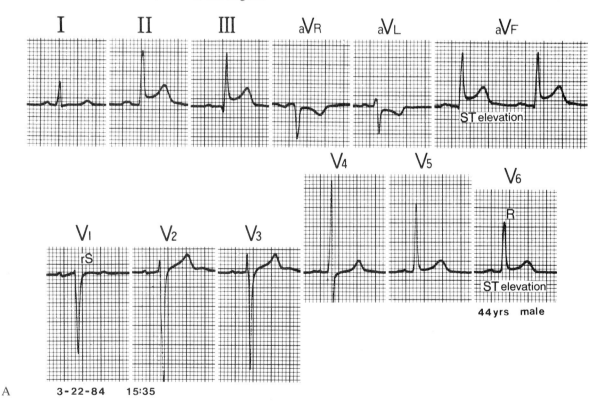

A   3-22-84   15:35

Fig. 25-15. A, This is an ECG of a 44-year-old man who developed epigastric pain after lunch. ST elevations are seen in II, III and aVF with reciprocal depression in aVL. There is no initial septal q wave in V_5 and V_6 which would indicate abnormal septal activity from acute involvement of the IVS. In addition, the r wave in V_1 is small, which suggests anteroseptal involvement.

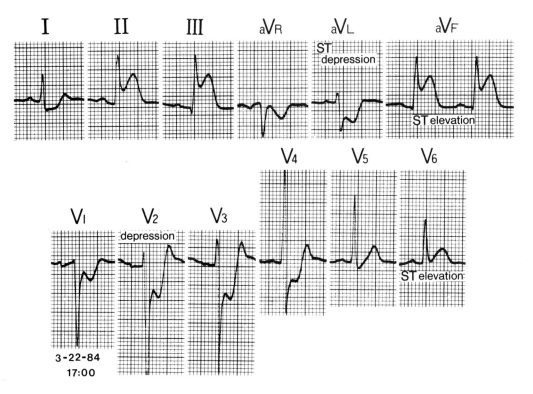

I II III aVR aVL aVF

ST depression

ST elevation

V4 V5 V6

V1 V2 V3

depression

ST elevation

3-22-84
17:00

B

Fig. 25-15. *(Continued)* **B,** His ECG 90 minutes after the initial tracing shows marked ST elevations in leads II, III and aVF with reciprocal ST depressions in aVL and V₁ to V₄ indicating involvement of both the inferior and posterior walls.

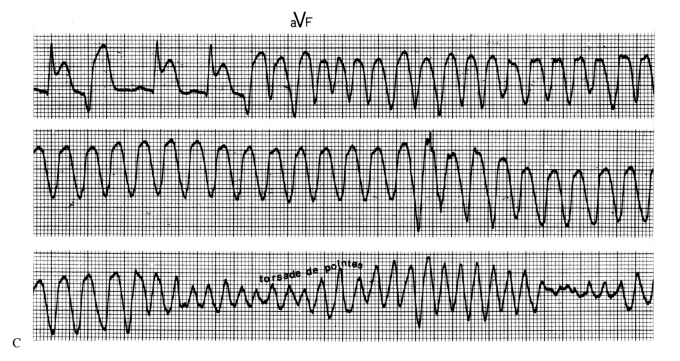

Fig. 25-15. *(Continued)* **C,** During the recording of his second ECG, the cardiac rhythm suddenly changed to ventricular tachycardia (VT) which became torsade de pointes.[*] The wide QRS complex during the VT shows distortion of the T waves, indicating superimposed P waves and therefore AV dissociation. This distortion of T waves is very important in distinguishing VT from supraventricular tachycardia (SVT) associated with the wide QRS of LBBB and/or the W-P-W syndrome.

[*] Torsade de pointes means "twisted coil of points." It is a multiform VT in which the QRS axis undulates over every 5 to 20 beats. It usually starts with a late premature QRS in a patient with bradycardia and a long Q-T interval which this patient did not have.

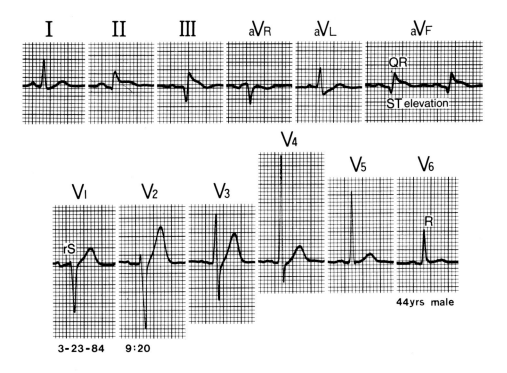

D

Fig. 25-15. *(Continued)* **D**, The VT resolved spontaneously. An ECG made the following morning shows residual ST elevations in the same leads as previously but with wide q waves. However, the previously noted precordial ST depressions have resolved.

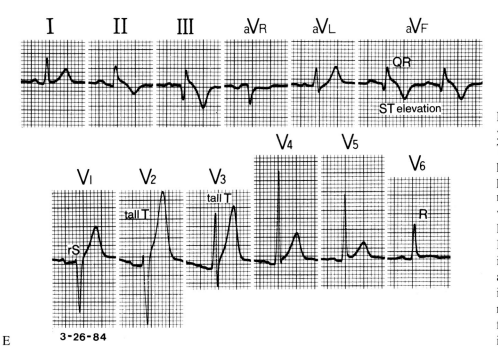

E

Fig. 25-15. *(Continued)* **E**, One year later, his ECG shows the tall T waves in V_1 to V_3 suggesting posterior MI in addition to the previous inferior MI. There was neither increased height of the r wave nor ST depression in these leads: this suggests the posterior MI is not recent. The tall T waves in the RV leads may represent an acute anteroseptal myocardial ischemia despite the patient remaining asymptomatic. No follow-up studies were possible in this case.

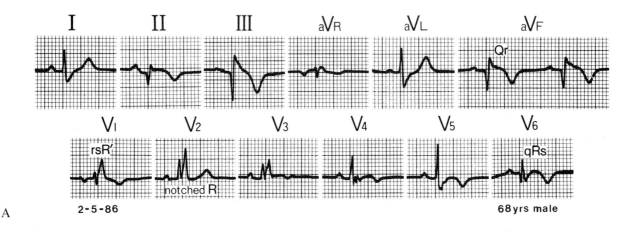

A 2-5-86   68 yrs male

Fig. 25-16. A, This is from a 68-year-old man with an acute MI. His ECG shows deep Q waves in leads II, III, aVF, and V₆ with slight ST elevations indicating an inferior MI of the q wave type. V₁ shows an rsR′ of RBBB which indicates IVS damage.

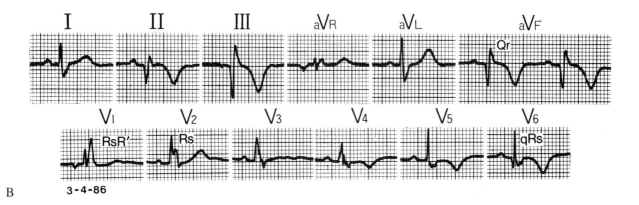

B 3-4-86

Fig. 25-16. *(Continued)* **B**, An ECG 1 month later shows increased amplitude of the initial r waves in V₁ and V₂, representing a possible reciprocal change caused by a posterior MI.

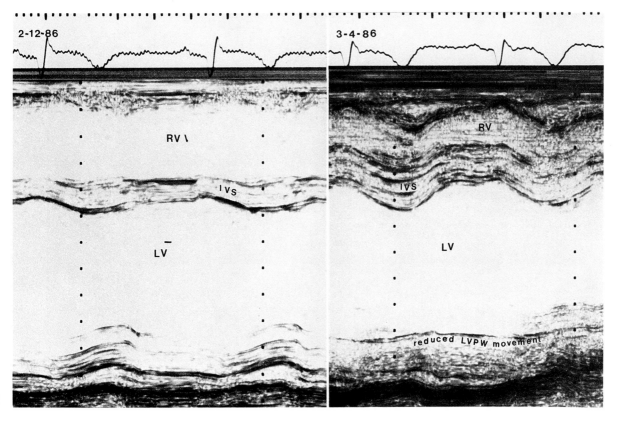

Fig. 25-16. *(Continued)* **C,** On the left, his M-mode echo 1 week after the initial ECG shows reduced thickness of both the IVS and LV with suppression of their movements, suggesting an MI involving these regions. On the right, follow-up M-mode echo made the same day as the second ECG shows improvement in the movements of the RV and IVS compensating for further suppression of the LVPW's movement. These echo findings seem to correlate well with the ECG changes.

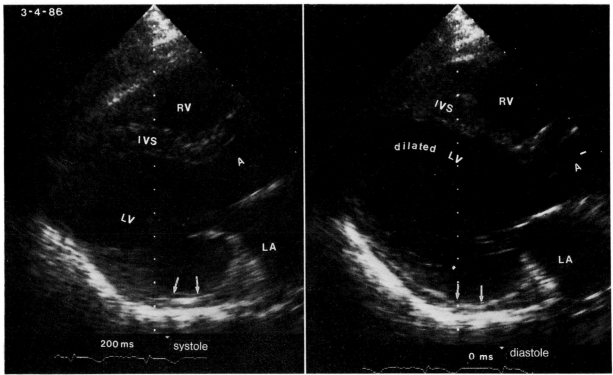

Fig. 25-16. *(Continued)* **D**, Long-axis echoes made the same day as the second ECG show marked thinning of the LVPW (arrows) below the level of the mitral ring and indicate a posterior MI. In addition, the apical portion of the LV shows reduction of its thickness and this region becomes dilated during diastole. This suggests the presence of an apical aneurysm caused by an anteroseptal MI in addition to the posteroinferior infarction.

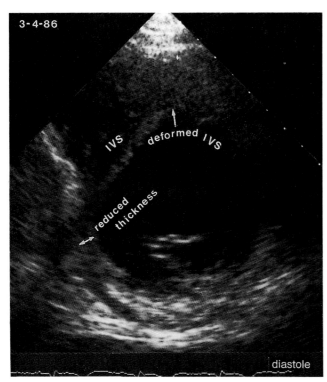

Fig. 25-16. *(Continued)* **E**, A short-axis echo on the same day as Fig. 25-16D shows marked reduction in the thickness of the medial aspect of the LVPW in addition to a deformity of anterolateral aspect of the IVS. The presence of RBBB also suggests an anteroseptal MI, and an increased amplitude of the initial r wave in V_1 may indicate a posterior MI. This hypothesis appears to correlate with the echo findings.

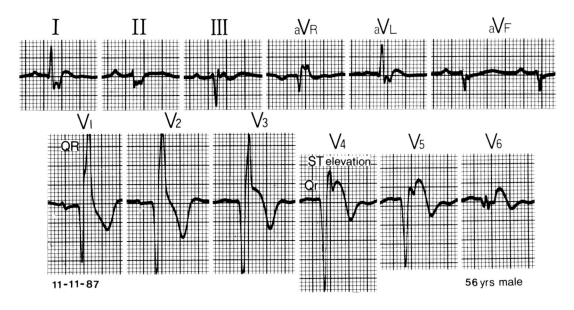

A

Fig. 25-17. A, This ECG from a 56-year-old man with acute chest pain shows a wide QRS complex of the RBBB type with Q waves in V_1 to V_6. ST elevation is present in leads I, aVL, and V_2 to V_6 which suggests an anteroseptal and lateral MI.

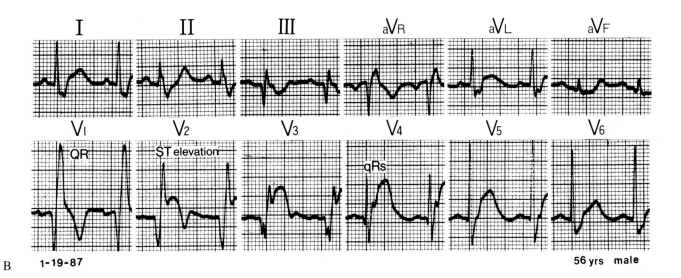

B

Fig. 25-17. *(Continued)* **B,** The patient recovered from his MI uneventfully; however, his ECG 10 months later shows ST elevations in leads V_3 to V_6 which strongly suggest a ventricular aneurysm.

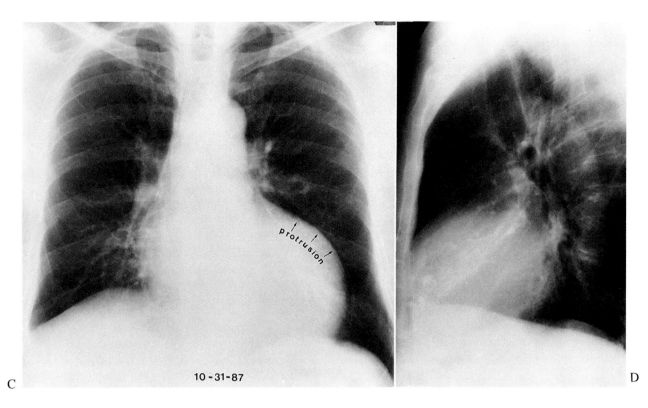

C   10 - 31 - 87   D

Fig. 25-17. *(Continued)* **C**, His frontal chest x-ray 9 months after the initial episode shows a protrusion of the upper segment of the LV suggesting an aneurysm, which correlates well with the ECG finding. **D**, His lateral projection is not remarkable.

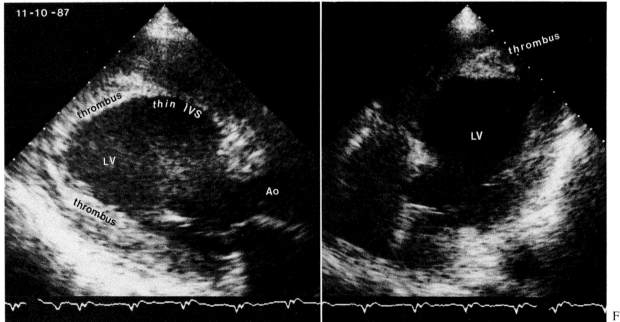

E   F

Fig. 25-17. *(Continued)* **E**, On the left, an echo in the apical two-chamber view of the same patient shows strong echoes attached to the inner surface of the LV cavity along the apical and posterolateral portions, suggesting the presence of a thrombus. The lower portion of the IVS is very thin. **F**, On the right, an apical four-chamber view shows a similar finding in the apical portion of the LV cavity. The apical portion of the IVS is obscure.

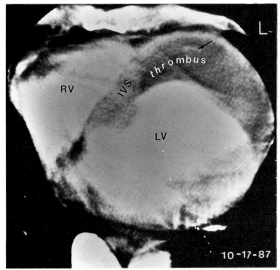

Fig. 25-17. *(Continued)* **G**, An enhanced cardiac CT section below the level of the mitral ring shows a large thrombus at the apex confirming the echo findings. Since the patient refuses surgical treatment, he is being followed medically.

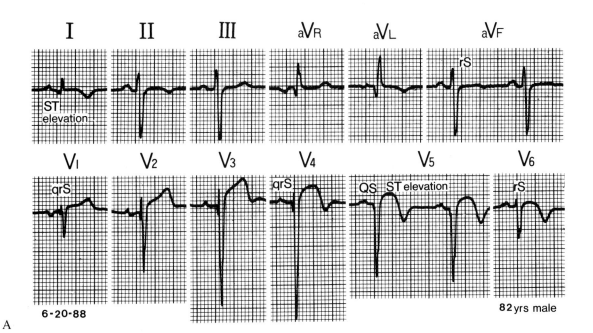

Fig. 25-18. A, This is from an 82-year-old asymptomatic man with diabetes mellitus. His ECG shows a qrS pattern in V$_1$ and V$_4$ and QS in V$_5$. The elevated ST and negative T waves in V$_5$ and V$_6$ indicate that he had a rather recent anterior MI.

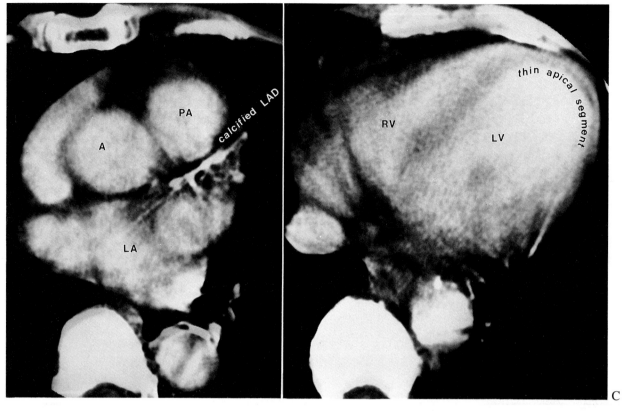

Fig. 25-18. *(Continued)* **B**, Because of his age, only a cardiac CT was performed. An enhanced cardiac CT section at the level of the aortic root shows a heavily calcified left anterior descending coronary artery (LAD). **C**, On the right, reduced thickness at the apical portion of his left ventricular wall is observed. There is no obvious aneurysmal bulge, but a large akinetic area can also be the cause of the ST elevation.

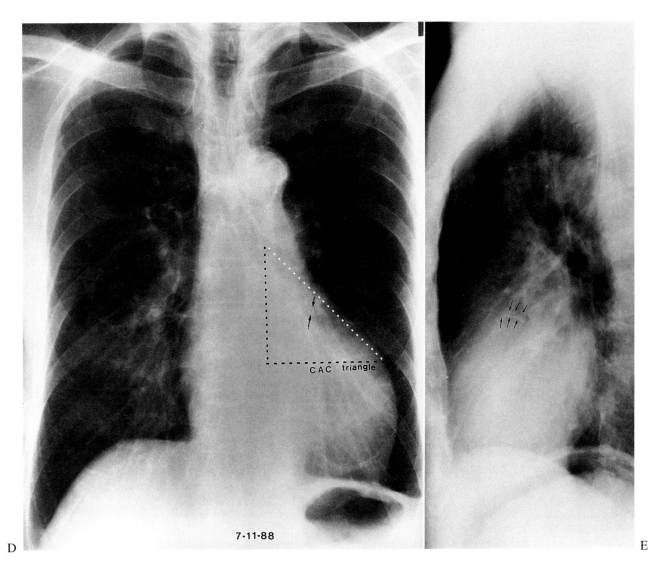

D

E

Fig. 25-18. *(Continued)* **D**, His chest x-rays show a calcified coronary artery in the coronary artery calcification (CAC) triangle.[*] **E**, In the lateral view, there is coronary artery calcification slightly above the center of the cardiac silhouette. The aortic valve is located in the center of the cardiac silhouette which is on the line between the bifurcation of the trachea and the sternodiaphragmatic angle.

[*] The coronary artery calcification (CAC) triangle is the area surrounded by the left vertebral border, a tangential line to the upper LV segment and a horizontal line from the upper LV segment line as indicated by dotted lines of white and black.

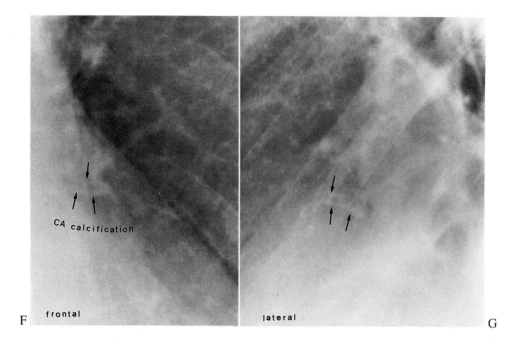

F frontal

lateral G

Fig. 25-18. *(Continued)* The coronary artery calcifications are better appreciated in magnified x-rays. **F,** On the right, a magnified frontal chest x-ray at the CAC triangle shows a pipe-like calcification which runs horizontally and is different from the pulmonary vascular distribution. **G,** In the lateral view, an identical pipe-like calcification is seen with distribution that is also different from that of the pulmonary vasculature.

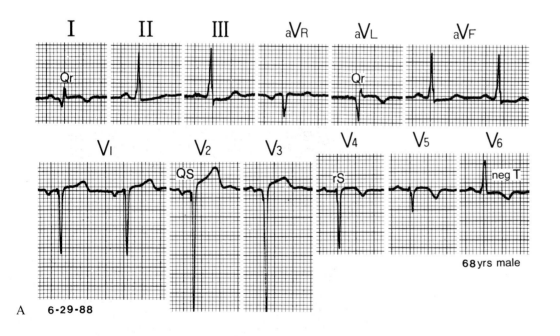

A   6-29-88

Fig. 25-19. A, This ECG is from a 68-year-old man who had an anteroseptal MI 2 years prior to the present visit. He complains of dullness in his right upper quadrant which was thought to be caused by cholelithiasis. His ECG shows a wide Q in I, a QS pattern in V$_2$ and V$_3$, and a poor r/S ratio in V$_4$ and V$_5$. These findings are compatible with an old anteroseptal and lateral MI.

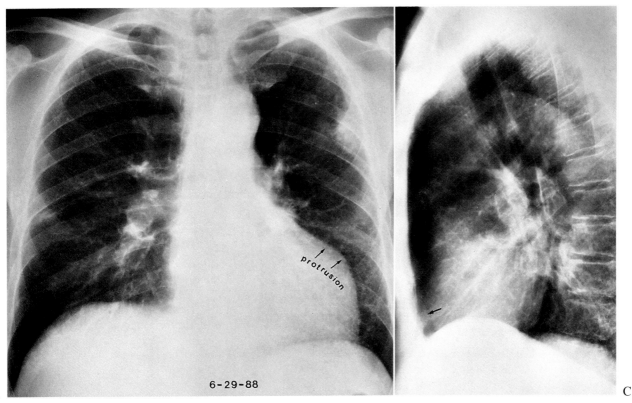

B

6-29-88

C

Fig. 25-19. *(Continued)* **B**, However, his frontal chest x-ray made the same day reveals a small protrusion at the upper portion of the LV segment suggesting an aneurysm. **C**, In the lateral view, an arrow indicates a fine anterior pericardial stripe confirming the absence of pericardial effusion.

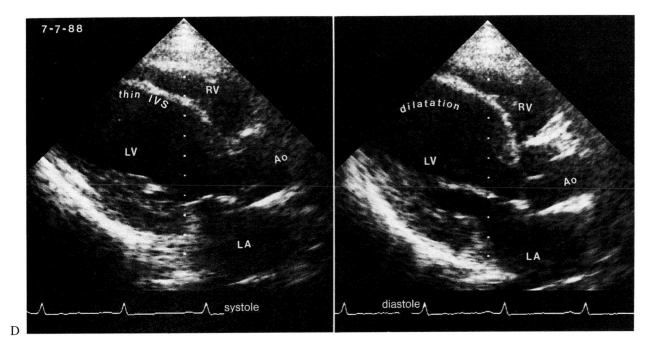

D

Fig. 25-19. *(Continued)* **D**, Long-axis echoes show very strong echoes at the IVS and LVPW towards the apex. These strong echoes suggest fibrotic changes from a previous MI. The thickness of the IVS is indeterminate; however, there appears to be aneurysmal dilatation of the LV cavity at the apex.

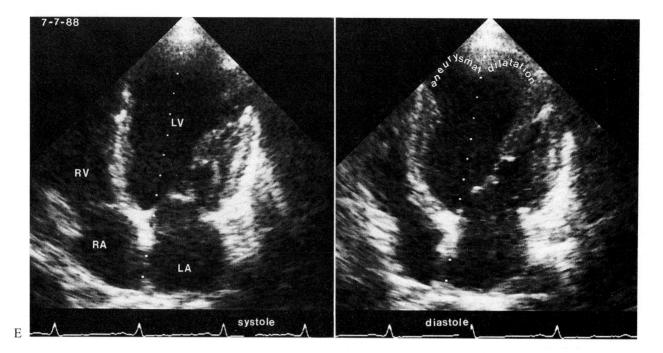

Fig. 25-19. *(Continued)* **E,** His echoes in the apical four-chamber view demonstrate the presence of an apical aneurysm more clearly during systole. There are strong echoes probably from fibrotic changes in the IVS and along the lateral wall of the LV.

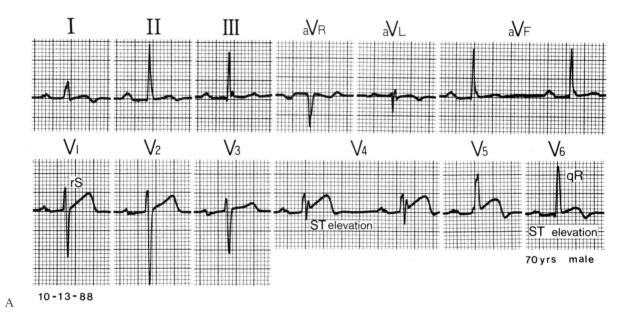

Fig. 25-20. A, This 70-year-old asymptomatic man demonstrates an interesting Doppler finding. His ECG shows a first degree A-V block and there are ST elevations in V_4 to V_6 which suggest anterolateral aneurysm. In addition, a relatively tall r wave in V_1 may indicate a posterior MI.

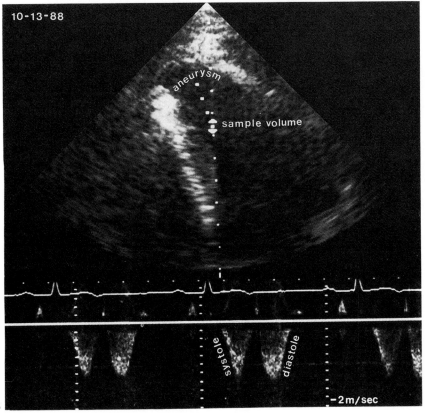

Fig. 25-20. *(Continued)* **B,** His Doppler echo in the apical four-chamber view shows an apical aneurysm and there are both systolic and diastolic flows away from the site of sample volume. The systolic flow suggests the normal blood flow directed toward the left ventricular outflow tract (LVOT) which is away from the site of sample volume. The diastolic flow, which is also away from the site of volume sample, suggests a turbulent blood flow from the aneurysm to the LV cavity. This is paradoxical flow. However, these blood flows are inaudible since their velocities are about 1.7 m per second.

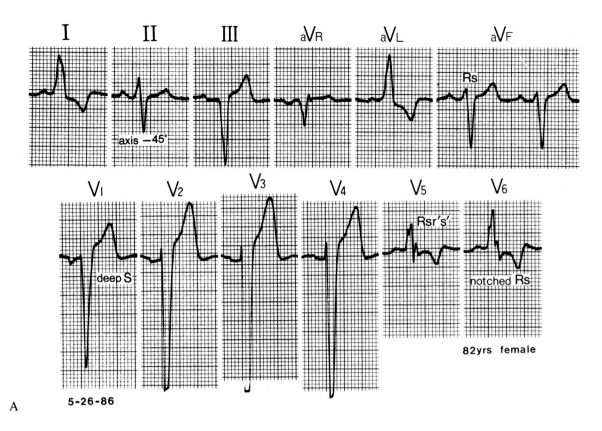

I   II   III   aVR   aVL   aVF

axis −45°   Rs

V₁   V₂   V₃   V₄   V₅   V₆

deep S   Rsr's'   notched Rs

82yrs female

A   5-26-86

Fig. 25-21. A, This is from an 82-year-old woman with hypertension. Her ECG shows wide QRS complexes with rS patterns over the RV and Rs in the LV leads indicating LBBB. The QRS axis is about −45°. In general, the LBBB includes the last portion to be activated in the LV wall, without an s wave in V_6. The s wave in V_6 is often a reflection of the LV intracavity potential that is transmitted to the epicardial leads due to a transmural MI. Other features of LBBB associated with MI include decreasing amplitude of the QRS and/or upright T waves in the LV leads. This unusual type of LBBB is also observed in some cases of dilated cardiomyopathy (DCM) particularly when it is associated with left-axis deviation as in the present case.

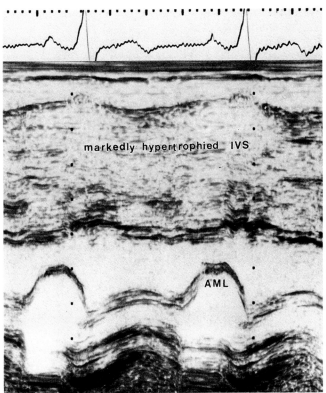

markedly hypertrophied IVS

AML

B

Fig. 25-21. *(Continued)* **B**, Her M-mode echo demonstrates marked hypertrophy of the IVS, with a decrease in size of the LV cavity. There is slight systolic anterior movement (SAM) preceding the opening of the mitral valve, and the opening is greatly suppressed. In summary, this is a case of LBBB associated with marked asymmetric hypertrophy. There was no evidence of MI as suggested by her ECG.

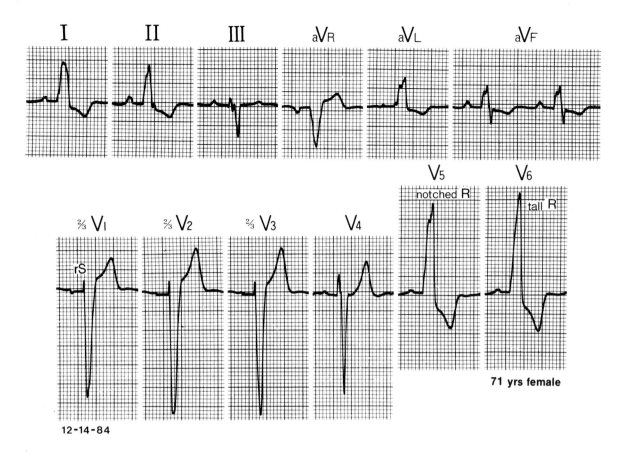

I II III aVR aVL aVF

V5
notched R

V6
tall R

⅔ V1 ⅔ V2 ⅔ V3 V4

rS

71 yrs female

12-14-84

Fig. 25-22. ECG from a 71-year-old woman with asymptomatic hypertension. During 6 years of follow-up her ECG remained unchanged, showing LBBB. The absence of the initial q wave in the LV leads is caused by septal activation either in simultaneous directions or from the RV to the LV side. However, the presence of r waves in the RV leads is caused by the initial activation of the RV. The initial upstrokes in V_1 and V_6 coincide with each other as measured by the P-R intervals in the same leads. This suggests that the RV activation must begin simultaneously with the onset of septal activation to produce the r wave in the RV and the R wave in the LV leads. The author's opinion is that in cases of LBBB, most portions of the LV are activated in a normal fashion except for a region which is activated by the blocked left bundle-branch. This delay in activation of the LV region is seen as notched R waves in the LV leads. However, from the beginning of the r to the nadir of the S wave, the RV leads remain the same in configuration and in duration after the development of the LBBB, indicating a fairly normal activation process in the LV wall. The width of the QRS is not so important, but when a qrS or a QS pattern is seen in V_1, a complicated LBBB must be suspected.

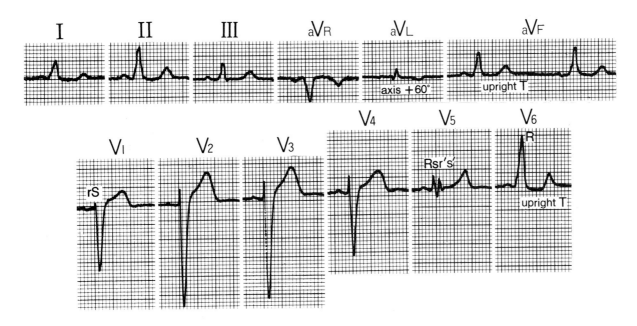

Fig. 25-23. ECG from a 71-year-old woman with asymptomatic hypertension. Her ECG shows wide QRS complexes without an initial q wave in the LV leads, indicating LBBB. However, the T waves in the LV leads are upright, unusual for LBBB and suggesting a LBBB complicated by a primary T abnormality. The QRS complex in V₃ shows an rsr's' pattern with the widest QRS complex. A similar QRS is also seen in Figure 25-20 suggesting that the last portion of the LV to be activated is near V$_4$ or V$_5$. In spite of the LBBB, Figure 25-22 does not show left-axis deviation, which is also inexplicable.

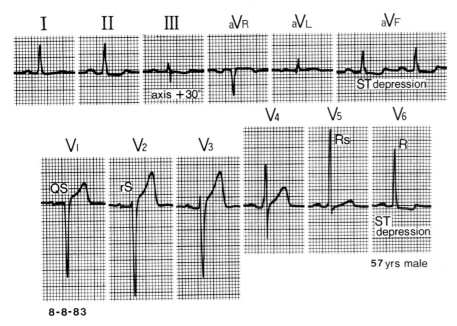

Fig. 25-24. A, ECG from a 57-year-old man with hypertension. His initial ECG shows a QS in V$_1$ and an R in V$_6$ indicating an abnormal septal activation despite his narrow QRS complexes. The definition of bundle branch-block includes a QRS of 0.10 and 0.12 seconds as incomplete, and those of more than 0.12 seconds as complete. However, the QRS complex in the present case is nearly 0.08 seconds or less and does not meet the previously mentioned criteria. Therefore, the term "partial LBBB" or "incomplete LBBB pattern" may be used to designate this abnormal septal activation.

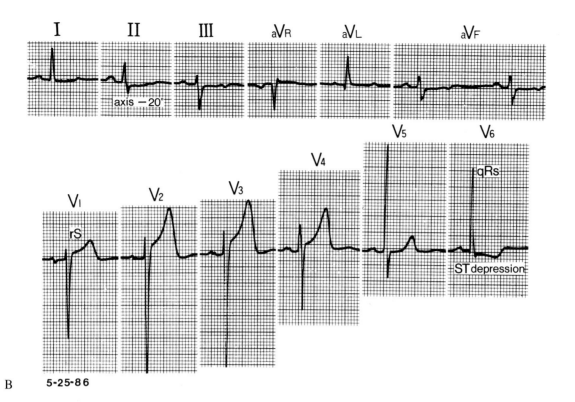

B   5-25-86

Fig. 25-24. *(Continued)* **B**, His ECG 33 months later shows the QRS axis to be −20° so that he now has an anterior divisional block (ADB). An rS in V₁ and a qR in V₆ indicate resolution of the partial LBBB.

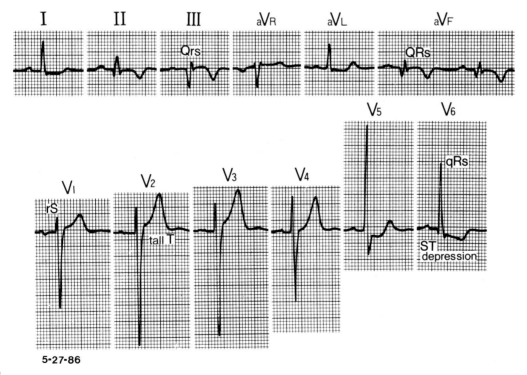

C   5-27-86

Fig. 25-24. *(Continued)* **C**, A posterior MI was suspected from the increased amplitudes of the R and T waves in the RV leads. Two days later, he showed a Qrs pattern in aVF and an increasingly marked R wave in V₁, indicating an acute posteroinferior MI.

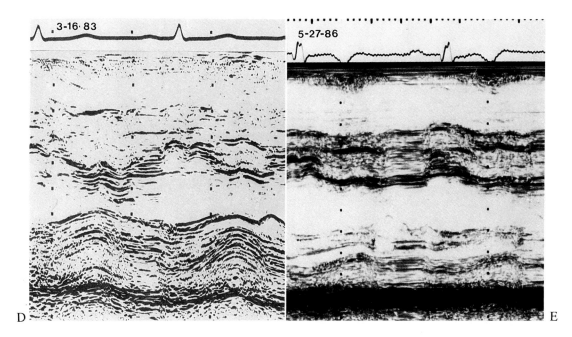

Fig. 25-24. *(Continued)* **D**, His M-mode echo on the left at the time of his initial ECG shows a normal left ventricular posterior wall (LVPW) movement. **E**, On the right, the tracing shows markedly reduced LVPW movement 33 months later, confirming a posterior MI. However, the anterior mitral leaflet is scarcely visible in the second tracing, indicating a slight difference in the direction of the echo beam. Therefore, accurate comparison of these 2 tracings is not possible. In summary, it is clinically important to recognize the absence of septal q wave in the LV leads, even without a wide QRS complex, since it may disguise the abnormality.

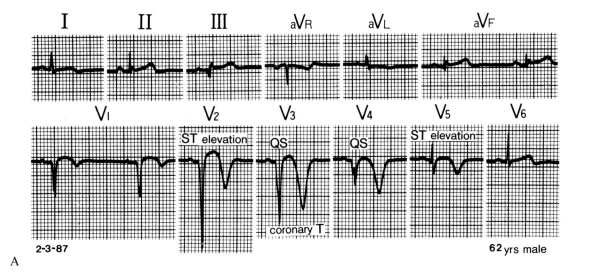

Fig. 25-25. A, This is from a 62-year-old man with an upper respiratory infection. The patient has no history of chest pain. His ECG shows a QS pattern in V_1 to V_4 and a q in V_5 with slight ST elevation and deeply negative T waves indicating a rather recent anteroseptal MI. With the ST elevation in aVF, one also should suspect an inferior MI is present.

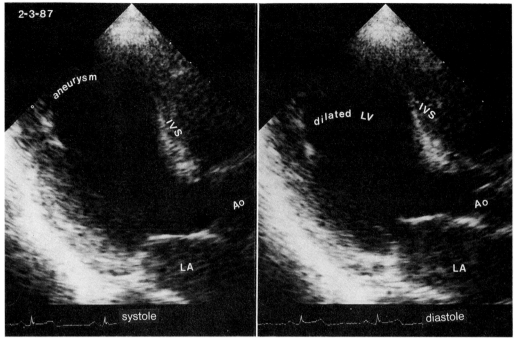

B

Fig. 25-25. *(Continued)* **B,** The echoes in the apical two-chamber view show aneurysmal dilatation of his cardiac apex with some smoke-like echoes observed in the video suggesting the presence of stasis. There is a reduced ejection fraction caused by hypokinesis of the apex.

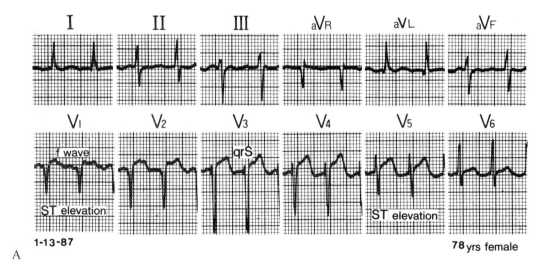

A

Fig. 25-26. A, ECG from a 78-year-old woman with palpitations showing AF at a rate of about 150. The QRS axis is $-30°$ with a QS in V_1 and an Rs in V_6. There are qrS patterns in V_3 and V_4. The absence of an initial septal q wave in the LV leads suggests abnormal septal activation; therefore, the QS pattern in V_1 and V_2 does not necessarily indicate the presence of MI. However, the qrS patterns observed in V_3 and V_4 are difficult to explain on the basis of partial LBBB. Since the RV cavity potential is qrS or QS and that of the LV is Rs in LBBB, the qrS in V_3 and V_4 is possibly caused by an RV myocardial infarction. The ST elevation in V_1 to V_6 seems to come from extensive myocardial injury, as in pericarditis; there is, however, no ST elevation in the extremity leads so that this possibility is most unlikely.

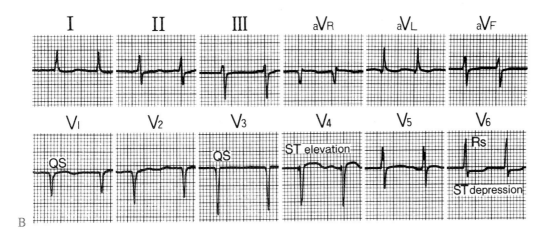

B

Fig. 25-26. *(Continued)* **B,** Her course was suggestive of an MI according to the results of her blood chemistries. Her recovery was uneventful, and an ECG about 2 months later showed resolving ST elevations with Q still present in V_1 to V_4.

Fig. 25-26. *(Continued)* **C,** Her M-mode echo the same day as her second ECG reveals reduced movements of the RV and IVS which correlate well with the ECG findings.

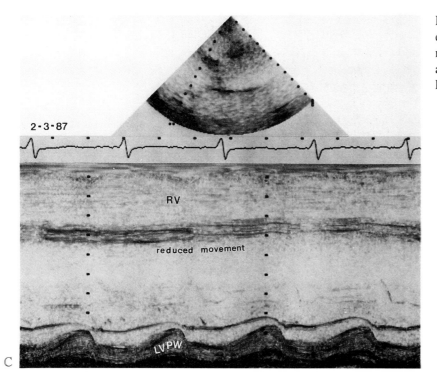

C

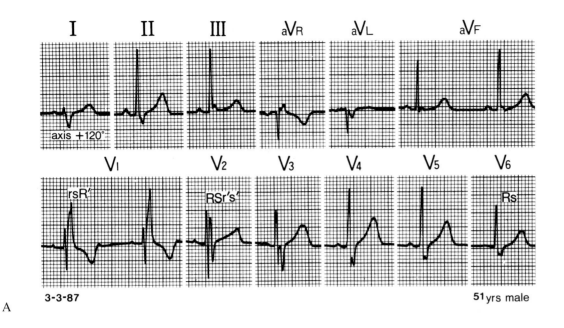

I II III aVR aVL aVF

axis +120°

V1 V2 V3 V4 V5 V6

rsR′ RSr′s′ Rs

A 3-3-87 51 yrs male

Fig. 25-27. A, This 51-year-old asymptomatic man was discovered to have an abnormal ECG at an annual physical examination. There is an rsR′ pattern of RBBB in V₁ with an unusually tall initial r wave. The QRS axis is nearly +120°, which is also uncommon in cases of RBBB. Therefore, the increase in the amplitude of the initial r wave in V₁ may come from a posterior MI and the marked right-axis deviation from a posterior divisional block.

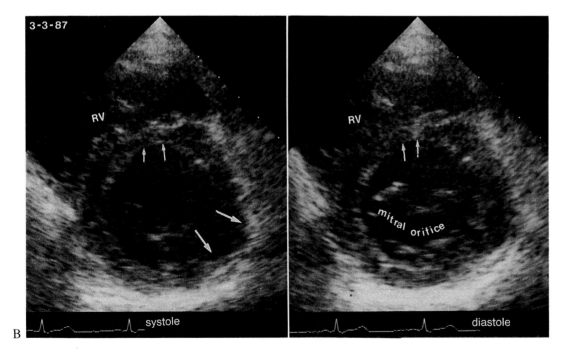

3-3-87 RV RV mitral orifice systole diastole

B

Fig. 25-27. *(Continued)* **B,** His short-axis echoes show thinning of the anterior portion of his IVS and the posterolateral aspect of the LV wall (arrows). This can be recognized in the video image, but it only appears as indentations in the illustrations.

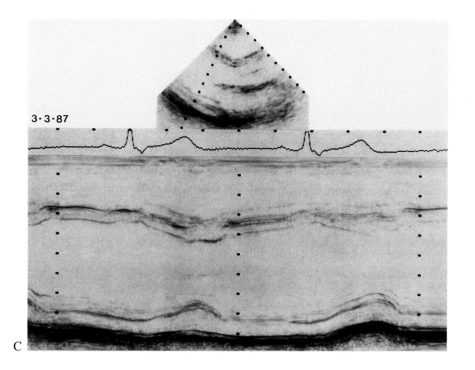

Fig. 25-27. *(Continued)* **C,** An M-mode echo of the same patient shows dilatation of the LV cavity toward the apex with reduced movement of the IVS, correlating well with the findings of the short-axis views.

Index